Inventing the Feeble Mind

Inventing the Feeble Mind

A History of Intellectual Disability in the United States

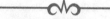

James W. Trent Jr.

Gordon College

OXFORD

UNIVERSITY PRESS

OXFORD
UNIVERSITY PRESS

Oxford University Press is a department of the University of Oxford. It furthers
the University's objective of excellence in research, scholarship, and education
by publishing worldwide. Oxford is a registered trade mark of Oxford University
Press in the UK and certain other countries.

Published in the United States of America by Oxford University Press
198 Madison Avenue, New York, NY 10016, United States of America.

© Oxford University Press 2017

First Edition published in 1995

Library of Congress Cataloging-in-Publication Data
Names: Trent, James W., Jr., author.
Title: Inventing the feeble mind : a history of intellectual disability in
the United States / James W. Trent Jr.
Description: [Second edition]. | Oxford ; New York : Oxford University Press, [2016] |
Includes bibliographical references and index.
Identifiers: LCCN 2015047794 | ISBN 9780199396184 (pbk. : alk. paper)
Subjects: | MESH: Intellectual Disability—history |
Institutionalization—history | Social Conditions—history | United States
Classification: LCC HV3006.A4 | NLM WM 11 AA1 | DDC 362.3/0973—dc23
LC record available at http://lccn.loc.gov/2015047794

1 3 5 7 9 8 6 4 2
Printed by Webcom, Inc., Canada

CONTENTS

LIST OF ILLUSTRATIONS

LIST OF TABLES

ACKNOWLEDGMENTS

In 1978, a librarian at Brandeis University assigned me to a carrel in one of the darkest aisles in the basement of Goldfarb Library where, one day not long afterward, I spotted a journal series with a set of curious names: *The Journal of Psycho-Asthenics* and the *Proceedings of the American Association for the Study of the Feeble-Minded*. That fortuitous assignment sparked inquiry into the history of an issue I have been interested in for more than four decades.

An earlier version of this book appeared in 1994 as *Inventing the Feeble Mind: A History of Mental Retardation in the United* States. Many people at several libraries and collections helped me find and use material for this edition. I am especially grateful to Joyce Lentz and Marvin Rosen of the Elwyn Institute. Elwyn's rich collection contains the archives of the American Association on Intellectual and Developmental Disabilities and the historical records of the Elwyn Institute. Martha Lund Smalley, archivist of the Divinity School Library at Yale University, was helpful in making the Henry Knight papers available. Several librarians at the Ohio Historical Society helped me use the Gustavus A. Doren manuscripts. Rue Moore, archivist of the Albany Medical College, located and provided a copy of William B. Fish's medical thesis on idiocy. Gene J. Williams of the North Carolina Department of Cultural Resources helped me find valuable material in the Records of the Departments of Social Services and Mental Health. Carolyn A. Davis of the George Arents Research Library of Syracuse University located Margaret Bourke-White's photographs of Letchworth Village, and Carol Johnson of the Library of Congress found material about Arnold Genthe's photographs, also of Letchworth Village. At the Illinois State Archives, M. Cody Wright provided invaluable assistance for the historical material on the Lincoln Developmental Center. Susan B. Case, rare book librarian of the Clendening History of Medicine Library at the University of Kansas Medical Center, located what I feared would be an unfindable photograph (Figure 3.1). At Southern Illinois University at Edwardsville, where I was a faculty member for seventeen years, I benefitted from Beverly Farm Records, and from the assistance of archivist Steve Kerber in the university's Louisa Bowen University Archives and Special Collections. I thank Kiyoko Lerner for permission to use an image of Henry Darger, and Joyce Scott and Lilia Scott for the image of Judith Scott.

Several people shared their own experiences in the matrix of intellectual disability, some in letters and some in person. Alex Sareyan of the Mental Health Materials Center helped me locate former conscientious objectors who had worked in state schools in the 1940s. Gordon C. Zahn, national director of the Center on Conscience and War, provided material on his work at the Rosewood State School during World War II. Muriel Pumphrey told me about her experiences with parents of intellectually disabled people in the 1960s. The late Emma Jane Nixon shared her experiences of nearly seventy years as a resident in public facilities for persons labeled mentally retarded. I am especially grateful to Gunnar Dybwad and Rosemary Dybwad for their authoritative remembrances covering seven decades in the field of intellectual disability. Their firsthand, yet critical, accounts of events were most helpful; their hospitality was also most appreciated. I appreciated conversations with Vici Riel-Smith about her experiences as a parent of a disabled child.

For the new edition, my colleagues and friends at the Perkins School for the Blind have been helpful with their historical records on the early years of the asylum movement. I am especially grateful for the assistance of Jan Seymour-Ford at the school's Hayes Research Library. I also thank the librarians and staff members of the John Carter Brown Library at Brown University, the Chapin Library at Williams College, the library of the Massachusetts Historical Society, the Boston Public Library, the Houghton and Schlesinger Libraries of Harvard University, and the library of the Maine Historical Society. I am grateful for my Gordon College colleague, Damon DiMauro, for deciphering and translating Edward Seguin's 1851 letter to Samuel G. Howe. Finally, I acknowledge a faculty initiative grant and a sabbatical leave from Gordon College, a Longfellow House fellowship, and a stipend from the National Endowment for the Humanities that allowed me to sustain the study and writing of the book.

I also enjoyed the support of colleagues and students at Gordon College: Juwan Campbell, Sybil Coleman, Margie Deweese-Boyd, Emily Fink, Ivy George, Daniel Johnson, Ashley Kang, and Judith Oleson. Finally, I remain most grateful for the support and many discussions held with Sue Trent, Mary Trent, Andrew Clark, and Rachel Trent. Friends and family made all the difference.

INTRODUCTION

In 1971, the *Chicago Sun-Times* received a Pulitzer Prize for one of the powerful photographs in its 1970 exposé of the Lincoln and Dixon state schools in Illinois (Figure I.1). For Jack Dykinga, the photographer, his images recorded moments of what he called "sheer terror." This message was a true one—his subjects were real victims—but it also reflected the limitations of Dykinga's gaze. We did not see in his exposé pictures of officials of the Department of Mental Health, the governor, legislators, or ordinary citizens—the creators and sustainers of state schools like Lincoln and Dixon and, in a sense, themselves casualties of the discourse and history that lay behind the gaze they gave to people they called mentally retarded and who, more recently, we call intellectually disabled people. We are doing bad things to intellectually disabled people, the photographs shouted out, and so, in the atmosphere of outrage and righteousness that followed the exposé, the Illinois General Assembly restored the funding to the schools that earlier in the year it had cut. For the time being, the circumstances of intellectually disabled people grew no worse.[1]

I came upon the *Sun-Times* articles around the same time I began working with the historical records of the Beverly Farm Foundation. This rich collection, given in 1988 to Southern Illinois University at Edwardsville where I was a faculty member from 1986 to 2003, included photographs of the Illinois State School and Colony at Lincoln dating back to the 1880s. One image in particular captured my attention (Figure I.2). Taken nearly a century earlier at the same institution, it was hauntingly similar to Dykinga's award-winning 1970 photograph. Both photos show a long, narrow room with three rows of beds and tall, undraped windows. Central in each photo is an "inmate" or a "resident" in bed. Although taken so many years apart, the images to me represent a continuity in the message they convey to the public: that of the utter helplessness of their subjects.

Yet, the photographs are also dissimilar. Jack Dykinga's 1970 photographs supplemented five articles by *Sun-Times* reporter Jerome Watson (1970*a–e*) whose titles made clear their perspective: "A Lingering Nightmare," "Neglect Grips School at Dixon," and "A House of Horror for State's Retarded." Watson and Dykinga were clearly outraged at the deplorable conditions they documented. In the 1880s, the photographer sought only to record the daily life of the Illinois facility. Accompanying the photograph of the inmate in bed were snapshots of pupils doing gymnastic exercises, participating in school assemblies, and engaging in other routine activities at the institution. The 1880s photographer set his gaze on the lone "inmate" in the dormitory not to expose the grim conditions at Lincoln, but to

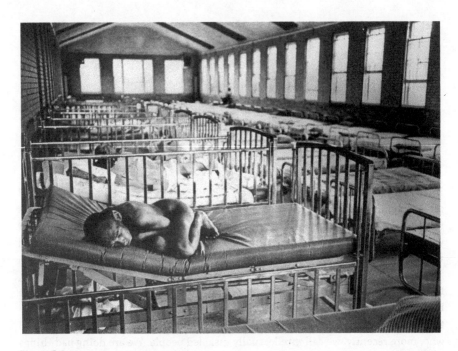

Figure I.1:
Ward of the Lincoln State School 1970. Pulitzer prize-winning photograph by Jack Dykinga of the *Chicago Sun-Times*. (Courtesy of the *Chicago Sun-Times*)

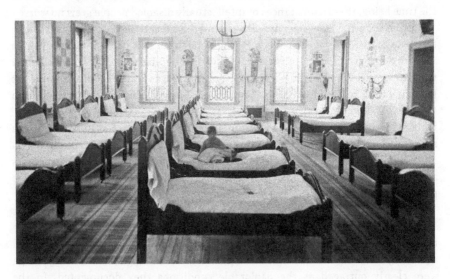

Figure I.2:
Bedroom of the Illinois Asylum for Feeble-Minded Children, ca. 1880. (Courtesy of Southern Illinois University at Edwardsville, Lovejoy Library, Beverly Farm Records)

show the humane care being given there. In 1990, as I looked at both photographs, the images appeared so similar, yet I knew from their contexts that the messages they intended to convey were not. Nothing had changed; yet something was very different.

This book describes and analyzes the history in the United States of what we have come to call "intellectual disability." Intellectual disability is a construction whose changing meaning is shaped both by individuals who initiate and administer policies, programs, and practices and by the social context to which these individuals are responding. Since it emerged as a social problem in the second quarter of the nineteenth century, educators, social reformers, physicians, psychologists, sociologists, and social workers have viewed intellectual disability in diverse ways: as a disorder of the senses, a moral flaw, a medical disease, a mental deficiency, a menace to the social fabric, mental retardation, and finally a disability. Constructed sometimes in the name of science, sometimes in the name of care, sometimes in the name of prevention, and sometimes in the name of social control, these views have accompanied and reflected shifts in the social, political, economic, and cultural order of the United States. Drawing on methods associated with intellectual and social history and a theoretical framework from social constructionism and critical sociology, I have concentrated my study on the fabrications and the gazes—pitying, fearful, knowing, preventing, controlling, and normalizing—of those in control of intellectual disability and on the larger context out of which these constructions emerged. In addition, I have tried to hear the voices of people whose lives were shaped by the gazes and the fabrications, to capture, however incompletely, their responses and to understand how so much apparent progress could cover so little real change.[2]

In Chapter 1, I discuss statements and images about "idiocy" in the colonial and early republican periods of the United States. During these times, Americans recognized that a particular family member or a person in their local community was slow to learn and to mature. But most inhabitants of these small towns neither rejected nor despised *their* local "idiots." From that overview, I study a shift in the 1840s from intellectual disability as a family and local problem to a social and state problem. I argue that, despite an emphasis on taking children out of almshouses and educating them for community productivity, by the late 1850s superintendents of "idiot schools" were already planning for custodial facilities, not for an "era of hope." Claiming the goal of productive citizenship, they began giving a narrow, institutional meaning to "productivity." Some felt compelled to do so by social and economic circumstances. Others, however, did so because they had begun to construct new images of the institution and its place in giving meaning to the "problem" of intellectual disability. In doing so, the superintendents also ensured their own survival and growing legitimacy. Even before the Civil War, care and control had assumed a curious linkage.[3]

I devote Chapter 2 to an analysis of the educational and social philosophy of Edward Seguin. The "apostle to the idiots," Seguin more than any other nineteenth-century figure shaped American interests in educating intellectually disabled people. Drawing on his French and American publications and also on recent

French secondary sources, I depart from previous histories of Seguin (e.g., Kraft 1961; Talbot 1964) to argue that American superintendents reshaped his educational views not to diminish the trend toward institutionalization but to facilitate it. I further suggest that, despite his warnings about large institutions, Seguin's preoccupation with technical problems undermined his vision of the outcome of the very educational system he had devised and thus undermined his warnings. By emphasizing the *methods* and *tools* of education while giving less attention to the *ends* of educating idiots, the advocate of productivity through education became, in the years after the Civil War, the mediator of disabling, unproductive institutionalization. This reduction of ends to means, I shall argue, continued to be an important (if rarely recognized) phenomenon in the history of intellectual disability.

In Chapter 3, I discuss the "burden of the feebleminded," a view of intellectual disability that burgeoned after the Civil War. Focusing on the growth of a "disciplinary matrix" of institutional superintendents in their own professional association and tracing their involvement in the National Conference of Charities and Correction, I stress the relationship of the superintendents' goals and aspirations to external forces in the nation. Although they usually had little control over these forces, superintendents of growing facilities were learning how to shape—if not have power over—policy and care.

In Chapter 4, "Living and Working in the Institution, 1890–1920," daily life in the turn-of-the-century institution is recreated, drawing on letters from intellectually disabled people and their relatives, institutional newsletters, memoirs and letters from superintendents, testimony from a 1909 Illinois House of Representatives' investigation of the Lincoln State School, and other institutional documents. I have tried here to present the perspective of inmates, attendants, and administrators. Many attendants were generous and kind to inmates under their charge, and many inmates and attendants built close relationships. When abuses occurred, however, superintendents used them as an opportunity to call for larger facilities and greater specialization of services. Superintendents and their philanthropic allies learned to use the threat of scandal to extract support from ever-stingy legislators. Troubles in the institution, therefore, took on several, often ironic, layers of meaning.

Chapter 5 focuses on the years 1908 to 1924, when intellectual disability was reconstructed as the "menace of the feebleminded." Although short-lived, this period was one of frenetic activity in the field of intellectual disability. I look most closely at the Committee on Provision for the Feeble-Minded. Involved not only in special education classes and institutions in the South but also with the intelligence testing, eugenics, and anti-immigrant movements of the period, the Committee played a brief (1915–18) but central role in shaping views on the "menace of the feebleminded." Although they would be discredited in scientific communities, the images of this "menace" would linger for five more decades in professional circles and in popular consciousness.

In Chapter 6, I look at the change in professional circles from the rhetoric of the "menace of the feebleminded" to what I call the "sterilization, parole, and routinization of mental defect." Opposition to the menace rhetoric came from sources both inside and outside the field. After 1920, the profession began to emphasize the adjustment and adaptation of intellectually disabled people to segregated services, whether in the community or the institution. This new emphasis was made possible, superintendents came to believe, by sterilization. It was made necessary by the Great Depression and World War II. Departing from the view (e.g., of Tyor and Bell 1984, Tyor and Zainaldin 1979) that superintendents faced the choice of "segregation versus sterilization," I argue that superintendents used sterilization for three different, although hardly distinct, purposes, but none of them competed with segregation. Looking at the Rome (New York) State School's efforts at community parole and the frustration of those efforts during the Great Depression and the war, I argue that the tool of sterilization and the policy of institutional parole became interrelated means for superintendents to preserve their institutions in the midst of fundamental social and economic stress.

Chapter 7 examines four overlapping events: exposés of state schools after World War II, the confessional literature of parents in the early 1950s and the founding of the National Association for Retarded Children, the rekindling of public (even popular) interest in intellectual disability in the 1950s and 1960s, and "the abandonment of the institution" after 1970. As I argue, the federal policy of deinstitutionalization resulted from an ironic convergence of developments: a combination of civil-libertarian and advocacy groups joined with state officials hoping to trim the ever-rising costs of state institutions.

In Chapter 8, I explore the period after the 1990 Americans with Disabilities Act. Ironies of the distant past are harder to see than are ironies of the moment: rather than merely weaving together policies of this period, I have explore what I call the "dilemma of doubt" by looking at intellectual disability as the convergence of contradictory meanings—extraordinary ability from disability, intelligence or function in definition, the self and its integration, the promise and costs of consequentialist-driven research and sterilization, and preventing disability through genetic testing and abortion. The chapter raises the issue of unstable meanings in a time of major social and established changes.

Throughout this book, I examine three central themes woven through the American history of intellectual disability. First, I claim that, in the history of intellectual disability, state schools became places where care became an effective and integral part of control. Furthermore, superintendents and social welfare agents did not move simply "from care to control," but also reshaped the contours of both care and control to ensure their personal privilege and professional legitimacy. Second, I hold that the tendency of elites to shape the meaning of intellectual disability around technical, particularistic, and usually psychomedical themes led to a general ignoring of the maldistribution of resources, status, and power so prominent in the lives of intellectually disabled people. Finally, I find that the economic vulnerability of these people and their families, more than the claims made for their intellectual or social limitations, has shaped the kinds of treatment offered them.

Throughout this book, I use words that in earlier times referred to intellectual disability and to people labeled intellectually disabled. These words—*idiot* and *imbecile, feebleminded, moron, defective, deficient, retarded, retardate,* and the like—are today offensive to us, yet they reveal in their honesty the sensibilities of the people who used them and the meanings they attached to intellectual disability. At various points in their history, these nouns began to be qualified: *defectives* became *mental defectives*, *imbeciles* became *high-grade* and *low-grade imbeciles*, *morons* became the *higher-functioning mentally retarded*. Later, the *mentally retarded* have become *mentally retarded persons* and *persons with mental retardation* and, in some circles, *persons with developmental disabilities* or *persons specially challenged*. In 2005, the American Association on Intellectual and Developmental Disabilities agreed to change the label to *intellectual disability*. In this process, essence has apparently been liberated from existence, being from descriptions of it. Behind these awkward new phrases, however, the gaze we turn on those we label intellectually disabled continues to be informed by the long history of condescension, suspicion, exclusion, and pity. That history is unavoidably manifest in the words we now find offensive, and so I have intentionally used them throughout the book (taking care to use words appropriate to the times under discussion, even when more than one word or group of words was being replaced by another). While our contemporary phrases appear more benign, too often, we use them to hide from the offense in ways that the old terms did not permit.

Social problems like intellectual disability are in fact social constructions—"modern myths," as James Gusfield (1989) has called them—built from a variety of materials: the desire to help and the need to control, infatuation with science and technique and professional status, responses to social change and economic instability. From the time people with the "thing"—intellectual disability—became social problems requiring help and treatment, the contours of this requirement have changed, sometimes dramatically. But the contours of our regard for people with intellectual disability has not. This and that must be done to and for them; this and that must be learned about them and said about them to ensure progress in treatment techniques, professional influence, institutional funding, or social control. It is important to understand that this image of intellectual disability as a "thing," the object of scientific understanding and intervention, conceals a history shaped by the implicit political choices of the mentally accelerated. In making care more scientific and professional, these political implications have been hidden, but they, more than our explicit "knowledge," have determined our fabrications of intellectual disability and the gaze with which we regard and control intellectually disabled persons (Rapley 2004).

I hope my book speaks to theorists and practitioners; to problem interpreters and to problem solvers; to social scientists, to humanists, to physicians, to caregivers, to neighbors, coworkers, religious congregations, and to families—all of whom in their own ways create and sustain this fascinating and peculiar history. History cannot predict the future. The lessons we can learn from it teach us about who we are now, about our own mythologies, and about the meaning of the gaze we cast on *miserable people* and on their apparent need for our help, our know-how, and our time. There are indeed aspects of the lives of intellectually disabled people (and mentally accelerated people, too) that require help from other individuals, but by looking at the intellectually disabled person, the Other, so obsessively, we fail to look at ourselves and examine the "screens of ideology" that shape and direct our obsessive gaze.[4] The problem of intellectual disability is a *social* problem because it is equally a problem of mental acceleration; it implicates our entire society. It is to us, the mentally accelerated, that I direct this book, in the hopes that it will stimulate self-reflection. And who knows? Perhaps out of this self-evaluation we may create a human solidarity based on what Richard Rorty has called "our sensitivity to the particular details of the pain and humiliation of other, unfamiliar sorts of people." This sensitivity, he reminds us, requires a "redescription of what we ourselves are like" (Rorty 1989, xvi).

NOTES

1. Five of the photographs are reprinted in Leekley and Leekley 1982, 80–83. The articles and photographs appeared in the *Chicago Sun Times* from Sunday, July 26 to Thursday, July 30, 1970 (Watson 1970*a–e*).
2. In the sociological debate between "strict constructionists" who give little validity to social constructors and the social contexts from which constructions emerge, and "contextual constructionists," who give validity to both, I am with the latter group. On this debate, see Best (1989), Rafter (1992*a*, 1992*b*), Spector (1985), Spector and Kitsuse (1987), Rapley (2004), and Troyer (1992). The clean Manicheanism of strict constructionists makes the historical analysis of the constructions they identify (like intellectual disability) nearly impossible. As Rafter (1992*b*, 39) has so aptly put it, "Unlike strict constructionists, who attempt to seal their studies of claims making activities off in an analytical vacuum, historians do not pretend that their work can be separated from the context in which they produced it." Contextual objectivity, as she notes, does not imply epistemological objectivity; sociological contextual constructionists, like many contemporary historians, hold to the relativity of knowledge.

   For writings that have criticized social constructionism, while still retaining an appreciation of its bias for knowledge as process, for epistemological construction and change, see L. Carlson (2010, 85–91), Goodey (2011, 1–12), Hacking (1999), Kittay (1998), and Rapley (2004).
3. Since the early 1970s, two distinct, although not internally consistent, groups of social scientists who use intellectual and social history to study deviant groups have emerged. The groups have quite differing outlooks on institutional care and control. One group, represented by such diverse critics as Allen (1975), Bellingham (1986), Bowles and Gintis (1976), L. Carlson (2010), deLone (1979), P. Ferguson (1994, 2013), Foucault (1973, 1979), Gould (1981), Katz (1968), Malacrida (2015), Margolin (1994), Nourse (2008), O'Brien (2013), Piven and Cloward (1971), Rafter (1992*a*, 1997), Reaume (2009), Rothman (D. Rothman 1971, 1981), Schweik (2009), Scull (1977*a*, 1977*b*, 1989), Sutton (1988), Tomes (1984), and Wolfensberger (1976), has emphasized a conflict and revisionist approach to a generally older "progressive" humanitarian view of the history of social problems (e.g., A. Deutsch 1937; Fink 1938; Scheerenberger 1983, 1987). The other group, including Cravens (1978), Dowbiggin (1997), Dwyer (1987), Grob (1973, 1977, 1980, 1985, 1990, 1991), K. Jones (1999), Miron (2011), Noll (1995), Patterson (1986), Rosenberg (1987), Shorter (2000), Sokal (1987), and Zenderland (1998), has emphasized a new humanitarianism by rejecting most or all the revisions of the conflict perspective. See also Trattner (1983).

The first group, employing intellectual history from a conflict, revisionist perspective, sees institutional policies and practices forced on groups of people who have intruded on the interests and values of powerful and usually conservative native populations. These policies and practices reflect the concerns of elites over changes in society brought on by the growing numbers or power of these interlopers. Thus, Irish immigration to the United States in the 1840s and 1850s produced anxiety among native-born Americans, who in response developed new and "progressive" ways of viewing and responding to social problems. Rooted in both their views and their responses was the aim of controlling "the Irish problem." Mental hospitals, penitentiaries, public schools, and public hospitals became institutional mechanisms for this nativist control. For the conflict revisionists, then, the history of a social problem becomes a history of control by elites over nonelites.

The second group, doing intellectual history from a consensus-based new humanitarianism, rejects this emphasis on social control. Instead, they view elite responses to social problems as, for the most part, sincere efforts by reformers and progressives to deal with distress. Often caught in a web of social forces that they were a part of but not in control of, elites and their purveyors merely devised rational responses that were shaped by both their own professional milieu and both the political and social realities of their time. Proper interpretations of their actions and motives must be limited, theorists in this group insist, to the times of the participants. For the new humanitarians, what must be avoided is the tendency of the conflict theorists to "read into" responses to social problems of the past a "presentist" perspective. Rather than trying to control groups of "outsiders," the elite problem-solvers combined humanitarian and scientific sentiment to care for people as best they knew how, even though from current prevailing views that care might be interpreted as control.

My study of intellectual disability rests in the conflict tradition. I argue that control and care merged as interrelated and interdependent factors in specialized services for intellectually disabled people (i.e., institutions, and special schools and classes). Although the message and meaning of care and control changed over time, care remained an important form of control. In the name of care, then, control was most effectively secured.

4. On "screens of ideology," see Scull 1989.

CHAPTER 1

Idiots in America

All colonial and post-revolutionary Americans knew feebleminded people. As members of their families and their communities, feeble minds were an expected part of rural and small-town life. Physically able simpletons found no great obstacle to day-to-day living, and obviously disabled idiots received care from various members of what were usually extended families. When a family broke down, idiots unable to care for themselves were placed with neighbors or in alms houses, and more able simpletons, especially those capable of breaking the law, might find themselves in local jails. Feebleminded people might be teased, their sometimes atavistic habits might disgust, but unlike the mad and the criminal, they were not feared.

A familiar nursery rhyme evokes the humor derived at the expense of the simpleton:

> Simple Simon met a pieman,
> Going to the fair;
> Says Simple Simon to the pieman,
> Let me taste your ware.
>
> Says the pieman to Simple Simon,
> Show me first your penny;
> Says Simple Simon to the pieman,
> Indeed I have not any.
>
> Simple Simon went a-fishing,
> For to catch a whale;
> All the water he had got
> Was in his mother's pail.

Simple Simon went to look
If plums grew on a thistle;
He pricked his finger very much,
Which made poor Simon whistle.

He went for water in a sieve
But soon it all fell through;
And now Simple Simon
Bids you all adieu.

Appearing in chapbooks of the late eighteenth and early nineteenth centuries, this rhyme embodied the good-natured reaction most citizens had to village fools (Opie and Opie 1951, 385). Often the unintentional buffoon and sometimes the brunt of mean-spirited jokes by townspeople, simpletons nevertheless usually found themselves protected by the generosity and familiarity of the locals.

The feebleminded were also the object of pity. "He could not run about like other young people," stated the American Sunday School Union's children's book, *The Idiot*, "sporting in the bright sunshine and the green fields, nor could he mingle in the games which others enjoyed." At his widowed mother's side as she sold fruit and sweetmeats in the town market, the idiot boy sang to himself, "pal-lal, pal-lal." Humble, obedient, and empty-headed, the lad endured the teasing and torments of local schoolboys. Upon the death of his mother, a hard-working widow, the idiot "was unhappy without knowing what had made him so." Sent to the almshouse, he died. "This tale of the idiot has been told you," concluded the moralist, "to soften your heart, and to excite in your bosom a kindly disposition towards the helpless and afflicted." Distributed widely, *The Idiot* became the possession of thousands of antebellum Sunday-schoolers (American Sunday School Union ca. 1840; Shaffer 1966).

Other images familiar to citizens of the colonies and later of the new republic portrayed feebleminded people as worthy of and receptive to Christian benevolence. In John Bunyan's *Pilgrim's Progress*, Mr. Feeble-mind from the town of Uncertain is simple and sometimes confused but sincere in his faith. In the company of other pilgrims, he is an equal, not a deviant. "I am a man of no strength at all of body, not yet of mind," admitted Mr. Feeble-mind,

but would, if I could, though I can but crawl, spend my life in the Pilgrim's Way. When I came at the gate that is at the head of the way, the Lord of that place did entertain me freely; neither objected he against my weakly looks, nor against my feeble mind. . . When I came to the home of the Interpreter, I received much kindness there; and because the hill of Difficulty was judged too hard for me, I was carried up that by one of his servants.

Recounting his survival from the capture of the giant of Assault-lane, Mr. Feeble-mind affirmed his resolve even in the face of adversity, "Other brunts

I also look for, but this I have resolved on, to wit: to run when I can, to go when I cannot run, and to creep when I cannot go. As to the main, I thank him that loved me. I am fixed: my Way is before me, my mind is beyond the River that has no bridge; though I am, as you see, but of a feeble mind." Later, Mr. Great-heart, a leader of the band, responded, "Come, Mr. Feeble-mind, pray do you go along with us, I will be your conductor, and you shall fare as the rest" (Bunyan 1856, 314–317).

Added to these humorous and compassionate images of idiocy was a romantic view linking feeble minds with nature and the "bliss of the lower order." As children of pure nature, feebleminded people were seen as a refreshing contrast to the worldly excesses of an artificial and increasingly mechanized world. In his 1798 poem, "The Idiot Boy," Wordsworth (1952) wrote of Johnny, an idiot sent by his mother, Betty, in the middle of the night to get the local physician for a sick neighbor. The boy and his pony became lost, never reaching the doctor. Despite the wilds of the night and the needs of the sick neighbor, he was unaffected:

> Who's you, that, near the waterfall,
> Which thunders down with headlong force,
> Beneath the moon, yet shining fair,
> As careless as if nothing were,
> Sits up right on a feeding horse?

When found, he remained unconcerned:

> And thus, to Betty's question, he
> Made answer, like a traveller bold,
> (His very words I give to you,)
> "The cocks did crow to-whoo, to-whoo,
> And the sun did shine so cold!"
> —Thus answered Johnny in his glory,
> And that was all his travel's story.

In his response to criticism of the poem, Wordsworth claimed, "I wrote the poem with exceeding delight and pleasure, and whenever I read it I read it with pleasure . . . the loathing and disgust which people have at the sight of an idiot, is a feeling which, though having some foundation in human nature, is not necessarily attached to it in any virtuous degree, but is owing in great measure to a false delicacy, and . . . a certain want of comprehensiveness of thinking and feeling" (DeSelincourt 1935, 295–296). Wordsworth acknowledged the poem as one of his favorites. He included it in the 1802 *Lyrical Ballads,* and it was thereafter widely read in England and America. Like many of Wordsworth's poems founded on the affections, "The Idiot Boy" portrayed a person innocent of the human manipulation of nature. Unconcerned even with sickness and death and the importance of his mission, the boy riding his pony was one with the sights, sounds, and movements of the night. His innocence and unconcern bound him closer than most to nature. "But where are we to find the best measure of [human nature]?" Wordsworth asked. "By stripping our own hearts naked, and by looking out of ourselves to[ward those] who lead the simplest lives, and those most according to nature; men who have never known false refinement, wayward and artificial desires, false criticisms, effeminate habits of thinking and feeling" (DeSelincourt 1935, 295). This intimacy with nature, even though arising from stupidity, gave the boy qualities most admired by Wordsworth and romantics of his day. For these critics of the "new order," even an idiot embodied ideals lost to people corrupted by an increasingly mechanized and commercial world.

In this milieu, American colonists and citizens of the early republic occasionally wrote about family members and neighbors who were intellectually disabled (P. Richards and Singer 1998; Wickham 2001a, 2001b, 2002, 2006, 2007). In early seventeenth-century Jamestown, Virginia, for example, Benomi Buck and his sister, Mara were orphaned after the death of their father, an Anglican priest. Benomi was only six years old. His father, anticipating his own death, appointed guardians for his children not only because of their ages, but also because the reverend along with his parish deemed Benomi an idiot. In doing so, Rev. Buck followed the guardianship rules in English Common Law (Wickham 2006).

Also following English Common Law, colonial Virginians distinguished idiocy from madness on the one hand and moral negligence on the other. Likewise, their counterparts in Puritan Massachusetts recognized that idiots, lacking the intelligence needed for salvation and faith, were nevertheless distinct members of God's good creation. Thus, unlike the morally depraved, who might claim that they did not know right from wrong, idiots were truly innocent of moral responsibility. Thus, in 1693, idiots became one of the "worthy poor" incorporated into the Massachusetts Bay Colony's new Poor Law. As such, the colonists regarded idiocy an impairment that would likely last for a lifetime (Wickham 2002).

Two decades later, Cotton Mather published his *Curiosa Americana* in which he recounted human and natural oddities and marvels in the New England colonies and their surroundings. One of his observations concerned the daughters of a Dunstable, Massachusetts man. The girls were nine and three years old. Mather's description shows that early eighteenth-century colonists had developed a discrete, and also shared, perspective about idiocy:

> [The girls] continued for several months after their nativity in the same circumstances of sensibility that other infants of their age use[d] to have. But anon they were taken with odd convulsive motions, which carried a little of an epileptical aspect upon them. . . . These fits anon left them wholly deprived of almost everything in the world, but only a little sight, and scent, and hunger. Nothing in the whole brutal world so insensible! . . . They never use their hand to take hold of anything. Was *idiocy* ever seen so miserable! (cited in Wickham 2002, 947)

In February 1774, Thomas Jefferson's younger sister, Elizabeth, died, probably succumbing to the elements after wandering away from home. The future president rarely spoke of his sister, either before or at the time of her death. Shortly after her death, however, he placed a clipping of the poem, "Elegy on the Death of an

Idiot Girl," into one of his scrapbooks. Family legend maintained that Elizabeth was "rather deficient in intellect" (Wickham 2006).

Another, if different, example of idiocy, this time beginning in the first decades of the early republic, appeared in the Cameron family of Orange County, North Carolina. Duncan Cameron was an attorney and wealthy planter. The second child and first son of Duncan and his wife, Rebecca, was Thomas Amis Dudley Cameron, born in 1806. Despite boyhood tutors and stints in Connecticut and New Jersey schools and a Vermont military academy, where the family hoped that the Northern winters would improve his constitution, Thomas continued to be a poor student. From family correspondence, however, it appears that Thomas was a happy boy, good-natured, and even a hard-working student. Yet, throughout this life, he had trouble reading and performing simple mathematical calculations. Although his younger brother, sister, and sister-in-law would eventually serve as his financial guardians, his adult life was rather normal, within the structures of antebellum upper-class Southern life. As an adult, he worked on the family's farms and, in 1831, was appointed the postmaster of Stagville, in what is today Durham County. He had numerous friends, regularly attended community activities, was an ardent supporter of the Whig party, and remained the favorite uncle to his nieces and nephews (P. Richards 2014).

Unlike Thomas Cameron, Bulkeley Emerson grew up with family members who, when he became an adult, made little attempt to integrate him into family matters. The youngest brother of Ralph Waldo Emerson, Bulkeley Emerson seemed to have grown normally until around the age of nine. His family placed him for a time in McLean Asylum in Charlestown, Massachusetts, and later with farm families in Littleton, where he boarded as a farm laborer and where he died in 1859 at the age of fifty-two. Waldo Emerson wrote affectionately of, and occasionally to, his younger brother, but as a busy member of the Concord and Boston literary circles, he had little time for his brother's care and education. On Bulkeley's granite gravestone in Sleepy Hollow cemetery, Waldo had inscribed, "Thou has been faithful over a few things," a reference to Jesus's parable of the talents (Beyer 2000; Bosco and Meyerson 2005, 6–7; see also P. Richards 2004).

On November 22, 1852, a petition requesting a pardon for the manslaughter conviction of twenty-six-year-old John A. L. Crockett arrived on the desk of Illinois governor Augustus C. French. Crockett was the grandson of David S. (Davy) Crockett's brother, William. At the time, Davy Crockett's fame at the 1836 Battle of the Alamo was well known to Americans. John Crockett's attorney, Springfield lawyer Abraham Lincoln, was not successful in winning Crockett's acquittal in Moultrie County Circuit Court. So Lincoln, along with John's father, Elliott Crockett, circulated among the leading men of Moultrie and Shelby Counties a pardon petition that would go to Governor French. Lincoln's petition justifies the pardon request as: "Crockett has been, from his infancy, only not quite an ideot [sic], being at least, of the very lowest grade of intellect above absolute idiocy. We, therefore, (several of us being jurors who sat on the trial) believing that his punishment can result in no public good, respectfully recommend that he be pardoned" (Lincoln 1852). The petition won the approval of the governor.

INVENTING IDIOCY

Although post-revolutionary Americans might feel humor, sympathy, benevolence, and even admiration for the familiar *local idiot*, after the panic of 1819, they began to view *idiocy* with a mixture of curiosity, anxiety, and, after the Civil War, fear. This change of perspective—from particular individuals to a general type—began with a major shift in the way Americans dealt with a host of so-called worthy dependents (widows, orphans, and disabled people) and unworthy dependents (the unemployed and criminals).

Before 1820, most dependent people (but especially the unworthy) were linked by what was believed to be their common moral frailty. Ignorance, idleness, intemperance, and prodigality—which led to hastily arranged marriages, gambling, frequenting the pawn broker, prostitution, and so forth—were associated with America's dependent populations (Society for the Prevention of Pauperism 1818, 3–6). Only their "worthiness" distinguished one dependent group from the other, and only the worthy received local public assistance. This help usually came in the form of so-called *outdoor relief*; that is, relief that respectable dependents received in their homes or in the homes of caregivers.

After 1819, the almshouse (or "indoor relief" as it was known) became the dominant model for both groups of dependents. As the economic crisis lingered into the early 1820s, pauperism increased, especially in the northeastern states. Committees in Massachusetts, New York, and Pennsylvania investigated the extent of unemployment and need. Josiah Quincy's 1821 report in Massachusetts called for the abolition of direct aid (or outdoor relief) in favor of more centralized and rationalized almshouses (Quincy 1821). John Yates's report in New York recommended that there be poorhouses and poor farms in every county in the state (Yates 1824). For the working poor (i.e., the unworthy), the report called for indoor relief requiring rigid, hard, even unpleasant work so as to discourage lengthy stays. For the worthy widow, orphan, or disabled person, indoor relief would, according to the Yates report, be a welcomed change from the exploitation often found in community homes.

Until their demise in the 1930s, almshouses accommodated many types of dependents, but, beginning with the depression of 1837, they especially began to house large numbers of one group of the unworthy poor: the unemployed. By the end of the depression in 1840, Americans had begun to view indoor relief as a place principally for the working poor. In large part, this change of perception was simply the result of widespread unemployment. But also states began to develop particular indoor relief for special groups of dependents, thus removing them from common almshouses (Axinn and Levin 1982, 41–57; Folsom 1991, 43–57; Trattner 1979, 47–76).

The first groups to receive special attention by purveyors of indoor relief were children and criminals. Orphanages, schools, and jails, of course, had existed before almshouses, but with the reforms of the 1820s the orphan asylum, the special state-operated school, and the penitentiary added new meaning to familiar problems.

Prior to the 1820s, orphanages had been places primarily for children whose parents had died or had abandoned them. The orphan asylum, however, sheltered a new and growing segment of the population: children whose parents, often in almshouses themselves or in debtors' prisons, could not afford to care for them. Usually operated by religious organizations or fraternal societies, orphan asylums had boards of directors made up of prominent citizens and benefactors. Certain that parental influence was just as damaging in the asylum as it was in the almshouse, the directors discouraged parental association with children. Although most orphan asylums took some delinquent children into their care, they almost always refused the admission of physically and mentally disabled children (P. Ferguson 1994, 21–43; D. Rothman 1971; D. Schneider 1938; Trattner 1979).[1]

The first specialized facilities to take such children were state-operated schools for the blind and the deaf and dumb that emerged contemporaneously with prisons and orphan asylums. Fueled by reports of the successful education of disabled children in France and England, Americans like Samuel G. Howe persuaded states to establish special schools. Always taking privately paying pupils, these schools also admitted poor students whose support came from the state (Edwards, 2012; Lane 1976; J. Trent 2012).

The penitentiary emphasized, at least at first, the self-reflective penitence of offenders on their road to personal reform and social amends. Penitentiary advocates believed that, segregated from the temptations of everyday life, offenders could change (D. Rothman 1971). Although Benjamin Rush (1812) and Isaac Ray (1838) had both noted the existence of the "moral imbecile," other penologists before 1830 showed little interest in this type of offender. Feebleminded lawbreakers, Rush, Ray, and others after them believed, were usually followers, unable to resist temptations whether outside or inside prison. At the same time, they were easily apprehended. Thus, under the watch of a new breed of prison reformers, more feeble minds began to appear in prisons and local jails (see, e.g., S. Howe 1848*b*; "Idiocy in Massachusetts" 1847; H. Knight ca. 1850–90).

Neither the orphan asylum, the schools for the blind and the deaf and dumb, nor the penitentiary drew attention specifically to feebleminded people. Yet, in the midst of economic stress and as part of the various institutional responses that endured after hard times had ended, a process of differentiating dependent people had begun.

The election of Andrew Jackson in 1828 marked the beginning of three decades of economic expansion, territorial annexation, and immigration, as well as the extension of political liberties (albeit only to white males). But growth and development were accompanied by economic, social, and political upheaval. Technological advances and imperial annexation gave Americans greater opportunities for commercial development, but two economic downturns (1837–43 and 1857–61) kept the rapidly growing population uncertain of its future. New England Unitarians began to challenge Calvinistic views of personal corruption. Romanticism imported from Europe but shaped to fit the American experience fueled a view of individual and social progress. The factory as the primary place for work began to remove the family from the center of production. Immigrants, principally from

Ireland and Germany and mostly Catholic, arrived in large numbers in the 1840s and 1850s. In response, nativist sentiment grew, especially in the Northeast and the West. Northern and Southern differences over the shape of the nation's political and economic future reached a crescendo. It was a period of faith in progress and fear of progress; a time for change and for controlling change (Folsom 1991, 17–82; D. Howe 2007; D. Reynolds 2008; Sellers 1991; Sklansky 2002; Wilentz 2005). This economic and social milieu provided the context for the development of idiocy as a recognized social construct.

In November 1844, John Conolly, chief physician to the county lunatic asylum at Hanwell, England, and a leading British proponent of moral treatment, visited two famous Parisian institutions, the Salpêtrière and the Bicêtre. In January 1845, he published an account of his visits in the *British Foreign and Medical Review*. After reviewing the use of small dormitory spaces and the absence of physical restraint at the Salpêtrière, he devoted the last section of his article to an overview of the school for idiots opened at the Bicêtre in 1842. Conolly's enthusiasm was unrestrained. Among groups of dependent people, he claimed, idiots had been the most neglected, even by enlightened progressives. In English asylums, officials left them "in total indolence and apathy." At the Bicêtre, however, under the teacher Edouard Seguin, even the most disabled idiots showed improvement in educational skills and moral rectitude.[2] Although warning against claims of curing all idiots, he added, "There is no case incapable of some amendment; that every case may be improved, or cured, up to a certain point [is] a principle of great general importance in reference to treatment" (Conolly 1845, 293).[3]

Howe, head of the New England Institution for the Blind in South Boston, and Samuel Woodward, superintendent of the Massachusetts Lunatic Asylum, already familiar with the work at the Bicêtre, read and circulated Conolly's article. Thoroughly involved in local and national politics, Howe, in April 1846, had himself appointed chair of a state commission "to inquire into the conditions of Idiots of the Commonwealth, to ascertain their numbers, and whether any thing can be done in their behalf" (S. Howe 1848*b*, 1). That spring the commission members examined "five hundred and seventy-four human beings who were condemned to hopeless idiocy" in sixty-three Massachusetts towns. Not unlike the reports of his friend, Dorothea Dix, who at the time was investigating conditions of the insane in Ohio, Kentucky, and Indiana, Howe's reports cited case after case of idiots "left to their own brutishness."

In February 1847, Howe received a detailed description of the French school in a letter from George Sumner, the younger brother of his close friend, Charles Sumner. Sumner's account of the work of Seguin and Félix Voisin, a physician and founder in 1836 of the treatment ward for idiots at the Bicêtre, included a thorough description of the educational techniques and philosophy employed at the school. Howe, who otherwise had little use for what he called French charlatanism, found in Sumner's letter a way to advocate for the educability of idiots. By May 1847, Howe's efforts convinced the Massachusetts legislature to appropriate funds for an idiot school. In October, Howe admitted his first idiot pupils to his school for the blind in South Boston (Donald 1960; Sumner 1876; J. Trent 2012, 151–154, 187–191; Waterson 1880).

About the same time, at Barre in western Massachusetts, Hervey B. Wilbur, a young teacher turned physician, read another British account of the education of idiots at the Bicêtre and a review of one of Seguin's recent publications ("Review of Edouard Seguin's *Traitement*" 1847; "Visit to the Bicêtre" 1847). After graduating from the Berkshire Medical School in 1843, Wilbur had moved seven times through four states, never quite able to settle into a stable and profitable practice. When he read and reread the articles in 1847, the unestablished doctor found his calling. The next year, he got married, settled down, and opened a private school for idiots in a modest house in Barre (Figure 1.1) (G. Brown 1884; Graney 1980; H. Wilbur 1881; "Wilbur, Hervey Backus" 1883, 1928).

In New York, Amariah Brigham reported the European successes in his annual report of the state lunatic asylum. He expressed the hope that New York would eventually open an asylum for idiots. Impressed by Brigham's report and Conolly's article, Frederick F. Backus, a physician and member of the New York State Senate, moved that information about idiots from the previous state census be referred to the Committee on Medical Societies, which he chaired. The committee issued a report in January 1846 containing census summaries and acknowledging the prevailing opinion that little could be done for idiots, but noting the educational

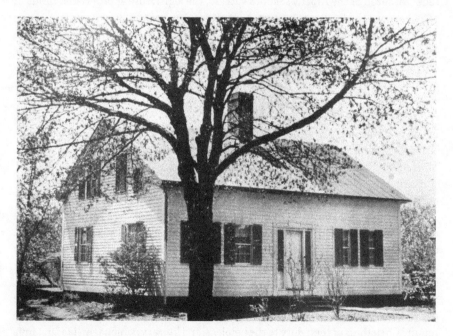

Figure 1.1:
Home of Hervey B. Wilbur and the first school for idiots in North America, Barre, Massachusetts, ca. 1850. (From the *Journal of Psycho-Asthenics*, 1897)

success in Paris (Godding 1883; New York Asylum for Idiots 1854; New York State, State Senate 1846).

By 1850, Wilbur's private school at Barre and Howe's publicly funded school in South Boston were teaching about a dozen idiots. Howe employed techniques learned from his nearly two decades of work with blind and deaf pupils, and both Howe and Wilbur used reports now readily available on Seguin's methods. With these techniques, success soon followed, and with success came the dissemination of information about their work. In newspapers and journals, primarily in the Northeast but also in the South and West, and in demonstrations before legislatures and civic organizations, the word got out.[4] In 1850, summing up the enthusiasm, John Greenleaf Whittier (1850), the New England abolitionist and poet, wrote to the *National Era* about Howe's efforts. The letter was later reprinted in his essay "Peculiar Institutions of Massachusetts" (Whittier 1854): "All the pupils have more or less advanced. Their health and habits have improved, and there is no reason to doubt that the experiment, at the close of its three years, will be found to have been quite as successful as its most sanguine projectors could have anticipated."

Impressed by these reports and with prodding by Backus, the New York Commission on Idiocy in 1851 hired Wilbur to direct an experimental school strategically located near the New York state capitol. Moving to Albany, Wilbur left his Barre facility to his assistant, George Brown, who, along with his wife, Catharine, and son, George A., would operate this first American facility for another six decades. Assured of the Albany school's success, the legislature appropriated funds in 1854 to move the facility to a permanent site at Syracuse.

Other states soon followed suit. In 1853, Philadelphia citizens began a private school at Germantown under the direction of James B. Richards, formerly a teacher at Howe's school. Facilities opened in Ohio in 1857, under R. J. Patterson, and in Connecticut, in 1858 under Henry Knight. After them, Kentucky opened schools under J. Q. A. Stewart in 1860, and Illinois under Charles T. Wilbur (Hervey's younger brother) in 1865. New York in 1868 opened a second school on Randall's Island in the city of New York (C. Brown 1892; "Brown, George" 1929; Kerlin 1892*b*; "Parrish, Joseph" 1904; Pennsylvania Training School for Idiotic and Feeble-Minded Children 1854; A. Potter et al. 1853).

During the 1850s, Howe and Wilbur, and later others, wrote additional journal and newspaper articles about their work (e.g., "A Chapter on Idiots" 1854; "Idiots" 1851; "Influence of Music on Idiots" 1857). In response, letters from parents and relatives of disabled children began to inquire about services. Despite this interest, the superintendents were convinced that legislators in particular and the public in general failed to appreciate the educational potential of idiots. To mobilize their crusade before lawmakers and the public, they solicited influential supporters. Senior legislators like Backus in New York and Norton S. Townshend in Ohio were petitioned to sponsor legislation, influential clergy like Samuel May were asked to remind Christians of their duty to the helpless, and literary personages like Dr. Linus P. Brockett were encouraged to write for the popular and professional press.

Added to these activities, superintendents began to make tours in states without idiot schools. Taking with them idiots transformed by their efforts, they attracted the attention of public officials and private philanthropists. In 1858, Grubb, a pupil at the Pennsylvania Training School, wrote to his relatives recounting such a trip to Trenton, New Jersey, with Isaac Kerlin, then the assistant superintendent of the facility:

> I have been to Trenton. . . . We showed the people what they could do; all the boys and me sung, and did the dumbbell exercises; sung geography, and did some sums. A whole lot of people was in, and ladies, and they stamped their feet. The Governor of New Jersey talked to us, and I made him a present of a smoking cap, that Lizzie M made. Next day we went to another hall, where there was a great many children, and some ladies and gentlemen; and we went up on top of a big State House, and saw the whole country. . . . Dr. Wm. A. Newell [the governor of New Jersey] took me into his room, and showed me a big pair of scales . . . and he took me into another room, and I saw, oh! A great large map of Massachusetts, as big as our new map of Pennsylvania. (Kerlin 1858, 54–55)

In demonstrations before legislators, in letters and articles in local and national publications, in cornerstone-laying ceremonies, and in the sharing of techniques and administrative trends, Howe, Hervey Wilbur, the Browns, and all the other early reformers assisted each other in creating a context for the emergence of idiocy as a social and cognitive construct (Connecticut General Assembly 1856; New York Asylum for Idiots 1854; Pennsylvania Training School for Feeble-Minded Children 1858). The common reference for this construction was Seguin's *Traitement* (1846*b*). Recalling her earliest days at Barre, Catharine Brown wrote, "When our helpless ones were safe in bed we sat down to read M. Seguin's *Traitement Moral, Hygiene, et Education des Idiots*" (C. Brown 1897, 140). Speaking to an audience of potential supporters in the late 1850s, Henry Knight claimed, "It was necessary to complete a theory of training which could encompass all the deficiencies of the vacuity called Idiocy. Such theory was to be found in the book of Dr. Seguin, *Traitement moral des Idiots,* not that the book was a perfect one, but because it was, and it is even now the only one" (H. Knight ca. 1860). With the arrival of Edouard Seguin on American soil in 1850, the newly developed group of advocates had "the apostle to the idiots" himself to add legitimacy to their social cause.

For Seguin, idiocy was a failure of the will. Training techniques mastered by Seguin were used to excite the will, to invigorate the muscles, and to train the senses, all leading to higher cognitive development. Idiots *unwilling* to exercise their senses were blocked from this higher development. Thus, the lack (or failure) of will was manifested as a functional blockage. Proper education through what he called physiological training, coupled with moral treatment, was the only successful way to break through this blockage. (I discuss Seguin's education system in Chapter 2.)

Pathologizing Idiocy

American reformers attracted to the philosophy and technology of Seguin's system of educating idiots were never completely satisfied with his definition of idiocy.

Departing from their French mentor, Americans during the period emphasized a definition of idiocy that took into account not only its moral and functional dimensions, but also its pathological, typological, and degenerative properties. These medical categories would become even more important in the late 1850s and after the Civil War as a medical model began to replace the educational model of the 1840s and early 1850s.

In his first annual report (while Seguin was residing at his Syracuse facility), Wilbur followed a definition that relied on Seguin's work:

> We do not propose to create or supply faculties absolutely wanting; nor to bring all grades of idiocy to the same standards of development or discipline; nor to make them all capable of sustaining, creditably, all the relations of a social and moral life; but rather to give dormant faculties the greatest practicable development, and to apply those awakened faculties to a useful purpose under the control of an aroused and disciplined will. At the basis of all our efforts lies the principle that the human attributes of intelligence, sensitivity, and will are not absolutely wanting in an idiot, but dormant and underdeveloped. (New York Asylum for Idiots 1852, 15–16)

Although Wilbur's definition included Seguin's emphasis on the will, it also presented different grades of idiocy, which Seguin's work had not emphasized (but would later include). By 1852, Wilbur had identified four types: *simulative idiocy* defined people whose development was merely retarded and who could be prepared for "the ordinary duties and enjoyments of humanity"; *higher-grade idiocy* defined those who would eventually enter common schools "to be qualified ... for civil usefulness and social happiness"; *lower-grade idiocy* applied to people who could become "decent in their habits, more obedient, furnished with more extended means of happiness, educated in some simple occupations and industry, capable of self-support under judicious management in their own families, or in well conducted public industrial institutions for adult idiots"; and *incurables* were idiots for whom education was a goal in itself (New York Asylum for Idiots 1852, 18–21). Going beyond Seguin, then, Wilbur defined idiocy to emphasize gradations of the condition. Idiocy became types of idiocies.

In his 1856 summary of the conditions of idiots in Connecticut, Henry Knight, like Wilbur, followed Seguin's definition: "Idiocy means isolation, solitude. The idiot is isolated from the rest of creation because he is deficient in means of perception and comprehension, action and reaction, feelings and willings" (H. Knight ca. 1860). In speeches to draw attention to his newly opened school, which despite concerted efforts failed to receive funding from the Connecticut legislature, by 1861 Knight added a new dimension to his definition. Idiots were passionate, filthy, self-abusive, animal-like, gluttonous, given to irrational behavior, intemperate, and possessed of all varieties of physical abnormalities. They were often the major attractions at circus sideshows, he added (H. Knight ca. 1860).[5]

Like Wilbur and Knight, Howe acknowledged the importance of Seguin's functional definition for the educational potential of idiots. Yet he departed from

Seguin's definition in his emphasis on physical abnormalities. Howe wrote in his 1848 *Report* that "without pretending . . . to scientific accuracy, idiocy may be defined to be that condition of a human being in which, from some morbid cause in the bodily organization, the faculties and sentiments in the bodily organization remain dormant or underdeveloped, so that the person is incapable of self-guidance, and of approaching that degree of knowledge usual with others of his age" (S. Howe 1848*b*, 20). Although Howe the educator acknowledged the functional outcome of underdevelopment, Howe the physician and phrenologist stressed more than Seguin the condition's pathology and etiology.

Fellow physician and champion of Seguin's methods in Connecticut, Linus Brockett also stressed a pathological basis. "We should define idiocy . . . as the result of an infirmity of the body which prevents, to a greater or less extent, the development of the physical, moral and intellectual powers" (Brockett 1855, 599; 1856*a*, 45). R. J. Patterson, the medical superintendent of the Ohio Asylum, stated: "Idiocy, though not a disease, may be regarded as that condition, in which, from the effects of physical disease in foetal or infantile life, or from defective organization of the nervous system, the intellectual and moral powers have never been developed, except in a slight degree. Idiocy, then, has a physical rather than a mental origin" (Ohio Asylum 1861, 12–13). In Virginia, John M. Galt, the medical director of the Eastern Lunatic Asylum, published his 1859 *A Lecture on Idiocy*. Quite aware of efforts to educate idiots in Europe and in the Northern states, Galt (1859) nevertheless stressed their medical classification, including both ordinal levels and nominal pathologies of idiocy. From the latter, he especially showed interest in cretinism and in Johann Jakob Guggenbuhl's work with cretins in Switzerland (Walsh 2012; Wickham 2006).

For these early reformers, the pathological emphasis was associated with a widely held view of degenerative and polymorphous heredity. Idiocy was related to many "sins of the father": intemperance, poverty, consanguinity (meaning marriage between cousins), insanity, scrofula, consumption, licentious habits, failed attempts at abortion, and overwork in the quest for wealth and power. "The vast amount of idiocy in our world," claimed Brockett, "is the direct result of violation of the physical and moral laws which govern our being; that often times the sins of the father are thus visited upon their children; and that the parent, for the sake of a momentary gratification of his depraved appetite, inflicts upon his hapless offspring a life of utter vacuity" (Brockett 1856*a*, 45–46). The physical and mental status of human beings could not only degenerate from generation to generation but could also take on varied and unpredictable forms. "There are thousands of parents," James Richards, then the principal of the newly founded Pennsylvania Training School for Feeble-Minded Children, wrote, "who have never had the least idea that they were at all responsible for the various infirmities with which their children are afflicted. Besides, transmission of disease is not always direct, nor is it always in the same form. There are many ways in which it may show itself, modified as it is by the thousand conditions in which the law may have been violated" (J. Richards 1856, 378).

A moral component was linked closely with this degenerative and polymorphous sense of hereditary idiocy. Leaders of the cause emphasized the education of younger children not only because children were thought to be more amenable to intellectual growth and development but also because, as Wilbur put it, "they are free from the confirmed habits which constitute, in the main, the disagreeable or repugnant features of the common appreciation of idiocy" (New York Asylum for Idiots 1852, 14). Few appeals to legislators or reports to the public failed to warn of the degenerative behavior of idiots left to their own devices. Few reports and demonstrations failed to indicate that even the most morally degenerate idiots could make remarkable progress under careful and intense training in special schools.

Like others of the period, Knight told Connecticut audiences about the nature and prevalence of idiocy. As was his custom, he paused in his address to bring out two or three idiots who demonstrated their abilities in reading, writing, handicrafts, and gymnastic exercises. With the audience primed, Knight told the sad life histories of each pupil. Before arriving at the special school, most had been "drivelling idiots" found in local almshouses or neglected by uncaring families. Given to making bizarre noises, masturbating frequently and in public, eating their own excrement, and abusing themselves, these transformed "worst cases" convinced audiences of the salubrious effects of careful and intensive education. They also reminded audiences of the consequences of inaction. Reformers thus added the threat of moral degeneracy to their developing construction of idiocy, which, by the end of the decade of the 1850s, was being given more and more public attention. Education, however, held out the promise of removing, or at least reducing, that threat (Goodheart 2004; H. Knight ca. 1860; McDonagh 2008, 257–265).

In addition to the educational, pathological, hereditary, and moral dimensions of the definition of idiocy was a concern for its incidence. The national census of 1840 had attempted to measure the extent of insanity and idiocy (Gorwitz 1974). Indeed, these data had provided impetus to Howe, Backus, Townshend, and Knight to begin their own statewide investigations. More carefully prepared and apparently more accurate than the national census, their investigations in Massachusetts, New York, Ohio, and Connecticut began to give policymakers a sense of what they believed was the prevalence of idiocy.

Several presuppositions affected their investigations. Howe, at the groundbreaking ceremonies of a new facility at Media for the Pennsylvania Training School, claimed that idiocy occurred randomly: "Idiots form a certain proportion of the population of every generation, in every large community" (Pennsylvania Training School for Feeble-Minded Children 1858, 42). Random occurrence, however, did not preclude the apparent contradiction that the lower classes, often immigrants and often given to degeneracy, seemed to produce greater proportions of idiots. "One of the most important [findings of the 1848 study] is that eight-tenths of the idiots are born of a wretched stock; of families which seem to have degenerated to the lowest degree of bodily and mental condition; whose blood is watery; whose humors are vitiated, and whose scrofulous tendency shows itself in eruptions, sores, and cutaneous and glandular disease" (S. Howe 1874, 11).

Their surveys of local physicians, clergy, and public officials and their own trips to assess conditions in almshouses and prisons led Howe, Knight, and Brockett in the late 1840s and early 1850s to estimate the incidence of idiocy at between one-ninth and one-half of 1 percent of the general population (Brockett 1855, 599). Although they suspected that the actual rate was higher, estimates of incidence during the pre-Civil War decades were much lower than those estimates made in the last two decades of the century and even lower than those of the 1920s. Indeed, many Americans identified as feebleminded during most of the twentieth century would not have been so viewed before the Civil War.

In their writings concerned with defining idiocy, leaders in the emerging field almost always brought up one type of defective, the *moral idiot*. More than any other group of feebleminded people, moral idiots (or moral imbeciles, as they began to be known by the 1880s) provided the underpinnings for the construction of feeblemindedness and for the shape of the custodial institution, both of which would linger for nearly a century. Following Benjamin Rush's initial identification in 1812 and Isaac Ray's more extensive treatment in 1838, Howe saw moral idiocy as a defect affecting "moral faculties of the mind" (S. Howe 1848b, 20–21):

> In the rank next above the idiot, stand those helpless creatures who are supposed to know right from wrong, and from whom are drafted almost all the tenants of our jails and prisons. It is a fearful question whether most of this class, though rising above the state of *mental* idiocy, are not still in a state of *moral* idiocy; whether by the necessity of the case, by the very question of our social system, they are not born in sin, nurtured in ignorance, and trained in depravity, so as to be certainly and necessarily predestined to the prison and the almshouse. (S. Howe 1874, 10)

Isaac Kerlin, at the time assistant superintendent of the Pennsylvania asylum and later its superintendent, was even more intent than Howe in exploring the linkage of idiocy and delinquency. He devoted sections of his 1858 book, *The Mind Unveiled; or, A Brief History of Twenty-two Imbecile Children*, to a study of Grubb, Neddie, and Alfred, all moral idiots and all males. Of Grubb, he wrote:

> He was a *moral* idiot, he recognized no obligation to God nor man, and having some appreciation of the value of money and property, nothing that could be appropriated, was safe from his reach. With this innate propensity, he had a good share of secretiveness too, so that the most disguised cross questioning rarely discovered the truth. His honest face, covered the most mature dishonesty. (Kerlin 1858, 48–49)

Of Neddie, a boy born to an "intemperate Irish mother," he claimed:

> Neddie's history reveals a sad and fearful state of morals, among the degraded classes of our large cities. His idiotcy [sic] and disease, may be traced directly to the want of nurture, in his early years; and it becomes a question of political economy, whether legal supervision, ought not to *seek out*, and correct the terrible abuses which, we are too certain, exist in the low abodes of squalid want and

vice . . . . Steeped and seethed in crime, from the moment they enter the world, and hardened as steel by brutality; what surprise is it, that before their tongues cease lisping, they commence swearing, and before men, they are murderers; and while we tolerate a nursery of crime, why wonder and regret, that annually our criminal records, expose such a large percentage of juvenile theft, outrage, arson, and murder? (Kerlin 1858, 98–101)

Combining a degenerative view of heredity with a concern for unsupervised idiots, Kerlin argued for a theme that would become increasingly important by the 1880s—idiots in general, but moral idiots in particular, were a class of citizens whose defects made them vulnerable to criminal exploitation and vice. Like Dickens's character Barnaby Rudge in the 1841 novel of the same name, moral idiots were basically good until mixed with the "wicked of our population, whose vicious conduct and habits [the idiot] eagerly imitated" (Kerlin 1858, 85; McDonagh 2008, 170–191).[6]

Moral idiots, then, were vulnerable to worldly temptations for which they could hardly be held responsible. "Abandoned to the irregular guidance of his own propensities—every ostlery and barroom open to his visits, and the corrupt and licentious his familiar associates—what limit could be set for his degradation?" (Kerlin 1858, 60). Foreshadowing a theme that would become familiar in his later writings on the subject, Kerlin noted that although the community created the "moral viciousness," it was also a victim of its creation. "They are known in their neighborhood as vicious idiots, or simpletons, and are cautiously avoided by those who wish to keep their families intact from sin. Association is a law of *their* nature, as of ours; they seek it where it may be found, and become the tools and imitators of the infamous" (Kerlin 1858, 60).

And what should be done for the moral idiot? Although of a "higher grade" intellectually than more common "simple idiots," moral idiots represented a greater problem for the social order as burdens, but also as potential threats. The moral idiot thus could benefit not only from schooling but also from character-building labor. "Confinement in a school-room," Kerlin (1858, 50) wrote of Grubb,

> was a new thing to him; its strict employments, to a boy whose home had been in the fields and on the streets, and who knew no government save his own will, was a new and irksome life; hence he was not kept regularly at his desk; if a load of hay came, Grubb helped stow it away; if corn in the field was to be husked, Grubb was employed—he was constituted cow-boy, boot-black, and errand-boy, and moderate compensation encouraged his interest, and ensured his punctuality. The school-room was a secondary matter for him, until he willingly sought it.

Though not at first attracted to the classroom, Grubb eventually began to learn, to say his prayers, and even to be the trustee of the institution's Sunday morning collection. Kerlin recounted how he was astonished by Grubb's interest in the multiplication tables and in his desire to be a storekeeper. Kerlin included a photograph of Grubb (Figure 1.2) in some copies of *The Mind Unveiled*.[7] In his best clothes, with his

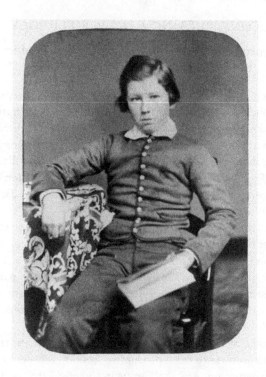

Figure 1.2:
Grubb, an inmate at the Pennsylvania Training School for Feeble-Minded Children, ca. 1857.
(From Isaac N. Kerlin's *The Mind Unveiled*, 1858)

hair neatly combed, he resembles other Americans photographed before the Civil
War. His right arm rests on a table covered by a patterned cloth. In his left hand,
Grubb holds a book, opened slightly by his thumb between the pages. Obviously
posed, the photograph showed a moral idiot transformed by the watchful guidance
of the asylum, no longer condemned by his natural frailty but amenable to learning.
With the book (presumably the *institution's* book) in Grubb's hand, the photograph
illustrated a vision superintendents like Kerlin were beginning to formulate: only
under the guidance, care, and restraint of the institution could moral idiocy be
controlled.

Before the war, moral idiots were, like Grubb, almost always male, and like him
they were portrayed as responding to the good efforts of the asylum to rescue them
from their moral degeneracy. When the superintendents wrote about this type of
idiot, their illustrations were of "boys" who had improved both intellectually and
morally under the tutelage of the institution. A decade after the war, the discovery
of female moral imbeciles, whose moral imbecility included the ability to bear illegitimate children, added a new urgency to the type. With their discovery, images
like those of Grubb and other male moral idiots began to compete with new and
more threatening images. In a few decades, the threat of a baby in the arm would
substitute for the promise of a book in the hand.

CONSTRUCTING A PLACE FOR IDIOCY

Burdensome Idiots, the Inconsistencies of Productivity, and Special Schools

The letters of grateful parents and the reports of demonstrations before legislative and public audiences made clear to teachers like Howe, Richards, Knight, and Wilbur their success in accomplishing what was previously unimaginable. Idiots were able to learn, and most educated idiots were able to become productive citizens. In 1851, John Greenleaf Whittier wrote of George Rowells, the son of his neighbor Jacob Rowells: "The change is almost like a resurrection of a mind from death" (*Villager [Amesbury Villager]*, March 6, 1851, letters from Jacob Rowells and John Greenleaf Whittier to Samuel G. Howe).

The first years in which specialized services were provided to idiots were filled with examples of the successes of schooling and of after-care community employment. But, by the 1860s, more than a few idiots began to use their training not to return as productive workers to their local communities but to remain as workers in expanding institutions. Although the original educational function of the institution would remain prominent, once in the institution, many feebleminded child-students would become feebleminded adult-workers.

Within a decade of the founding of the first schools, then, the education of idiots with all its promise to train productive workers was becoming a means of institutional perpetuation. As I shall argue in Chapter 3, by the 1880s, the shift from a focus on external, community productivity to an internal, custodial function for education had become explicit (P. Ferguson 1994). By the 1890s, this shift would move from being a dominant theme among superintendents and their social welfare supporters to becoming social policy in most of the states with institutions.

Although this new perspective on productivity would become most apparent after the Civil War, glimpses of it appeared even before the war. By the late 1840s, then, superintendents of idiot schools had begun to feel the pressures to retain educated pupils and to admit students whose eventual discharge, they believed, was unlikely. Howe, the superintendent to express the strongest opposition to long-term custody, for example, was not without inconsistencies brought on by what he called "necessity" (Pennsylvania Training School for Feeble-Minded Children 1858). In short, his words and actions did not always match. Thus, in the name of education for productivity outside the institution, Howe began (ironically enough) to shift the focus of education and productivity to the institution itself. Superintendents less troubled by custodialism, of course, could make the transition more gracefully than Howe. How was the original policy of educating idiots for community productivity reconciled with the emerging policy of educating them for institutional growth and perpetuation?

Typical of progressives of his generation, Howe acknowledged the burden of feeblemindedness to the family, community, and state, but he claimed that the responsibility for the burden rested with a public indifferent to the laws of heredity, to the loss of productivity caused by untrained defectives, and to the expense of caring for pauper idiots. Indeed, Howe saw public indifference to a host of social problems as a great threat to the republic. Burdensome idiots, he stressed, were unproductive citizens. In their idleness, they were apt to become lawbreakers or burdens to citizens whose productivity had to be expended in their behalf. It was in the self-interest of all citizens, he claimed, to train idiots not only to relieve them of their unproductive inactivity but also to relieve productive citizens of one more social burden: "This class of persons is always a burden upon the public," he wrote in 1848.

> There are at least a thousand persons of this class who not only contribute noth-
> ing to the common stock, but who are ravenous consumers; who are idle and often
> mischievous, and who are dead weights upon material prosperity of the State....
> [T]hey generally require a good deal of watching to prevent their doing mischief,
> and they occupy [a] considerable part of the time of more industrious and valuable
> persons.... Many a town is now paying an extra price for the support of a drivel-
> ling idiot, who, if he had been properly trained, would be earning his own liveli-
> hood, under the care of discreet persons who would gladly board and clothe him
> for the sake of the work he could do. (S. Howe 1848*b*, 51–52)

Basic to Howe's view, then, was the assumption that idle idiots were unproductive in two ways. They were themselves unproductive, adding nothing but mischief to the common good. They were also unproductive because, in their idleness, they required supervision from people whose productivity was lost in their care. This dual emphasis on greater productivity—for the idiot and for the caregiver—reappeared throughout Howe's writings and in the writings of other superintendents and legislative advocates of the period (e.g., in addition to Howe, see H. Knight ca. 1860; J. Richards 1854, 1856).

Linked to this dual emphasis was the importance of education in the asylum. To show that a burdensome, unproductive idiot properly trained in a special facility could become a productive, law-abiding worker was a crucial task for superintendents seeking private and public funds. George Brown (of the Barre home) and Knight, along with Howe, enjoyed repeating the story of two idiots who had graduated from the Pennsylvania Training School, one to find employment in a factory in Maine and one in a factory in New Hampshire (S. Howe 1874; Knight ca. 1860; Pennsylvania Training School for Feeble-Minded Children 1858, 55). In a speech given throughout Connecticut in the 1850s, Knight (ca. 1860) stressed productivity as a central rationale for training. "Why should Connecticut erect an asylum for the Education of Idiots?" he asked rhetorically. "Laying aside humanity it would be economic. Being consumers and not producers they are a great pecuniary burden to the state. Educate them and they will become producers." Even as late as 1866, Seguin (1866, 295–457), in his *Idiocy*, devoted a lengthy appendix to cases of idiots who after receiving proper physiological education became productive citizens, some even giving their lives in service to the Union army.

To offset these success stories, the superintendents were never reluctant to report tales of families financially ruined by an idiot child in the household. Kerlin wrote:

> Several examples have occurred, such as this: the heads of a family had been so preoccupied with their unfortunate child, that a broken down constitution for the mother and an entire disastrous interruption to the business of the father, had resulted. The State came in at this crisis, and assumed the charge of the child: the insufferable weight removed, a new life was infused into the household; business became again possible, health was restored, and after a few years the child is on the "pay list," and the family is prosperous. This is the strongest *economical* [Kerlin's emphasis] argument our statistics show, for the extension of our work to all and every condition of the class under consideration, providing ample schools, receptacles and asylums in all parts of the State. (Pennsylvania Training School for Feeble-Minded Children 1869, 15)

The goal of education was productivity, and superintendents assumed that educated idiots, freed from inactivity and no longer a burden to their family, would return home to be productive and upright citizens in their communities. Without education in the institution, however, the likely consequences were not promising for idiots, families, or communities.

A critical element of this assumption was the superintendents' insistence that the education of idiots could effectively occur only in a school segregated from family and community. Neither the home nor the common school was seen as an appropriate setting for an idiot's education. In the homes of the poor, idiots were neglected and allowed to develop "degrading and loathsome habits . . . eat[ing] the most filthy and disgusting garbage they can find . . . addicted to constant motions of the head, tongues, or lips . . . [and] to vicious and malicious practices"; if moral idiots, they were led to the "inevitable degeneracy" of crime (Connecticut General Assembly 1856, 12–14). In the homes of the well-to-do, they were overly indulged and left to become pampered social embarrassments (S. Howe 1848*b*, 33–35; Kerlin 1858, 28; New York Asylum for Idiots 1861, 18). Neglect and overindulgence were both the bane of proper education.

In the common school, teachers were unfamiliar with the habits of idiots. When confronted with idiot children, they lost valuable time needed for normal children (Kerlin 1858, 68). Idiot children, too, institutional authorities believed, needed companionship with people like themselves. Normal children were apt to tease and frustrate them. Confinement in the common school ensured that any gregariousness they might have would wane (H. Knight ca. 1860). Only special schools, in which teachers like themselves were sensitive to the needs of such children and companionship was assured, could release idiots from their idleness to become productive and upright people.

The first generation of American superintendents, then, while justifying the need for special schools on educational and socioeconomic grounds also justified the need for their own special knowledge and skills. On the one hand, neither the family nor the community school could properly educate idiot children. On the other, both the family and the community found themselves burdened by an idiot child—the family by loss of productivity and the community by distraction from educating normal children. Special schools freed families and public schools from the burden of caring for and educating feebleminded children, and they provided legitimacy for special teachers.

If the home and the common school were improper places for educating idiots, so, too, the almshouse and the prison were the likely refuge of idiots educated outside the idiot school. Degenerate because of neglect or overindulgence, a burden to family and community, uneducated idiot adults languished in permanent pauperism in local poorhouses. Led to vice and corruption, uncontrolled by kith or kin, moral idiot adults became the prey of criminals and the perpetrators of crime.

By insisting that the proper education of idiots could occur only in special facilities and that the fate of the improperly trained was the almshouse or prison, the first generation of reformers justified the creation of their schools and, of course, their positions in them. Ironically, however, they were also leaving themselves vulnerable to social and economic pressures, none of which they predicted at the outset of their efforts but which soon began to turn their special schools into custodial havens. After the panic of 1857, local officials facing growing unemployment coupled with heavy immigration began to pressure superintendents to take, not discharge, idiots: a pool of unemployed workers with able minds was available to fill jobs. In a short time, superintendents like Howe, Parrish, and Hervey Wilbur found that more than a few discharged pupils placed in community jobs or with their families were returning to their former schools (e.g., New York Asylum for Idiots 1864; Pennsylvania Training School for Feeble-Minded Children 1873). Thus, the purpose of the school began to shift from returning productive idiots to their communities to keeping them in the special school.

Having widely publicized their educational successes, which they insisted could have occurred only in special schools, the superintendents also opened themselves to calls for expanding the size and mission of their schools to include pupils whom they previously had not considered eligible for admission. Especially after the Civil War, most schools began both to admit children and adults with multiple problems and to retain adult graduates. At first, the stated policy of all schools had been to admit only improvable idiot children, so-called simple idiots, who were free of complicating physical and moral disabilities. Superintendents hoped such idiots, like their common school counterparts, would receive training and leave school to become productive citizens, thereby giving up their places for younger pupils. Most state authorizations assumed such a course, and most schools, therefore, explicitly excluded epileptics, insane idiots, and other "incurables" and prohibited the admission or retention of adult idiots. The model followed was an extension of the common school, not unlike that extension envisioned by schools for the blind and the deaf and dumb.

By 1871, when Pennsylvania changed its statutes to allow adults into idiot training schools, most institutions, despite legislative prohibitions, had long been admitting them. Some epileptics were also among the earliest pupils at the Pennsylvania school (Kerlin 1858). The Ohio facility began to admit and retain adult idiots as early as 1861, even though legislative authorization did not come about until 1898 (Ohio Institution 1899, 5–11; Pennsylvania Training School for Feeble-Minded Children 1858, 61–62). Even Hervey Wilbur, who publicly insisted on the exclusive admission of "simple idiots" to the New York Asylum, allowed some "improvable" epileptics to remain at his facility (New York Asylum for Idiots 1861).

Most superintendents found "worst cases" with multiple disabilities to be a mixed blessing. As I noted earlier, such cases, if they improved, could melt the hearts of the stingiest legislators. In their efforts to get initial funding, superintendents and their advocates in the antebellum years were eager to show the remarkable successes that occurred even in educating idiots whose physical, intellectual, and moral capacities were extremely limited (e.g., Brockett 1856a, 1856b; J. Richards 1854). Although careful to avoid claims for cures, the superintendents in their enthusiasm in the heady days of the late 1840s and early 1850s no doubt achieved remarkable change in several cases. Success came, however, only through tedious, individualized training. For superintendents like Wilbur and Brown following Seguin's model, this meant the creation of a family-like environment and minute-by-minute involvement with the pupil in the classroom, at the table, in the kitchen, and in the bedroom (C. Brown 1897; L. Richards 1935, 176–177). Frank Knight Sanders recalled his boyhood visits to his uncle's Connecticut school:

> During my early years I shared the daily life of the institution. The household was a real family. The pupils were always known as "the children." The whole staff assembled with the Doctor's family at meals and all with the children at morning prayers, which were led by Dr. Knight. He knew each child by name. With unfailing tenderness and professional cunning he individualized the treatment of each one. (Sanders 1927, n.p.)

Letters from pleased and often astonished parents lent credence to these successful transformations (Schwartz 1956, 145–146; J. Trent 2012, 188; C. Wilbur 1870–81). But the very successes used to get additional funding helped to make future successes less likely. More funds to enlarge the schools to meet greater demand meant more pupils who inevitably had more unique problems that were less likely to receive unique attention. Larger schools especially had less time to provide the individual attention needed to improve the condition of exceedingly disabled pupils. Once the schools began to grow, the promise to legislators to send productive pupils back to their home towns was best fulfilled by concentrating on the most capable, who were more likely to leave the facility. "Worst cases" might get funds, but "higher-grade cases" ensured future funding. Even into the 1860s, Wilbur dismissed "confirmed epileptics" and those "unimprovable after a fair trial" (New York Asylum for Idiots 1861, 9, 16–17). Yet on the rolls of his school and in descriptions in his annual reports were what could only be described as "worst cases."

To be sure, the first superintendents were eager to admit pupils who might benefit from the training offered at their schools. Also they were quite willing to discharge students who had successfully completed a course of study. From their earliest years, however, superintendents, despite legislative restrictions, admitted pupils whose limitations were great and whose eventual release was doubtful. The admission of *custodial* cases, then, began not from outside pressure but from the desire of superintendents to acquire legislative and public support and enhance their own legitimacy. As their schools grew, however, they had less time for the intense training necessary for "worst cases." When external pressures did begin to develop after the panic of 1857 and the Civil War, superintendents (with varying degrees of reluctance) persuaded legislators to change the restrictive admission policies that most schools had never rigidly enforced. By the dawn of the war, superintendents were increasingly faced with two groups of unproductive clientele: institutionally trained idiots unable to find or keep employment in their home communities or unable to live with their families, and "asylum-grade" idiots who often had multiple disabilities.[8]

Most superintendents thus found themselves preaching the educational function and purpose of their facilities while preparing the way for custody. This split between rhetoric and reality continued into the 1870s, when most reformers began, cautiously at first but by the 1880s with more vigor, to acknowledge the need for custodial preparation alongside educational programs (P. Ferguson 1994).

In 1857, nine years after his optimistic *Report* of 1848, Howe, still the leading champion of education over custody among the heads of state schools, addressed the cornerstone-laying ceremony at the Pennsylvania Training School. Wilbur, Seguin, Joseph Parrish (a local physician who had replaced James B. Richards as superintendent of the Pennsylvania School in 1856), and Kerlin were in attendance and could not have been unaffected by the new tone of caution in his words:

> Do all that we may, we cannot make out of the *real idiot* a reasoning and self-guiding man. We can arrest the downward tendency to brutishness which his infirmity entails. We can teach him even some elementary truths; and, what is more important still, we may draw out and strengthen his moral and social faculties, so as to make them lessen the activity of his animal nature; but, after all, he must ever [have] a child-like dependence upon others for guidance and support.

He went on, "They can indeed be made less burdensome, but not materially productive. They are idiots for life" (Pennsylvania Training School for Feeble-Minded Children 1858, 43). After nearly a decade of practice and pressure, Howe insisted that a new goal was necessary. The goal of education for idiots could no longer be *productivity*. In his 1848 *Report*, the explicit goal had been the reintegration of productive idiots into communities. By 1858, "humanity" itself had become a new and more realistic purpose. We must *care* for idiots, Howe now claimed, not because we expect them to be productive, but because we are obligated to serve the weak. Put another way, education in itself is the goal. With education as an end rather than a means, especially within growing institutions, superintendents like Howe could warn about custody even as they were turning their schools into custodial facilities.

In the later years of his life, Howe spoke about the evils of congregating disabled people in large institutions—a phenomenon beginning even before his death in 1876. Yet his own facility in South Boston expanded during his tenure there. Although Howe de-emphasized lifetime custody in large congregate dormitories, the facilities that housed his schools for the blind and feebleminded gathered more and more pupils, some of whom spent their whole lives there. Laura Bridgman, his most famous pupil, arrived at the facility in 1837 and died there in 1889. As early as 1840, Howe had anticipated the necessity of providing a work department for blind graduates unable to find employment outside the institution. Some years later, he reluctantly opened a workshop at the Massachusetts school for unemployable graduates (J. Trent 2012, 65–66; F. Williams 1917).

Thus, Howe, the most vigorous opponent of custody among the earliest superintendents, would reconstruct community productivity for an institutional context. Like the others, he abandoned the hope of returning educated and productive idiots to their local communities because he could not find work for them "on the outside." Others more at ease with the contradictions of custody would shift their perspectives as well as their policies. Without work, educated idiots needed care, and the need for care necessitated new rationales for the special school.

From School to Asylum

In 1873, Isaac Kerlin criticized Hervey Wilbur for continuing to insist that the New York Asylum for Idiots was an educational facility (Pennsylvania Training School for Feeble-Minded Children 1873). Despite Wilbur's protests in his next annual report, Kerlin's criticism was a correct one (New York Asylum for Idiots 1874). Wilbur might remind his board that "the large institutions are to be deprecated" (New York Asylum for Idiots 1874, 19). Nevertheless, he emphasized in the same report the need for classifying idiots to determine "special needs," and, as he had from his first year as superintendent, he advocated expanding the size of his facility. When in 1878 he helped Josephine Shaw Lowell open the Custodial Asylum for Feeble-Minded Women in Newark, New York (which I discuss in Chapter 3), the first American custodial facility explicitly for idiots, he was only postponing the coming of custody to his own Syracuse school. Henry Knight, who in the 1850s had stressed productivity as the goal of educating idiots, joined the others to write and speak about the burden of feeblemindedness as a rationale for obtaining public funding to expand his school to include idiots who could not return to their homes (Goodheart 2004; H. Knight 1877; Rose 2008, 25–63).[9]

Expansion remained on the minds of most superintendents. In a letter to R. J. Patterson in 1860, Parrish advised the Ohio superintendent:

> I am decidedly of opinion that a farm is desirable. We occupied eight acres in Germantown, and as you know, removed to this locality, which is a farm of sixty acres, including ten acres of woodland in the rear of our buildings. Our present number of children is sixty-seven, and out of that number we can find twelve working boys, and when our household increases to twice its present size, have no doubt at all that we shall find it desirable to add to our acres likewise. (Ohio Asylum 1861, 10)

During the same year, Wilbur advised Patterson: "The education given to idiots, in the main, should be a practical one. You will observe that a farm enables the Institution to provide profitably for a certain number of adult idiots, who are beyond the school-attending age." He added, "I have to-day at least forty boys at work about the place." He concluded by noting the financial consequences of attempting to operate a school without a farm: "Where there is only land enough for [a] play-ground, there can be no work for the large boys. The consequence is that it takes twice the number to care for such children out of school hours than in. Thus, the proportion of teachers to attendants will generally be less than one to two" (Ohio Asylum 1861, 10–11). Wilbur's advice to Patterson suggested that, despite his claims to the contrary, he anticipated custody for some idiots. The farm attached to the school provided work for those idiots.

In his 1861 annual report, Wilbur left the door open for custody: "Whenever, in the farther experience of the institution, it shall be deemed advisable to extend the limits of age in the reception of pupils, it can be done" (New York Asylum for Idiots 1861, 15). By planning for an adult population, Wilbur anticipated custody. Following the advice of his colleagues, in 1860 Patterson became one of the first superintendents to acknowledge the necessity of planning for custodial clients. "A farm is needed," the Ohio superintendent claimed, "with its stock and implements, as means of education, while it would also diminish to some extent, the expense of support. A farm would also provide for the permanent retention and profitable employment of a certain number of adult idiots who would else be obligated to find homes in county infirmaries, jails or lunatic asylums" (Ohio Asylum 1861, 9).

Patterson, like the others, saw that trained idiot teenagers and young adults, instead of finding employment, were just as likely, if not more likely, to be reinstitutionalized locally in the almshouse, the jail, or the lunatic asylum—the very institutions from which reformers had sought to remove them. However, communities began to resist adding idiots to their growing poor rolls; the economic downturn that began in 1857 and lingered until the first war years had swelled community poorhouses and initiated a greater concern for pauper children (Stansell 1986, 198–216). Indeed, as we have seen, most local officials began to pressure the state schools to take more idiots out of their communities. Given economic hardship, even productive idiots were losing their jobs. Some returned to the state asylum; others to the poorhouse. Families unable to deal with the downturn were likewise unwilling to reintegrate a family member who might have been away for as long as a decade.

By 1860, these pressures—hardly resisted by the superintendents—resulted in the expansion of the schools. Although smaller than the growth that occurred after the war, this expansion was significant. The Pennsylvania and Connecticut schools, both inaugurated as private facilities, began to grow as they took on publicly supported charity pupils. The New York facility, having moved in 1851 to what was then the small town of Syracuse, expanded as institutional officials bought and rented more land. The Pennsylvania school moved from its rented house in Germantown to a farm outside of Media, and the Ohio facility found spacious land in Columbus. In rural western Connecticut, Knight began to purchase more land for his growing school. Even Brown added to his land holdings at his small private school at Barre, Massachusetts (Sanders 1927; Seguin 1870*b*, 1870*c*).

More land meant more buildings. From the earliest days of their activities, superintendents were calling for additional buildings to carry out more specialized functions. As early as 1852, at the ground-breaking ceremony of the Syracuse facility, Wilbur had expressed pride in his new medical building, school building, student dormitory, and living quarters for his staff (New York Asylum for Idiots 1854). In their 1856 recommendation to the Connecticut legislature, Brockett and Knight insisted that Howe's decentralized institution lying on "low and wet" ground in South Boston was not an appropriate model for the projected Connecticut asylum. Instead, they insisted, a Connecticut facility should be centralized with a full-time superintendent who would administer a "main edifice, contain[ing] school-rooms, dormitories for pupils, attendants and teachers, and a full suite of rooms for the accommodation of the Superintendent and his family, a wash-house, a gymnasium, barns, etc." (Connecticut General Assembly 1856, 15–21).

More land, more buildings, and more pupils, of course, required superintendents, not teachers, to oversee them. Howe, Wilbur, and Richards had begun their work with idiots using educational approaches. Their earliest professional writings on the subject had appeared in educational journals. Although the former two were physicians, Howe had gained his international reputation as a teacher of the blind, and Wilbur had followed in his father's footsteps to become a teacher before taking up medicine. Both focused on the *education* of idiots. The next group of superintendents—Parrish and Kerlin in Pennsylvania, Patterson in Ohio, Brown in Massachusetts, and Knight in Connecticut—were all physicians. Although committed to education, they, along with Howe and Wilbur, soon became administrators of growing schools. Eventually, the education of idiot pupils was left to others as institutional structures expanded. Even in the earliest years of the special schools, superintendents were lobbying to ensure that the dominant institutional model would become the asylum, a model that would accommodate not only their educational interests but also their concern for professional status. The case of Richards's tenure at the Pennsylvania Training School illustrates this point.

James B. Richards arrived in Germantown, then some distance from Philadelphia, in 1853. He was thirty-six. Born to missionary parents, he had become caught up in the progressive Unitarianism of Theodore Parker and the abolitionism of William Lloyd Garrison. As a young man, he became a teacher at the Chauncy Hall School in Boston. Attracted to Horace Mann's educational reforms, Richards was known as a patient and devoted teacher. In 1848, Mann recommended Richards to Howe, and that summer Howe sent Richards to Europe to study methods for teaching idiots. There he became familiar with the efforts at the Bicêtre and likely met Seguin. On his return to Boston, he took over the primary responsibility for educating idiot pupils newly admitted to Howe's facility. All indications are that his work there was successful. Perhaps because of his association with Garrison and other radical abolitionists, or maybe due to his conflict with the school's matron, Richards left Howe's employment in 1852 (Kerlin 1887*b*; J. Trent 2012, 179–180; T. Williams 1887).[10]

In fall 1852, he turned up in Philadelphia to start a small private school for idiots. In February 1853, he met with prominent Philadelphia citizens to propose a larger facility supported by public funds and private subscriptions. Included in the group were Alonzo Potter, Episcopal bishop of Pennsylvania; James Barclay, a prominent attorney; and Alfred Elwyn, a physician and local philanthropist. By the end of the year, Thomas Kirkbride, superintendent of the state lunatic asylum, joined the group. In September, they appointed Richards principal of the new school at an annual salary of $2,000 plus living expenses. They rented two houses in Germantown for eight pupils. Richards estimated quarterly expenses for the pupils of $1,200 but receipts of only $900. With this projected deficit, it is not surprising that problems began to develop. In October, without Richards's approval, the board of directors appointed a female matron. They also restricted Richards's term to a single nine-month (although renewable) appointment. Finally, contrary to their own restrictions and Richards's warnings, they agreed to admit one child and, in November, admitted two more children over the age of twelve (Pennsylvania Training School for Feeble-Minded Children, *Minutes*, September 21, 1853, October 13, 1853, November 4, 1853).

By summer 1854, financial and administrative problems had thoroughly strained Richards's relationship with his board. At its August meeting, the board voted to require Richards to submit a detailed inventory of "any and all articles of Furniture, or utensils of whatever kind, that have been purchased [and] . . . also to state whether in the knowledge of the Principal, there are any articles purchased for the Institution (other than customary monthly requirements) for which payment has not been made by the Treasurer under warrant from the Board." They also insisted that Richards submit monthly requests for reimbursement of *educational* expenses (Pennsylvania Training School for Feeble-Minded Children, *Minutes*, August 9, 1854).

Despite receiving its first legislative appropriation, the board continued to express concern throughout 1854 about Richards's purchase of specialized teaching equipment. In 1855, the school moved its seventeen students to Woodland Avenue in Germantown. In November, Richards requested reimbursement in the amount of $92.71 for a "rocking boat" used for physical exercises for his pupils. The board objected to the expense of the strange item and feared the liability it might incur: "Altho no accident has heretofore occurred from its use, the committee [on finances] would not be surprised at any moment to hear of serious or perhaps fatal consequences being produced by it. They therefore recommend that use of it by the pupils be at once discontinued" (Pennsylvania Training School for Feeble-Minded Children, *Minutes*, December 7, 1855). The board also objected to Richards's hiring of a teacher without its authorization. By January 1856, the board had recommended "a change in the administration of the school" (Pennsylvania Training School for Feeble-Minded Children, *Minutes*, January 18, 1856).

A committee of board members including Kirkbride was appointed to study a new administrative structure for the growing school. In February, it recommended that the managerial functions of the school be separated from the educational functions. The committee also insisted that Richards stop requesting reimbursement for teaching supplies and submit requests in advance for board approval. The tone and content of the recommendations left little doubt that the directors were frustrated with Richards's emphasis on teaching and his apparent disregard for proper institutional administration. Richards was primarily interested in his pupils. The board was interested in maintaining the facility, in having it operate efficiently, and in seeing it grow (Pennsylvania Training School for Feeble-Minded Children, *Minutes*, February 1, 1856).

In March 1856, a new twist developed. Edward Seguin, at the time residing at Wilbur's facility in Syracuse, was appointed "head of the institution." The appointment, made with no involvement from Richards, proved to be short-lived. By the next month, Seguin had resigned because of the board's equivocation over his authority—the same problem that had plagued Richards. At that time, too, Seguin had no medical degree.

In May, Richards left Germantown–but not before the directors had appointed their first *superintendent*, Joseph Parrish. The authority they had so resisted giving Richards and Seguin they immediately turned over to Parrish (Pennsylvania Training School for Feeble-Minded Children, *Minutes*, March 4, 1856; April 4, 1856; April 19, 1856; May 7, 1856).

It is clear from the board minutes of this period that the directors were interested in having a superintendent, not a teacher. They wanted someone with authority to shape services to their liking, whose focus was not exclusively on educational matters, and who could direct people and institutions. Parrish, a native Philadelphian and a respected doctor from a family of respected local physicians, fit their image of an appropriate administrator. In July, Parrish persuaded his friend Dorothea Dix, who up to this point had shown little interest in idiots, to help him secure a new legislative appropriation to put the institution on sounder financial footing. By December 1857, the cornerstone of a large facility on farmland near Media had been placed. When Parrish, the physician-superintendent, replaced Richards, the educator-principal, the change meant more than a substitution of titles. Parrish represented a vision of a new context for "educating" idiots—a context that resembled an asylum more than a school. With this new and enlarged direction, the once small school, now an asylum, drew the financial support of some of eastern Pennsylvania's most prominent citizens. Josiah Dawson, a thrifty Quaker land dealer, gave a most generous $6,000 donation, and John P. Crozer, a wealthy mill owner, gave $2,000 ("Life Subscribers and Donors" 1859).[11]

This vision had begun to develop not after an extended period of institutional history but within a few years of the founding of the first schools. Champions of services for feebleminded people were not willing to restrict their emerging facilities to the model of the common school. Although they continued to draw upon the tools and techniques of educators, their vision of the future was modeled after the lunatic asylum with its dependence on medical practice, medical institutional structure, and medical paradigms. For nearly thirty years, Richards would be the last educator who was not also trained in medicine to exert leadership in the field. It would be almost fifty years before educators would again take up an interest in idiocy

(Pennsylvania Training School for Feeble-Minded Children, *Minutes*, June 6, 1856; July 13, 1856; Pennsylvania Training School for Feeble-Minded Children 1858).

The medicalizing of idiocy completed the constructing of a place for idiocy. The idiot asylum modeled after the lunatic asylum had competed with the model of the common school even from the beginning. Howe, in 1848, had praised Seguin's educational achievement but had been quick to add that because Seguin was not a physician, his views on idiocy were incomplete (S. Howe 1848*b*). In his first annual report, Patterson at the Ohio Asylum (never named "School") insisted that medicine had become the primary profession for developing and sustaining services for idiots both in the United States and in Europe (Ohio Asylum 1858, 29). In the same year, Parrish at the Pennsylvania Training School, in a letter to Patterson, noted that his new facility would be "a home—a hospital—and a school" (Ohio Asylum 1858, 37). Likewise, Kerlin noted that all pupils at the Germantown facility went through daily medical inspections in the "medicine room" (Kerlin 1858, 140). At the Syracuse school, Wilbur required that all applications for admission include a certificate from the family physician. As he related to Seguin around 1864, "The selection of pupils is usually based upon such [a] certificate" (Seguin 1864, 16–17).

In growing facilities like those in Pennsylvania and Ohio, too, medical superintendents began to hire assistant physicians, the former in charge of the growing institutional bureaucracy and the latter in charge of the institutional infirmary or hospital. Increasingly, the annual reports contained the language of medicine alongside the language of education. By 1857, Parrish was referring to his pupils as *inmates*, a term more familiar to prisons and asylums than to schools (Pennsylvania Training School for Feeble-Minded Children 1858).

Also around that time, superintendents began describing their inmates in terms of their pathological symptoms and hereditary traits. Often these descriptions emphasized the idiots' "atavistic and recapitulatory characteristics." Kerlin pointed out the "marked elongation" of the tongue of one moral idiot and said that another looked "more swinish than human" (Kerlin 1858, 25, 30).[12] Before the late 1850s, superintendents had emphasized the hereditary flaws of the parents "visited upon the children." After this time, they began to classify hereditary traits identified in the feebleminded people themselves. In his speaking tour of Connecticut to gain support for his efforts, Henry Knight described a family thus:

> In the town of Coventry there is a family of five persons. All of them are congenital idiots. The father is sixty-five years of age. The mother sixty years. They have three daughters. A low grade of idiocy—but they can speak, feed, and dress themselves—cannot count—can do some work—"all of a very bad breed"— Intemperate, lustful, brutish and filthy. All [are] paupers except one daughter who lives in a private family. One daughter is pregnant illegitimately of course. She is a common strumpet. Her father was found by the postmaster having carnal intercourse with her a few weeks ago. (H. Knight ca. 1860)

With this change, too, came a gradual shift from associating hereditary flaws with defects in the social structure to associating them with defects in the person.

Eventually, in the writings of the superintendents, the victim of hereditary flaw became the perpetrator of such flaw. After the war, with the publications of the writings of two British superintendents, J. Langdon Down (1866, 1867) and William W. Ireland (1877), who both stressed the pathology of idiocy, American superintendents had an even firmer medical basis upon which to carry on their work (Fish 1879).

Just as medical terminology, themes, and treatments began to enter the language of superintendents and to replace an emphasis on education, so, too, did they pervade the professional relations of superintendents in charge of idiots. Even before the founding of the Association of Medical Officers of American Institutions for Idiotic and Feeble-Minded Persons in 1876, superintendents were expected to be physicians, institutions were expected to have hospital facilities, and inmates were expected to need a type of medical care particular to feebleminded people.

Of course, to provide doctors, hospitals, and specialized care, institutions needed to be sufficiently large to operate efficiently. As early as 1856, Brockett had supported the British trend of constructing institutions to accommodate four hundred inmates. Increasingly unwilling to resist the growing requests from local officials and parents, superintendents even before the Civil War had reminded legislators that the most efficient way to provide training and care for idiots—especially pauper idiots—was in large facilities (Connecticut General Assembly 1856). Not surprisingly, these expanding institutions with their medical facilities and supervision meshed well with the growing emphasis on custodial care. A sick idiot fit a custody model better than did an educated and productive one.

CONCLUSION

In the 1840s, local idiots became a concern of reformers and state officials because of three factors: the census, reports of idiots in jails and almshouses, and reports from Europe about the successful education of idiots. The national census of 1840 identified idiots, along with other dependents and deviants. Already concerned with several of these groups, reformers of the time were ready to see in the census an abundance of American idiots. When Howe reported their frequent appearance in almshouses and jails, reformers linked their perceptions of the abundance of idiots with a concern for their care. In the almshouse or jail, according to reformers, idiots were mistreated, neglected, or, worse, led to public vice and personal corruption. Reports from Europe, however, indicated there was hope for the local idiot. Education in special schools away from corruption, neglect, or overpampering could free idiots from their natural deficiencies and transform them into productive citizens. In the special school, too, reformers insisted, idiots, like the blind and the deaf and dumb before them, could return to their homes better off than they had been when they arrived at the school.

Soon, however, superintendents found that educated idiots could return to families or to community employment only when economic conditions were good. They might talk about their successful transformations of "driveling idiots" into productive workers, but, by the late 1850s, superintendents found that returning lower class students to local communities was increasingly difficult. There simply were not jobs for them, and local almoners were not eager to add them to their already swelling rolls. Feeling the pressure to house more and more unemployed and unemployable idiots, superintendents looked to the state for support. Indeed, the very survival of the institution began to depend on public aid. To convince state officials that their schools needed state support and, thus, to ensure the survival of their institutions, superintendents saw the need to broaden the function of their facilities. Although education continued to be emphasized and educational techniques were discussed and shared, after the Civil War, the goal of returning productive, law-abiding workers to their homes or communities was becoming less central to the operations of the enlarging facilities. Even as some inmates (primarily from professional and upper class families) were educated and discharged, the new goal of the institutions was becoming self-perpetuation. Well-behaved idiots remaining in public institutions would soon replace productive idiots returning to their home communities.

Like the shift from local to state responsibility for many groups of the disabled poor—the mad, the blind, the deaf, and the delinquent—care for feebleminded people became part of a response to rapid changes in the social and economic fabric of American life. Superintendents guided that response, to be sure, within the limitations imposed by these emerging changes. Yet that response soon solidified into a uniform vision of the asylum. In this vision, medicine, not education, would dominate, and physician-superintendents would, in turn, create a familiar milieu in which to establish and maintain their own professional legitimacy. They were not the victims of social forces they could not control nor were they forced to shape their institutions in ways that were fundamentally contrary to their original intent. They constructed not only institutions but also meaning, defining the public's understanding of idiocy and, in the process, ensuring their professional status and survival.

NOTES

1. There were a few exceptions to this exclusion. In 1817, for example, officials at the American Asylum for the Deaf in Hartford admitted a blind and deaf idiot (Turner 1856). Two decades later, an idiot child was left at the Massachusetts Asylum for the Blind. In neither case was much effort made to educate these children, with Howe in Massachusetts, for example, preferring to examine their phrenological anomalies.
2. After he immigrated to the United States in 1850, Edouard Séguin anglicized his first name and dropped the accent from his surname, thus becoming Edward Seguin. He used this spelling for the remainder of his life. After his death (and occasionally before it), some American writers employed the French spelling. I use the anglicized version throughout this work.
3. Also in 1840, Norton S. Townshend, a physician, legislator, and later prominent abolitionist from Ohio, observed the work done in Paris to educate idiots. In 1843, under the auspices of the Massachusetts Board of Education, Horace Mann likely

visited Edouard Seguin's school at his Paris home on the rue Pigalle (Seguin 1880c, 207). The next year Samuel Woodward, superintendent of the Massachusetts Lunatic Asylum, in a letter to the *Boston Advertiser*, claimed that idiots could be educated. He based his claim on the work done in Paris. At the beginning of the following year, he wrote Samuel G. Howe urging him to begin a school for idiots at his asylum for the blind. Between February and March 1845, Howe wrote four letters published in the *Advertiser* claiming the educability of idiots and the proper role of public support for their education. At about the same time, at the initiation of William M. Awl, superintendent of Ohio's lunatic asylum and a founder in 1837 of the state's school for the blind, the Association of Medical Superintendents of American Institutions for the Insane at their inaugural meeting in Philadelphia in 1844 set up a committee of Awl and Amariah Brigham and Samuel White, both of New York, to study the care of idiots. In 1846, at the association's second meeting, the committee issued its report, which called for the development of idiot asylums (Pelicier and Thuillier 1980, 27–28; Pelicier and Thuillier 1996, 1–9, 160–186; Schwartz 1956, 137–139; Trent 2012, 146, 150–154).

4. See "The Bicêtre Asylum" 1848; "Education of Idiots" 1847; "Education of Idiots" 1849; "Education of Idiots at the Bicêtre" 1847; S. Howe 1848a, 1848b, 1848c; "Idiocy in Massachusetts" 1847; "Idiocy in Massachusetts" 1849; Schwartz 1956, 137–146; "Tuition of Idiots" 1848; "Visit to the Bicêtre" 1847.

5. In 1842, the same year that Samuel G. Howe confirmed Dorothea Dix's claim that blind and deaf people, the insane, and idiots were congregated with criminals, debtors, and paupers in Massachusetts prisons and almshouses, P. T. Barnum opened his American Museum in New York City and began exhibiting a variety of freaks, many of whom were the same sort noted by Knight in 1860.

   On the place of feeble minds in the circus sideshow and the county fair, see R. Adams (2001); Bogdan (1988, especially chapter 5); Bogdan (2014); Bogdan, Elks, and Knoll (2012); Krentz (2005); and R. Thomson (1996). Bogdan (1988) tells the stories of several people exhibited in circus side shows as "wild men" (and occasionally "wild women"). Most, although not all, became attractions after the Civil War. Even in the twentieth century, such people as the "dean of freaks," whose stage name was Zip, attracted the attention of more than 100 million sideshow viewers. William Fish (1879), in his medical thesis at the Albany Medical College noted: "The so called Aztec children exhibited in this country a few years ago were microcephalic Idiots." Interestingly enough, his clinical descriptions of microcephalic training school inmates were not dissimilar to the descriptions of sideshow barkers. Fish wrote of one such inmate, "T. M. . . . is active, fond of notice, dances well, and save when asleep, is constantly in motion, reminding one by his darting quick movement of a humming bird, is a little disposed to be quarrelsome, is fond of gymnastic exercise, . . . [and] in attempting to whistle makes a noise like the peep of a chicken." These sentiments, memories, and visions Fish would take with him to the Illinois Asylum in 1884.

   Krentz (2005) reviews the life of Thomas Wiggins, commonly known as "Blind Tom," who was born a slave in Georgia in 1849. From reports of the time, Wiggins was both blind and cognitively disabled. Because of his skill at playing classical music on the piano, he became a figure in the sideshow carnivals and later on the stages of leading American theaters.

6. Barnaby, like Kerlin's Grubb, Neddie, and Alfred, was a child of nature. But unlike Wordsworth's idiot boy who interacted only with nature, Dickens's Barnaby became the easy victim of unsavory and artful companions. Caught in the Gordon riots,

he was used by the riot leaders to participate in mob actions. Unable to appreciate Gordon's jingoistic motives, Barnaby became a tool of the plotters. Arrested and condemned to die, he was rescued and returned to his mother. Back with her, although he still rambled, he had protection from the world's temptations (Dickens 1871).

7. After reviewing several copies of *The Mind Unveiled*, I discovered the book's printer had included different sets of photographs in them. Each copy also had engravings, but these were the same. For example, in a copy at the University of Minnesota, I found the photograph of Grubb I have included here. In a copy at the University of Kansas Medical Center, Grubb was in a group portrait with other men labeled moral idiots.

Eric Carlson, in his introduction to Sander L. Gilman's (1976, xiv) edition and reprints of Hugh W. Diamond's famous 1850s photographs of patients at the Surrey County Lunatic Asylum and essays by Diamond and John Conolly, suggests that Kerlin's *The Mind Unveiled* may have been the first book to use psychiatric photographs. Like Kerlin's use of the book in Grubb's hand, Diamond placed objects in the hands of some of his patients to symbolize one of their diagnostic characteristics. In one engraving of a photograph, a woman with "religious melancholy" has her arm propped on prayer books. In another, a woman who obsessively steals has a basket in her arms. In a third, a woman holds a chicken, symbolizing her delusions. Unlike Diamond's "face of madness," Kerlin's "face of moral idiocy" included a promise of controlling nature through moral training and care.

8. All histories of intellectual disability, which generally stress a seamless web of scientific and intellectual advances (e.g., Clausen 1967; Kanner 1964; Milligan 1961; Scheerenberger 1983, 1987; Sloan and Stevens 1976), describe a brief period in which students in idiot schools received education and individual care. These histories appear to take up the perspective first developed by Walter E. Fernald (1893) and later repeated as a common litany by succeeding generations of superintendents. According to this ongoing tradition, in the 1870s, the focus of services for feeble minds shifted from education and individual care in small schools to custodial care in large facilities. It did so because superintendents lost faith in their ability to educate their pupils. Even more critical analyses have taken this perspective for granted (Hollander 1986; Sarason and Doris 1969, 209–329; Tyor 1977; Zigler, Hodapp, and Edison 1990). These critics are correct to hold that the custodial perspective began to become more overt in the 1870s. My reading of the period, however, suggests that the seeds of custodialism were apparent even before the Civil War. Economic recession in the 1850s began the first of several cycles that made educated feeble minds unproductive in the community. Also, economic hard times outside the institution motivated families with feebleminded children to look to the idiot school as a source of relief. I take exception with Tyor's claim that, "Earlier improvements which had seemed so encouraging, were due to the combined influence of the natural process of growth and entry into the therapeutic environment of the school. The effects of both factors diminished with time. Except for a few cases, there were no continued improvements after the age of puberty" (Tyor 1977, 476). Tyor, I believe, too easily accepts the superintendents' rationale for the so-called failure to improve. Many did not show "improvement" because they could not find work; faced with hard times, they were unable to support themselves. Others did not "improve" because their relatives or communities could not afford to keep them.

Superintendents began to doubt the efficacy of education not because of misgivings about physiological education or because their pupils failed to learn. Their doubt was the result of unstable economic conditions that left their pupils trained but unemployed. Of course, when they looked back on such times, they constructed a rationale that tended to "blame the victim." As such, they interpreted the trend toward custodialism as a product of demand on the one hand and their pupils' failure to learn on the other. Philip Ferguson (1994) has called the phenomenon "chronicity," or the tendency of authorities to emphasize the chronic "incurable nature" of their clientele to justify ongoing institutional "treatment."

9. In his excellent study of the work of Henry Knight and his son, George Knight, in Connecticut, Goodheart argues, I believe too strenuously, that George "departed from his father's emphasis on education and assimilation to embrace eugenics and segregation of the mentally retarded" (Goodheart 2004). Although Goodheart's claim is accurate, the elder Knight had lost his optimism about the transformative effects of education even before the beginning of the Civil War. With the economic downturn of 1857–61, and followed by his educated pupils' inability to find gainful employment in local communities, he was forced to adopt institutional segregation before his son George took over the Connecticut facility.

10. Howe never aligned himself with the Garrisonian radicals and did not become widely known as an antislavery proponent until after the passage of 1850 Fugitive Slave Law and the 1854 Anthony Burns affair (J. Trent 2012, 181–202).

11. Other donors included John A. Brown, $500; Alfred Cope, $1,000; Jasper Cope, $1,000; Joseph Harrison, $1,175; George P. Parrish, $250; Thomas Remington, $500; Richard Ronaldson, $500; J. N. Sharpless, $500; and Dr. George B. Wood, $600.

12. These atavistic and recapitulatory sentiments penetrated the views and fears of parents, too. Darthula Buckner explained her request to admit her son, Mayo, to the Iowa Home for Feeble-Minded Children: "He rolls his eyes and makes a peculiar noise in exact imitation of Blind Boone. I do not wish to send him to public school for he will not protect himself. . . . I think he needs special management and I am unable to undertake it. Have talked to our doctor, A. W. Fees, and he thinks so too." While pregnant with Mayo, Buckner had been frightened by Blind Boone, a traveling minstrel who rolled his blind eyes in a bizarre way. When Mayo, who had unusual musical abilities like Boone, began to roll his eyes, Buckner became convinced that Mayo's behavior was the result of her fright during pregnancy. Mayo Buckner, whose I.Q. in 1958 was 120, spent nearly seventy years in the Iowa facility (Wallace 1958). I shall say more about Mayo Buckner in Chapter 7.

CHAPTER 2

༶

Edward Seguin and the Irony
of Physiological Education

E dward Seguin (né Edouard Séguin) was a man of contradictions. Seguin spent
his adult life as a free thinker, yet Pope Pius IX commended him, calling him
"the apostle to the idiots." Generous and open-minded toward what he saw as the
sweetly disposed idiot, he spoke harshly of the more capable imbecile. Committed
to the principles of moral treatment, around 1840, he was accused of mistreating
children at his private school on the rue Pigalle and, in 1843, of "abominable" practices at the Bicêtre. A champion of the rights of women, the name of his first wife,
the mother of his only child, remains unknown. A sharp critic of medical elitism
among the Paris alienists, he insisted in America that physicians should control
all teaching of idiots. Although he criticized what he called the pathological and
"mentalist" views of idiocy, the study of neurology influenced his own physiological perspective in the last two decades of his life. Generous with friends and colleagues, he was obsessed with being known as the discoverer of the first successful
system for educating idiots and tolerated no pretenders to that fame. Although he
published and lectured widely on educational and medical topics, earning great
praise and loyalty, our understanding of his personal life is filled with gaps and un-
answered questions. Along with the breadth of his writings and their importance
in the formation and development of social programs and policy in nineteenth-
century America, these contradictions in the life and thinking of Edward Seguin,
what Pelicier and Thuillier (1980, 10) have called a "terribly discreet biography,"
make him an interesting study.

Several excellent investigations have focused on the antecedents, philosophy,
and methods of Seguin's physiological system (Boyd 1914; Bourneville 1880,
1895; Fynne 1924; H. Holman 1914; Kraft 1961; Pelicier and Thuillier 1980,
1996; Simpson 1999, 2000; Talbot 1964, 1967; Thuillier 2011). Contemporary accounts of Seguin's work were also numerous (Atkinson 1880; Brockett 1858, 1881;

Bourneville 1880; Conolly 1845, 1847; Dana 1924; *New York Times* 1880*a*; "Séguin, Edouard" 1888; "Séguin, Edouard" 1915; Sumner 1876; H. Wilbur 1881). Seguin's system was affected by changes in his personal life, by changes in his professional commitments, and, in the milieu of American institutional development (which he initiated as the intellectual mentor to the first generation of superintendents), by changes in the American view of idiocy. His legacy, with all its contradictions, reflects even today the ironies in our social constructing of intellectual disability. It is his influence on that construction—never divorced from his views on education, idiocy, or medicine—that deserves a fresh consideration.

A "TERRIBLY DISCREET BIOGRAPHY"

Edward Seguin was born in the small provincial town of Clamecy in the district of Nièvre in 1812.[1] During his teens, he studied at the college d'Auxerre, up the road from Clamecy, and later at the lycée Saint-Louis in Paris. In Paris during his student days, Seguin, like many others of his generation, was influenced by Saint-Simonism, a quasi-religious socialism adopted by Henri Saint-Simon in his *Nouveau Christianisme* (1825). Under the "citizen king," Louis Philippe, what to some appeared to be a bizarre philosophy and to others a threat to traditional institutions was more or less tolerated. In 1831, at the age of nineteen, he was listed as a "third-degree" member of the doctrinal school of Saint-Simon (Talbot 1964, 10).

In 1837, Seguin began a course that he would follow for the remainder of his life. Guersant, a physician at the hospital for incurables (Salpêtrière) and a friend of his father, introduced Seguin to Jean-Marc Itard, the famous teacher of the Wild Boy of Aveyron. In the twilight of his career and a year from his death, Itard, who had also studied medicine with Seguin's father, apparently was impressed with the young provincial. After Itard's death in 1838, Seguin found a new mentor in Jean-Etienne Esquirol, the most influential French alienist of the period. A champion of Pinel's moral treatment and of Gall's phrenology, Esquirol (1818, 1838), like his two mentors, had consistently denied that idiots could be cured or their conditions improved. In 1839, with Esquirol, Seguin published his first text, *Résumé de ce que nous avons fait depuis quatorze mois* (Esquirol and Seguin 1839). In it and in an accompanying volume (Seguin 1839), he summarized his first efforts to educate an idiot boy. Publishing with Esquirol was a professional feat for Seguin, but securing his begrudging admission that idiots could learn was an even greater accomplishment.

Between 1838 and 1844, the philosophical underpinning and methodology of Seguin's work with idiots evolved. In 1840, Esquirol died. Having worked with two of the most famous and influential alienists in France, Seguin began developing his own system of teaching idiots—a system made legitimate by his association with Itard and Esquirol but never subject to their review or rebuttal. It was an envious position for a man of twenty-eight about to launch an independent career (Pelicier and Thuillier 1980, 1996; Talbot 1964). Appointed head teacher of the class of idiot children at the Salpêtrière in 1840, Seguin that year also began to take private pupils in his home, a necessity because he worked for little or no salary at the Salpêtrière (Brockett 1881).[2]

In 1842, he published the first part of *Théorie et practique de l'éducation des enfants arriérés et idiots*, a summary of his work with the idiot class at the hospital for incurables. In November 1842, in recognition of his success and growing fame, Seguin was offered the leadership of a larger class of idiots at the Bicêtre, where he would work under Félix Voisin, a disciple of Esquirol and, like him, a phrenologist. Voisin, who employed moral treatment and phrenological principles, had moved the idiot school at the hospital on the rue de Sévre to the Bicêtre. In 1843, Seguin published the second part of *Théorie et practique* and *Hygiène et éducation des idiots*, his first systematic treatment of his educational principles. As a volume of the *Annales d'hygiène publique et du médecine légale* series, *Hygiène et éducation* further enhanced Seguin's already growing reputation. In February 1843, a commission of the Academy of Sciences issued a report praising Seguin's accomplishments (H. Holman 1914; Pelicier and Thuillier 1980, 1996; Talbot 1964).

Although his beginnings at the Bicêtre held much promise for the thirty-year-old teacher, problems between Seguin and the medical authorities soon began to develop. A year after he began work there, Bicêtre officials fired him. At the close of 1843, forced to discontinue his medical studies and with an infant son, Edouard Constant, less than a year old, the teacher of idiots was without work and in disgrace among the French medical establishment.[3]

Little is known about Seguin's life between 1844 and his emigration to the United States in 1850. We know that in 1844 he reopened and expanded his private school. (Although Conolly wrote of Seguin's work at the Bicêtre, it must have been at this private school where he observed Seguin's educational practices in November 1844. This school was probably also the source of George Sumner's information for his letter to Howe in 1847.) In addition, during part of this time, Seguin was also busy writing. He published his three most influential books, *Traitement moral, hygiène, et éducation des idiots*, his magnum opus, and *Images graduées à l'usage des enfants arriérés et idiots* in 1846, and *Jacob-Rodrigues Pereire, premier instituteur des sourds et muets en France* in 1847, which together totaled more than one thousand printed pages. In the three texts, Seguin solidified his philosophy and methodology of educating idiots. These works would ensure his notoriety among British and American social reformers.

Although Seguin had a following of American admirers at the time of his emigration, there is no evidence that he sailed for America with a promise of work from any of them.[4] In 1850 or 1851, he took up residence in Cleveland.[5] Seguin's early years in the United States were probably difficult. Beginning in the late 1840s, the Ohio Medical Society had begun to limit its membership to physicians trained in approved medical schools and to discourage the practice of medicine by "unscientific" practitioners. Seguin's name never appeared in the society's membership listings of the period (Ohio State Medical Society 1856). It is likely that, without credentials and with his limited use of English, his attempts to practice medicine were frustrated. Dana (1924) noted the family's financial stress during this period.

The first concrete reference to Seguin in America was in a letter from Howe to Mann dated January 21, 1852, reporting Seguin's forthcoming employment at Howe's school. By March, however, Howe was writing to Charles Sumner that he could "hardly keep" Seguin; apparently, the two men cared little for each other (L. Richards, ed. 1906–09, 362, 367–368). In addition to their conflicting personalities, Seguin's intellectual heritage among French sensualists like Condillac conflicted with Howe's reliance on phrenology (J. Trent 2012, 150–153). By the end of 1852, Seguin appeared at Wilbur's school in Albany, where he stayed until 1860. He then moved to Mount Vernon, New York, and in 1861 graduated from the University Medical College of New York. Around this time, his wife died. Finally settling down, he spent the remaining twenty years of his life in New York City, occasionally visiting the Syracuse and Barre schools and traveling to Europe (Brockett 1856a, 1881; Burrage 1923; Dana 1924; *New York Times* 1880a; H. Wilbur 1881).[6]

"NOT TO TEACH THIS OR THAT, BUT TO DEVELOP HUMAN FUNCTION"

During the past six months [i.e., since August 1846], I have watched with eager interest the progress which many young idiots have made in Paris, under the direction of Mr. Seguin and at the Bicêtre under that of Messrs. Voisin and Vallée, and have seen . . . nearly one hundred fellow-beings who, but a short time since, were shut out from all communion with mankind, who were objects of loathing and disgust, many of whom rejected every article of clothing, others of whom, unable to stand erect, crouched themselves in corners, and gave signs of life only by piteous howls, others in whom the faculty of speech had never been developed, and many whose voracious and indiscriminate gluttony satisfied itself with whatever they could lay hands upon, with the garbage thrown to swine, or with their own excrements; these unfortunate beings—the rejected of humanity—I have seen properly clad, standing erect, walking, speaking, eating in an orderly manner at a common table, working quietly as carpenters and farmers, gaining by their own labor the means of existence, storing their awkward intelligence by reading one to another; exercising towards their teachers and among themselves the generous feeling of man's nature, and singing in unison songs of thanksgiving. (Sumner 1876)

George Sumner's report of Seguin's work intrigued American social reformers like Howe and Wilbur because it appeared to answer the fundamental question: Can human deficiencies, especially deficiencies that affect human intelligence, be reclaimed? In the 1840s, there was room for both optimism and pessimism in answering this question. In Europe and America, schools were successfully training the deaf, dumb, and blind by focusing on their other senses. Success, however, came by overcoming one failed sense; a failed mind was another matter. The mind, after all, was the seat of all the senses. How could one train the senses in the absence of a mind? For Seguin's second mentor, Esquirol, reclaiming the mind of an idiot had been a doubtful, if not impossible, prospect. In 1818, in an article on idiocy in the

Dictionnaire des sciences médicales, he had painted a hopeless picture for the treatment and cure of idiocy, and, in his 1838 *Des maladies mentales*, published about the time he coauthored his report with Seguin, he had reaffirmed that hopelessness. The most one could do for idiots was to care for them in a humane and orderly manner and provide moral treatment, which at least would not exaggerate their otherwise downward degeneracy and at best might result in some improvement in their habits.

In this context of success and hopelessness, Seguin began to educate idiots and to develop a theory of physiological education. This theory drew on several intellectual antecedents. Locke, and closer to Seguin's French roots, Abbé de Condillac, had raised questions about the nature of humans, their ability to think, and about what it meant to think in the context of adaptation to the environment. Condillac, departing from the Cartesian emphasis on the mind's separateness from the senses and emphasizing the mind's unique capacity to utilize and generate ideas, had posited a radical "sensualism," a view that the senses were the agents of ideas. Seguin's first mentor, Itard, had absorbed Condillac's writings and had remained a sensualist despite the mediating influences of Abbé Sicard and his use of signing with the deaf. Itard's labors with the Wild Boy of Aveyron had been an effort, in addition to other personal and professional goals, to demonstrate the theoretical claims of Condillac. From Itard, then, Seguin had absorbed both the Condillacan emphasis on the senses as the starting point for the development of the mind and the Sicardan method of translating that emphasis into signing techniques for educating deaf-and-dumb students. From Esquirol, Seguin was exposed to a view of moral treatment whose antecedents in France went back to Pinel, as well as to a naturalistic view of the mind in which mental deficiencies were permanent.

After working with idiots for nearly ten years, Seguin began studying the techniques of Jacob-Rodrigues Pereire, the grandfather of two of his fellow Saint-Simonians. Pereire's emphasis on educating the deaf and dumb to communicate through touch would modify and reinforce Seguin's departure from Itard's and Sicard's emphasis on education through sight. From Pereire, too, Seguin developed a new appreciation for Rousseau's claim that notions mediate between senses and ideas. From the Saint-Simonians, Seguin drew on a "Christian socialism," a Utopian vision of the potentiality of educating idiots and, albeit vague and incomplete, of reintegrating idiots into the mainstream of society. Finally, beginning with his work with Wilbur, Seguin was influenced by his experience in the United States. These influences, including his work at Syracuse and Randall's Island, his medical credentialing, and his comparative studies of American and European institutions in the last years of his career, shaped Seguin's mature vision of educating idiots, a legacy— not one he would have completely anticipated or chosen—to future generations of American superintendents and social reformers (Lane 1976, 51–95; Netchine 1970– 71; Netchine-Grynberg 1979; Pelicier and Thuillier 1996; Talbot 1964, 1–52).

When the first generation of superintendents read his definition of idiocy in the late 1840s, they must have thought it a curious, although from all reports, encouraging, definition. After all, Isaac Ray (1838), the only American of the period to attempt a systematic study of idiocy, had emphasized the pathological and hereditary deficiencies of the condition in the context of the law. Most American reformers had not given serious thought to educating idiots. Even a quintessential progressive like Howe in the 1830s had believed that phrenology offered the only hope for their improvement.

Seguin's definition, however, opened the door for their education. "Idiocy," he proposed, "is a disorder of the nervous system in which the organs and faculties of the child are separated from the normal control of the will leaving him controlled by his instincts and separated from the moral world. The typical idiot is one who knows nothing, thinks nothing, wills nothing, and can do nothing, and every idiot approaches more or less this summum of incapacity" (Seguin 1846*b*, 107). While avoiding the potential accusation that he was not dealing with "real" idiots—there could be no question from his definition that he believed he was referring to real idiots—Seguin focused his definition on the separation of the normal functioning of the nervous system from the will. Because of this separation, idiots were instinctual creatures given to all the bad habits and disgusting behaviors for which they were known. These habits and behaviors, however, were not, as Esquirol, Ray, and others had claimed or implied, the result of an irrevocable flaw of nature. The flaw—and there was a flaw—was a result of the separation of the will from the senses. The behavior of idiots was not the natural outcome of idiocy but rather the outcome of an unnatural flaw. Idiots, then, were not as Pinel and Esquirol had claimed "devoid of understanding and heart" because of an absence of mind, nor was their condition, as Gall claimed, the result of overly small, overly large, or malformed skulls (Sumner 1876, 61). Idiocy was the result of a flawed interaction of the will and the nervous system that affected the mind. Although Seguin acknowledged that several physical factors could complicate the condition of idiots, they, like all other human beings, had sensations, perceptions, and mental capacities. Their inability to control these sensations, perceptions, and mental capacities was the result of the arrested development of the will, which, according to Seguin, likely occurred before, at, or shortly after birth. Many factors—poor maternal nutrition, maternal emotional stress, sensory deprivation of the infant—could produce children in which the interaction of the will and senses remained dormant and unordered. This arrested state made idiots appear brutish and their condition hopeless. But this was an appearance only, unsubstantiated by attempts to teach them.

SEGUIN'S PEDAGOGY

Idiots could be taught. Seguin's definition implied that idiots were educable, and more importantly, the results of his efforts demonstrated that they were. Even Esquirol was forced to acknowledge that idiots under Seguin's tutelage "appeared" to have learned. In his first three publications (Esquirol and Seguin 1839; Seguin 1839, 1842) describing case after case and analyzing strategies for educational intervention, Seguin emphasized empirical results. Idiots were learning. In *Hygiène et éducation* (1843 [1980]) and especially *Traitement* (1846*b*), and in his writings about Pereire's work (1847), Seguin began to formulate and expand the theoretical underpinnings of his successes. What he called physiological education had three emphases: muscular or physical education (*activity*), education of the senses (*intelligence*), and moral treatment (*will*).

Seguin's physiological education relied on touch to awaken the senses, the will, and the mind of the idiot. The dominant characteristic of all idiots was the dormancy of their senses. Along with an undeveloped will, their senses atrophied in states of confusion and inactivity. For the dormant senses to come under the control of the will, both senses and will had to be awakened. Idiots, instinctual, undirected physical masses—demonstrating what Freud a half-century later would call polymorphous perversity—did not want their state of dormancy changed. Indeed, often pampered by well-meaning but ignorant parents, most idiots settled comfortably into their own dormancy. For this reason, it was usually necessary, Seguin claimed, for the teacher to push idiots to awaken their senses, and the first level of awakening had to be the muscular. Drawing on the theories and practice of Francisco Amoros (1834, 1848), the famous French physical educator and his contemporary, Seguin insisted that idiots could not exercise their senses and thus their will if their bodies were so neglected that sensual activities were frustrated or impossible (Seguin 1843 [1980], 63–68).

To carry out physical exercises, Seguin employed various types of gymnastic equipment, often devising such equipment to meet the needs of a particular pupil. Some children benefited from dumbbells, rope ladders, swings, balancing bars, and the like. Other children, capable but unwilling, required the continual guidance and motivation from a teacher even to stand on their own. Whether complex or simple, however, Seguin insisted that exercises meet the individual needs of the pupil and be undertaken only after careful planning based on experimentation. The exercises should never emphasize repetitious motions in the belief that repetition itself led to learning. If a movement or exercise was repeated, it must be done so, Seguin urged, to reach a specific and planned goal. Here, Seguin departed from Itard, who had stressed repetition as a means of learning. Too, avoiding rote exercises facilitated the overcoming of the idiot's "negative will," which, Seguin insisted, was the principal impediment to idiots' learning. Physical exercises, therefore, must be stimulating and exciting, drawing always on the idiot's desire for pleasure, enjoyment, and companionship with other idiots (Seguin, 1866, 71). Seguin also underscored imitation as an effective tool for exciting the will. The pupil's imitation of the teacher or of educationally advanced idiots was for Seguin preferable to endless repetition based on the Condillacan notion of direct sensual learning (Seguin 1843 [1980], 68–76).

In strengthening their muscles and developing their coordination, Seguin prepared idiots for the second part of his physiological system, the education of the senses. In the normal child, the senses developed in the following order: touch, sight, hearing, taste, and smell. Seguin assumed that, with some possible variations depending on the needs of the particular child, they developed in the same order in the idiot. Thus, he initially concentrated on touch.

Although influenced by Itard and thus Condillac and Locke, Seguin rejected their view that ideas grew from the immediate experience of the senses. He thought that repeatedly pouring ice water and hot water over an idiot's hand to stimulate the sensations of cold and heat was a foolish practice, part of an educational methodology based on flawed assumptions derived from Condillac's theoretical system. Seguin held that notions mediated between sensations and the knowledge gained from experiencing those sensations. Notions were names or categories of names for objects, experiences, and feelings. For example, a child might identify two objects on a table as a key and a hammer. This distinction reflected the child's notions of the objects "key" and "hammer." These notions in themselves, however, did not lead to ideas. Notions were things that the teacher imposed on the child. Ideas, unlike notions, could not be imposed. Ideas were the result of reflection, which in turn was stimulated by curiosity. When an idiot could reflect upon the relationship of the key to a lock and the hammer to the joining of two boards by a nail, then the idiot had ideas.

Notions required the training of the senses; ideas required the awakening of the "curious" will. Notions were passive; ideas were active. Ideas were dependent on notions but went beyond them by means of deduction and induction. Thus, teachers could build, manipulate, and impose notions, but they could only try to stir the curiosity of pupils to explore and develop ideas for themselves. Seguin insisted that physiological education developed both the senses and the mind in what he called a synergetic relationship. By breaking through the idiot's "negative will," the teacher could excite the will, the fundamental starting point in the interrelated linkage of the sensually derived notions with the mentally derived ideas. With this explanation, Seguin divorced his method from one of the main tenets of the Condillacan tradition, that ideas proceed directly from the senses, which to him was nearly as flawed as the Cartesian view that ideas were independent of the senses. The distinction between notions and ideas, Seguin believed, was an important correction to the sensationalist tradition. Incorporating this distinction, he began his second phase of physiological education: the educating of the senses (Seguin 1843 [1980], 120–123; see also Netchine-Grynberg 1979).

From Itard, from his study of Rousseau and Pereire, and from his own work, Seguin learned that physiological education of the sense of touch must emphasize the handling of objects of different textures, temperatures, weights, sizes, shapes, and elasticities. Often shocked by their tactile experiences, idiots were brought into an awareness of the sensations derived from the objects touched. Aware of the sensations, idiots became conscious of the object. In their new state of consciousness, their wills were piqued. They began to choose to touch and experience objects. At the same time, consciousness of touch awakened their other senses, especially sight and hearing. Under the guidance of the physiological teacher, they were given exercises in sensual association. For example, the teacher might play music while pupils swung to and fro on a swing and experienced pressure on the soles of their stockinged feet as they gently hit a wall in front of them (Seguin 1843 [1980], 76–80).

Although Seguin used music in sensual association, his principal use of it was to "educate the ear." He believed idiots were gifted with a musical faculty. Even if their other senses remained dormant, idiots would "seize rhythms," singing or chanting tuneless or wordless songs. Seguin's training of the ear involved three types of exercises. First, pupils were taught to differentiate general sounds, such as those made by falling objects, moving objects, and stationary objects emitting regular sounds. Second, they were taught specific sounds; here, he emphasized using musical notes. Finally, they were taught to be sensitive to feelings by learning to hear the joy, pain, and fear in people's voices. Initially, exercises for developing the ear, Seguin believed, should rely on hearing without cues from the other senses. Then, as the ear learned, the other senses could become involved in the hearing exercises (Seguin 1843 [1980], 81–84).

Speech was closely associated with hearing. Most idiots did not speak, Seguin believed, because they had no need to. The "organ of speech" thus atrophied, which further impeded idiots' ability to speak. While drawing on the work of Itard and Abbé Sicard's use of signing with deaf students, Seguin was also attracted to the work of Pereire, who, in what became and continues to be a fierce debate with the advocates of signing, stressed oral communication. Seguin was aware, of course, that in most cases idiots' inability to speak was not the result of hearing impairment. Lack of will and weak muscles were the principal factors in idiots' muteness or tendency to speak incoherently. With this in mind, Seguin utilized many of the techniques of Sicard and Pereire toward a rather different purpose (Seguin 1843 [1980], 84–88).

First, Seguin believed idiots had to be taught how to mimic their teacher. Watching the teacher's movements, idiots felt their own mouths, running their fingers over their lips, then touching inside their mouths. Careful attention was given to mastication; idiots were led to greater consciousness of the movements of chewing. Finally, Seguin prepared various exercises for the tongue, sometimes using a wooden knife to control motion in the mouth. After gaining some control of the mouth, an idiot began a second phase of exercises that emphasized the voice. Moving from simple labial consonants followed by a vowel—*ma, pa, do*—to more complex three- and four-letter syllables—*cha, bri, spra*—Seguin exercised the idiot's voice. Again, imitation of the teacher was important (Seguin 1843 [1980], 88–91).

Seguin believed the senses of smell and taste were not important in the development of the intellect but were important in daily life. The idiot, he claimed, should be able to appreciate variations in smell and taste. Because in an uneducated state they were often incontinent and not otherwise conscious of proper hygiene, and because they usually ate their food quickly, often barely chewing it, their senses of smell and taste were obviously primitive. Moving from strong and prominent smells and tastes to delicate and subtle ones, Seguin introduced his pupils to wide varieties of scents and flavors, always emphasizing those that idiots were likely to experience in refined living (Seguin 1843 [1980], 80–81).

The formation of ideas, Seguin believed, was most often associated with the sense of sight. For this reason, sight was the final sense to be educated. However, as he noted again and again, the senses were linked; thus, except in those exercises in which the pupil was blindfolded, an idiot's visual sense was educated when any of the other senses were educated. Sight was last in physiological education because of its association with the higher cognitive skills: reading, writing, arithmetic, and the traditional arts and sciences (Seguin 1843 [1980], 91–93).

Seguin also graduated the exercises for strengthening the visual sense, progressing from the simplest exercises to more complex academic subjects. First, pupils were taught to distinguish different colors, forms, sizes, and the like. Teachers encouraged pupils to "train the eye" by drawing, often stimulated by music. In the United States, through the influence of Wilbur, Seguin was attracted to Pestalozzi's system of object training from which he incorporated the use of everyday objects in miniature form into his own system of sight training. Pupils would look at and touch miniature objects, of, for example, a typical nineteenth-century bedroom, and would learn to identify the objects and create new arrangements with them. Seguin also associated sight and touch in his reliance on drawing. Pupils first learned to draw straight lines and eventually were able to form the letters of the alphabet.

Seguin insisted that drawing precede writing, which should precede reading. The combination of touch and sight necessary to write drew on more primary sensual skills than did the combination of hearing and sight necessary to read. After reading came practical grammar, the training of memory, arithmetic, and natural history. According to Seguin, these traditional academic subjects were best learned as the outcome of the education of the senses. He was quick to point out in virtually all his writings that his system of physiological education, with its emphasis on the active involvement of pupils in the development of their own sense receptors, was far superior to those in practice in Europe and America. Classical education—with its reliance on rote memorization of dead languages and about dead civilizations; its insistence on quiet, nontactile lessons in which fear dominated the teacher–pupil relationship; its separation of the sexes; its virtual denial of the pupil's need for physical exercise and training; and its disregard of the practical—ensured that idiots would not be educated and that the abilities of many normal children would not be developed (Seguin 1843 [1980], 93–136; 1866, 112–129):

> Away, then, with books! Give us the Assyrian and Jewish mode of instruction. The representative signs of thought were painted, engraved, sculptured in deepness or in relief, sensible to the eye and to the touch; the tables of the mosaic laws appear in the midst of thunder and of the lightning's flash; in the same way, the symbols, under which is concealed the modern mind, should appear to the idiot, under these histories and powerful forms, so that seeing and feeling all at once, he will understand. (Seguin 1856, 150–151)

The final component of Seguin's physiological education was moral treatment. He defined moral treatment as "the systematic action of à will upon another, in view of its improvement; in view for an idiot, of his socialization" (Seguin 1866, 148). This definition, with its emphasis on the teacher's authority in activating the will of the pupil to arrive at a level of social functioning compatible with the remainder of society, was central to Seguin's interpretation of what was, at the time of the development of his physiological system of education, a familiar treatment concept. From Pinel to Seguin's contemporaries, Voisin and Leuret, moral treatment had become widely accepted, if not always practiced, by French alienists. Seguin's modifications developed along two lines.

First, from his own work with idiots, whose dormant wills had to be forced out of their lethargy, Seguin saw that the application of moral treatment required the authority of the teacher over the pupil. Merely making the idiot's learning environment congenial and nonthreatening, a fundamental precept of the alienists' understanding of moral treatment, was, in Seguin's view, necessary but deficient. Pleasant environments did facilitate the training of idiots, but they were no substitute for the direct involvement of the teacher: "Idiots do not seem to possess that natural curiosity—mother of the beautiful and of all progress—but the teacher can excite it in him" (Seguin 1856, 150).

Moral treatment, then, was grounded not so much in treatment as it was in education. Idiots might have physical problems amenable to medical treatment, but idiocy itself was not a medical condition. Instead of treatment, then, idiots needed education, and moral treatment, normally applied to the treatment of lunatics, had to be adapted to the training of idiots. Furthermore, Seguin warned, when pity activated moral treatment (a not uncommon occurrence in the case of idiots), great harm could be done. "*Pauvres enfants*," a well-meaning reaction to the sight of idiots, became a damaging condescension, reducing them to "*le dernier rang des animaux*" (Seguin 1843 [1980], 139).

SEGUIN'S SOCIOLOGY

Maintaining authority over idiots during their education, then, was necessary to overcome the undeveloped linkage between the will and the senses. This authority, however, must never be for its own sake but to arouse idiots' curiosity as a means to their socialization. Socialized idiots could attain independence (Seguin 1843 [1980], 137–142). Here emerged Seguin's second variation on moral treatment. Influenced by Saint-Simonism, Seguin held (although he did not fully develop) a view of the potential of idiots for independent citizenship. The goal of their education, then, was independence. This independence should not be private and idiosyncratic (Seguin knew that "idiot" derived from the Greek *idios*, meaning a "private person"). Rather, idiots must acquire an independence grounded in relationships with other citizens: "changing his *negative* will into an affirmative one, his will of loneliness into a will of sociability and usefulness; such is the object of moral training" (Seguin 1856, 151). Chained to primitive habits and appetites, subservient to behaviors that fellow human beings found unpleasant, under the control of indolence and insouciance, idiots were not free because they had no chance to socialize with fellow human beings. As *idios*, they were only "free" to remain separated from humanity. To lose this "private freedom," this "will to loneliness," Seguin insisted, was to gain the only freedom available to human beings, the freedom of association (Seguin 1843 [1980], 142–171).

Such association could take place in a variety of social settings and activities. First, idiots should, he believed, regularly visit museums, churches, theaters, and parks (Seguin 1866, 243–244). They should learn social graces, including proper table manners and the ability to carry on small talk (Seguin 1864). Second, they should be trained to do useful work and to maintain day-to-day skills and habits. This, he emphasized, was especially necessary for those idiots whose families were poor and therefore unlikely to care for them after they reached maturity. Useful work most likely meant manual labor, for example, on a farm or in a small shop: "The majority profit more by the physiological than by the mental training; they are decidedly poor scholars, and are only proficient in kindness, honesty, and love of labor proportionate to their power" (Seguin 1870*b*, 183; see also 1870*a*). The more well-to-do idiots, he believed, could return home, where, as educated idiots, they could contribute to the daily activities of their families and communities.

Thus, Seguin retained a broad and impressionistic vision of freedom of, and through, association, an abstract goal flowing quite naturally from his Utopian Saint-Simonism in what otherwise was a detailed and even painstaking educational system. Implied but never fully developed in his system was the sense, understood by Americans since the time of Jefferson, that education transformed individuals—in this case, idiots—into free men and women, interacting as citizens in a wide variety of social and political arrangements. When the group of American reformers in the 1840s observed or heard about Seguin's successes and read about his methods and theories, they were likewise prepared to believe in the democratizing potential of education, and the United States seemed the perfect place to test and demonstrate that potentiality. If even idiots could be educated to be citizens and fully participating members of society, then surely none could deny the power and potentiality of education. Seguin's faith in education never waned, although his predictions about outcomes for idiots would moderate. This moderation would reflect the contribution of Seguin's American experience to his mature thought.

"ATTAIN A RESPECTABLE MEDIOCRITY"

After the 1850s, Seguin increasingly attempted to build a neurological basis for his system of physiological education. Remaining ever suspicious of craniometry, Seguin, under the influence of his son, Edward Constant, one of the founders of American neurology, began to frame physiological education in neurological categories and language. This framing emphasized what he called the *synergy* of the nervous system, the fluid and interactional relationship of the brain with the other parts of the nervous system. By the end of his career, positing a "poly-energy" of the nervous system, Seguin (1877, 1880*a*, 1880*b*) claimed that the brain could be developed by training such peripheral nervous centers as the hand and the eye. "We are so used to locating idiocy in the brain," he wrote, "that the idea of an *idiotic hand* seems, at first enunciation, like a grammatical blunder. But . . . we must recognize the power of the million of peripheric brains to give the impulse as well as to receive it" (Seguin 1880*b*, 122–123). Coming close to claiming a multicentered nervous system, Seguin left himself open for criticism, which in at least one *New York Times* (1880*b*) review he received.

Although his neurological thinking was unusual even by standards of his own day, it represented his attempt to provide a medical grounding for his educational system. As a teacher among physicians in Paris, Seguin had found the need for such a grounding less important than as a physician in the rapidly growing New York medical community, in whose professional associations he remained an active, if marginal, member. By 1860, his Parisian hostility to the medical establishment and to medical constructions of idiocy began to wane.

His growing dependence on a medical paradigm also affected his views on the idiot institution. In *Idiocy* (1866, 173–195), he described the ideal institution. Located "on high ground and well drained," the main structure would have sleeping quarters and dining areas on the second floor and educational facilities on the first. All facilities would be small and homelike. The classrooms and gymnasium would be well stocked with learning equipment, musical instruments, and military drill apparatus. Outdoor activities, weather permitting, would be encouraged.

A physician would head the institution. Assisting him (and in this period, only men were superintendents) would be a steward in charge of maintaining the facility. The medical superintendent would supervise the teachers, most of whom would be well-trained women; keep detailed records on the educational progress of the students; and provide them medical care and treatment. He would be the principal liaison between the institution and parents and the public. He would maintain good relations with his board of trustees and the state legislature but always assert his leadership, not answering at every turn to the board, nor to any under his supervision. Above all, Seguin stressed the superintendent's "absolute understanding of children" and his qualifications as a physician (1866, 195). Only a medical man could fully appreciate the educational needs of idiots while also providing the necessary diagnostic skills to separate the simple idiot, who was amenable to training, from the idiot encumbered by other disabilities, who was not.

The matron and attendants, Seguin stressed, would be loyal and have good dispositions. These women should be "very kind, gay, attractive, endowed with open faces, ringing voices, clear eyes, easy movements, and affectionate propensity toward children" (1866, 190).

At the Bicêtre, he had worked with a class of around one hundred idiots, many of whom were multiply handicapped. Based on his experience there, Seguin insisted that only young idiots who were free from epilepsy, paralysis, and insanity could be effectively educated. Higher functioning and usually older imbeciles, too, should never be mixed with idiots. Like Kerlin, Seguin (1866, 51) considered imbecility as a separate category of mental disability and offered little hope for helping the imbecile: "The imbecile [is] self-confident, half-witted, and ready to receive immoral impressions, satisfactory to his intense egotism.... [T]oday he is an imbecile, tomorrow he may be a criminal."

In an 1864 article, Seguin showed his admiration for American institutions. In the United States, idiots in publicly supported facilities were trained for the most part by females, whom he believed made better teachers. Pupils were young and educable, with postadolescents and the physically and emotionally disabled usually excluded. For example, when Seguin had visited and spent time in the 1850s at Wilbur's facility in Syracuse, he had found a small but growing school where, for the most part, only "simple idiots" without other complicating problems were admitted.

A third positive feature of American institutions was the integration of both sexes in the classroom and gymnastic activities. Finally, he observed approvingly, "In no American asylum has the idiot been set to work, as idiots and insane persons have been elsewhere, as a machine to make money with; here he has been regarded as a child, who needs exercise and to educate and develope [sic] his own functions" (Seguin 1864, 4–5). Compared with his experience in France and his observations of British institutions, Seguin concluded that American facilities were superior, although, by the 1860s, he began to acknowledge the need for long-term institutionalization in the United States, especially for those older pupils discharged from the institution but without means of support and for the "unimproved and unimprovable" (1866, 52–54, 172).

These sentiments were echoed in *Idiocy* (1866), where he reaffirmed his confidence in American institutions. He noted, however, that the five American institutions receiving full or partial public support were all different, especially in their architecture and pupil population. In 1870, he reported on his 1869 tours of Wilbur's public facility at Syracuse and Brown's private school at Barre to the New York Medical Journal Association and published a version of his report in the popular *Appletons' Journal* (Seguin 1870b, 1870c). At both schools, he found dedicated officials who utilized physiological education for the improvement of their charges, but in other respects the schools were different. Syracuse, as might be expected, was the larger, and classes there were held in groups. Barre had both group and individual instruction. Syracuse pupils, selected from a large applicant pool, were required to show potential for educational improvement. Some idiots at Barre, however, were taken as custodial cases. Syracuse had one large educational and residential building; Barre had several smaller buildings, including private apartments for pupils with servants. The sexes were educated together at Syracuse, apart at Barre. "Though I had expected to find a marked difference," Seguin (1870b, 185) remarked, "between a State and a private institution, yet the contrast was even greater than I had anticipated."

Seguin's report contained revealing observations, some foreshadowing developments in social policies in the 1880s. The first was Seguin's ambivalence toward private schools. As a student of Saint-Simon, Seguin had little use for old-order class distinctions that kept ordinary people in traditional, prescientific social arrangements and less use for the wealthy whose fortunes added nothing to social progress. Of them, he remarked, "How many of these [pupils at Barre] are offshoots from some kind of aristocracy, miserable sprouts dried up with paralysis, softened by imbecility, shaken by the St. Vitus's dance, epilepsy, and what else that may befall haughty and empty families for believing themselves above the brotherhood of man, the universal family of patient workers, God alone knows" (1870b, 184). Yet, going back to his days on the rue Pigalle, Seguin knew that physiological education, free from the demands made on it by public sponsorship, was best carried out in the private setting. Thus, despite compromises to the tenets of physiological education made at Barre, Seguin wrote approvingly of it, and he seemed to accept as inevitable that the wealthy preferred to have their children, even their idiot children, educated separately. The wealthy who needed it could also afford custodial care for their children. Finally, in a footnote to his report, he acknowledged that, at Syracuse, "exceptionally, a few old pupils who are without property or friends anywhere, are allowed to stay on the farm or in the laundry, where they make themselves useful and happy, and are paid what their work is worth. This is a paternal, not yet legalized, arrangement" (Seguin 1870b, 182; 1870c, 12).

As the virgin field was about to experience a major shift in its concept of idiocy and in the social policy affecting feeble minds, Seguin's observations in 1866 and again in 1869 anticipated two trends: the growth of custodial care and the growth of care based on socioeconomic differences. The emergence of custodial care would affect two groups of idiots. Many educated idiots would be unable to find work except in the institution, and many severely disabled idiots would find a place in institutions that had previously excluded them. The growth of custodial care in public institutions after the 1880s ensured the proliferation in (and after) the 1890s of private schools where idiots from well-to-do families, like their working-class counterparts, would find a perpetual haven. Ironically, then, although the private school in large part inaugurated custodial care, the growth of custodial care for the lower classes in public facilities fostered the burgeoning of private facilities after the 1880s.

In a concluding section to his New York Medical Journal Association article, but omitted from the *Appletons'* article, Seguin (1870c, 21–22) qualified his enthusiasm for Syracuse and Barre by sounding a warning against institutional growth.[7] The qualification, however, did not fail to allude to the already growing class distinctions among schools for feebleminded Americans:

> I do not feel at liberty to leave this subject, so deeply interesting to me, without calling attention to the happy distribution of labor and proportions of the American institutions for idiots. The State schools for the poor; the private ones for the rich; sufficiently large to give scope to the genius of a manager, not so large as to reduce him to the condition of a steward. . . . Let us hope that the State institutions for idiots will escape that evil of excessive growth, which has already overtaken other establishments of similar character, in which patients are so numerous, that the accomplished physicians who have them in charge cannot remember the name of each; where to superintend practically means building, repairing, laying pipes for air, gas, heat, water, in the houses, in the grounds or fields, or under the Legislature. The man whose eminent capacities would be engrossed by these and similar cares could not easily be also the father, the physician, and teacher of idiots. (Seguin 1870c, 21–22)

In the last decade of his life, Seguin became concerned with the growing size of American institutions and with their willingness to compromise their original educational emphasis. In 1866, he claimed that no institution with more than 200 students (of which 150 attended school and 50 worked on the institution's farm) could provide good education and care. In larger schools, pupils were merely "kept at the lowest ebb of vitality" (Seguin 1866, 186). His travels to British public institutions, most of which were larger than those in the United States, further convinced him that greater size was an impediment to students' development: "The advantage of large institutions for the classification of the pupils, for their general entraînement in group and general exercises, for the prosecution of scientific inquiries, hardly compensates for the consequences of the sequestration of the pupils from the world, its habits, manners, and dealings" (Seguin 1880c, 94–95).

Seguin's discomfort with directions in the growth and outlook of the idiot institutions grew deeper in his last years. Yet there was little he could do. In reaction, he founded his private school in Manhattan, where "the children of endless siestas and satieties, or of moneyed and sensualistic indulgences" received the best of physiological education from the master himself (Seguin 1870b, 184; Seguin Physiological School 1896). Agreeing to be the first president of the Association of Medical Officers of American Institutions for Idiotic and Feeble-Minded Persons in 1876, he sat through its first meetings listening to papers describing the complexities of institutional management and supervision from superintendents who clearly projected the growth of their asylums. At these meetings, too, the dominant themes of classification, heredity, and pathology must have made the old Saint-Simonian wonder about the future.

CONCLUSION

A technological genius not unsophisticated in translating his methods into theory, Seguin could only vaguely answer the question: Education to what end? Since his time, the methods, tools, and theoretical foundations for educating intellectually disabled people have changed surprisingly little. Indeed, many of the techniques demonstrated by Seguin for successfully educating disabled people have now been available for nearly 170 years. Better understanding of physical therapy and learning theory has led to improvements in education, subtleties in equipment have allowed easier access to learning, and medical advances have made for healthier learners. Yet, Seguin's physiological education remains amazingly contemporary. Neither his technical advancements nor his educational theories remain wanting.

Despite his faith in the progress of society to recapture its weakest members, Seguin, like Howe and Hervey Wilbur, began to regard education as an end in itself. Interestingly, some of his contemporary admirers spoke more readily about what he rarely acknowledged: that is, the outcome of educating idiots. George Sumner summarized in his 1847 letter to Howe his understanding of Seguin's expectations: "Although their intelligence may never perhaps be developed to such a point as to render them the authors of those generous ideas and great deeds which leave a stamp upon an age, yet still, they may attain a respectable mediocrity and surpass in mental power the common peasant of many European states" (Sumner 1876, 63). That same year, an anonymous reviewer of *Traitement* made a similar observation: "An idiot . . . becomes if not restored to society, at least restored to his family, his bad habits are corrected, he is more obedient, more active, in better health, and affectionate to those who have given him their affection and support, whilst others have been enabled to read, write, speak and occupy themselves readily in many manual occupations" ("Review of Edouard Seguin's *Traitement*" 1847, 4). Seguin had seldom in his writings been so forthcoming about the outcome of education.

"Attaining a respectable mediocrity" back on the family farm or in a local small shop would, after the Civil War, become less and less likely for educated idiots. In a growing and increasingly industrialized nation, communities did not need idiots, even educated ones. Indeed, their presence was a hindrance to the social and productive order. What became necessary—as Seguin feared—was a shift of the respectable mediocrity from the community to the institution itself. Ironically, Seguin's physiological education, rather than impeding that shift, would facilitate it. Even before his death in 1880, superintendents were using his educational technology to build their facilities and his name to honor their enterprise.

NOTES

1. During Seguin's youth, the town's principal industry was lumbering. His father Jacque Onesime, whose second Christian name he shared in some records with his son, was born in 1781 and was a physician. His medical thesis dealt with fever, a topic that would interest his son a half-century later. The Seguin family was well to do at and after Edouard's birth in 1812 (Pelicier and Thuillier 1980, 10–11). In 1832, Seguin began to read law, and, at the time of the marriage of his sister, Antoinette Constance, he listed himself on the civil rolls as a lawyer. In 1843, at the age of thirty-one and while working at the Bicêtre, he enrolled in the Faculté de médecine but did not finish his course of study (Pelicier and Thuillier 1980, 11–12). Contrary to the reports of his American contemporaries, he never claimed to be a physician until he arrived in the United States.

2. In February 1841, he sued the concierge of the building on the rue Pigalle where he held private classes. Seguin's suit, which demanded damages of $20,000, alleged that the concierge had falsely told the parents of Seguin's pupils that Seguin had mistreated their children, hitting them, and even throwing one child out the window (*Gazette des tribunaux*, February 4, 1841, 241, cited in Pelicier and Thuillier 1980, 13, n. 2). Despite this embarrassment, Seguin maintained the support of the medical establishment at the Salpêtrière.

3. The reasons for his firing are somewhat unclear and complex yet revealing. Both Seguin's contemporary Brockett (1858, 1881) and later his biographer Talbot (1964, 11, 36) suggested that his political activities led to his downfall. Their suggestion is unlikely. Even Karl Marx found a haven in Paris during this period. Pelicier and Thuillier (1980) argue convincingly that Seguin's contemporaries (and later his biographers) exaggerated his political activities during the period. It is more likely that Seguin moved to the United States in 1850 because of financial problems caused both by his dismissal from the Bicêtre and by a general economic downturn as a result of the Revolution. Although no doubt Seguin was affected by the turmoil of the period and cared little for Louis Napoleon, personal problems exacerbated by politics, rather than political vulnerability, motivated Seguin to leave his native land to move to a country where he knew he had admirers interested in his educational system. Pelicier and Thuillier (1980, 24–25) have developed a more convincing scenario.

In reaction to the Academy of Science's report, Voisin and Etienne Belhomme, a phrenologist and alienist of the time, challenged Seguin's claim to priority in the successful training of idiots, as they had previously challenged each other's similar claims. As founder of the treatment efforts for idiots at the Bicêtre, Voisin soon came to view the young teacher as a bit of an upstart, resenting Seguin's notoriety. Belhomme was offended by Seguin's lack of humility in making his claim to priority. Also, both Voisin and Belhomme, in the tradition of Esquirol and Gall, were phrenologists. Convinced that their "mentalist" approach to the treatment of idiocy was futile, Seguin began what would be a life-long attack on phrenology and the subsequent science of cranology. Even in 1843, when his attack was measured and mild, it produced tension at the Bicêtre.

In addition to these factors, there were differences in policy. For example, Seguin opposed the integration of idiots with epileptics and lunatics, a position he would hold throughout his career but one opposed by Voisin (and incidentally by Conolly). Likewise, he opposed the use of inmates at the Bicêtre for institutional labor, especially in the name of treatment. Work as treatment had value, he claimed, but labor to maintain the institution, even if done in the name of treatment, was a perversion. This, too, would become a position that he would stress later in his career. Finally, there is the matter of the "accusations abominables" reported by Bourneville (1895, 167). Shortly after Seguin's firing, an investigation occurred at the Bicêtre. Reports of cruelty and ill-treatment appeared. In his absence, Seguin was associated (justly or unjustly) with these reports (Conolly 1847; Pelicier and Thuillier 1980, 20–21; Semelaigne 1894, 189–192, 334–338).

Goldstein (1987) and Castel (1988) have both written important accounts of the development of French psychiatry after the Revolution. Goldstein argues that the earliest psychiatrists were interested in legitimizing their professional status in the midst of volatile political and institutional struggles in nineteenth-century France. They shaped a French view of madness around that legitimation. Castel argues that, after 1789, French alienists added medical authority to madness. Previously, it had been seen as a matter of law. As a medical phenomenon, madness required medical treatment by medical authorities. Alienists were part of a bourgeois way of controlling mad people. Incarceration was relabeled "treatment," a post-revolutionary rationale. Nineteenth-century France could justify incarcerating mad people and thereby deprive them of rights guaranteed to other citizens because the nation was providing them medical care.

Interestingly enough, although both authors discuss important specialists who overlapped with Seguin, neither mentions the French alienists' interest in idiocy nor in Seguin's work. It was, nevertheless, in this milieu that Seguin's ideas and methods emerged. It would take Bourneville in the last quarter of the century to reappropriate Seguin for French psychiatry, although this rediscovery of Seguin may have had more to do with Bourneville's admiration for Seguin's son, Edward (né Edouard) Constant Seguin, and the emergence of American neurology than it did with Seguin.

4. Seguin's American connections date back to his earliest days at the Salpêtrière. In 1840, Norton S. Townshend, an Ohioan who had just completed his medical training at the New York College of Physicians and Surgeons, was sent by the college as a representative to temperance societies in Europe and by the Anti-Slavery Society of Ohio as a delegate to the World Anti-Slavery Convention in London. While on his journey, Townshend spent the summer and fall in Paris observing medical practices and investigating institutions in the city. It is likely that he met or at least heard of

Seguin before returning to Ohio in 1841. In 1853, incidentally, Townshend, then a member of the Ohio Senate, introduced the bill that culminated in the establishment of the Ohio State Asylum for Idiots, on whose board of trustees he served for more than twenty years ("Townshend, Norton Strange" 1897).

In 1843, Horace Mann, who between 1837 and 1848 was the secretary of the Massachusetts State Board of Education, visited Seguin at his private school on the rue Pigalle. Mann, who was on his honeymoon with his second wife and for part of the trip traveled with Samuel Gridley Howe and Julia Ward, also newlyweds, was probably introduced to Seguin through George Sumner. It is unlikely the Howes met Seguin at this time, but no doubt they at least became familiar with him as a result of Mann's visit (H. Mann 1891 [1844]; "Mann, Horace" 1893; M. Mann 1937; Seguin 1880c, 207).

In 1846, while living in Paris, George Sumner visited Seguin, whom, according to Seguin, he had known since 1842, and provided a detailed and critical account of Seguin's educational philosophy and methods. In 1848, James Richards visited Paris to learn techniques for training idiots at Howe's school soon to open in South Boston. It is unclear whether he met Seguin at this point, but it is likely he did (S. Howe 1848b; Schwartz 1956, 142; J. Trent 2012, 150–153). Added to these visits were the accounts of Seguin's work made popular in American medical and social reforming circles by John Conolly; Backus, Wilbur, Knight, Awl, and Woodward were all intrigued by these reports.

5. His settlement there may have been the result of his association with John Strong Newberry. Newberry, one of the first graduates of the Cleveland Medical College in 1848, had studied in Paris in 1849 and 1850. He returned to Cleveland about the time Seguin settled there, began a medical practice, and, in 1852, published a translation of Seguin's account of the origins of the training of idiots (Seguin 1852a). Earlier, in August of that year, Seguin (1852b), having returned to Cleveland, had written Howe (in French) about what Seguin indicated was Howe's willingness to translate the *Traitement*. Seguin's use of English was minimal, whereas Howe had spoken French through much of his time in Greece during its revolution. In any case, there is no indication that Howe ever carried out the translation (Seguin 1852b). Newberry took up the challenge instead.

   Although there is no reference to Townshend in Seguin's writings, Seguin and he would be associated again in New York in the 1870s, when, as the president of the New York Academy of Sciences and then a renowned geologist, Townshend provided Seguin a forum for lecturing on garden schools (*New York Times* 1878, 5; Seguin 1878a). His earlier association with Townshend may have prompted Seguin's move to Cleveland ("Newberry, John Strong" 1899; "Newberry, John Strong" 1934).

6. In 1863, Seguin was instrumental in organizing the School for Defectives, known also as Idiot House, on Randall's Island. He consulted at that school for the next seventeen years (Burrage 1923; *New York Times* 1880a). During the winter and spring of 1864–65, he worked on his book *Idiocy*. When Philip Gillett, superintendent of the Illinois School for the Deaf and Dumb, visited him at Syracuse in 1865, he noted that Seguin agreed to become the superintendent of the yet unopened Illinois asylum "at a moderate compensation." Gillett had second thoughts about offering the position to Seguin, both because of his problems at the Pennsylvania School and because of his "desidedly [sic] foreign accent" (Experimental School 1865–70, 17–29).

   In 1866, Seguin, with the aid of his son, then interning at the New York Hospital, published *Idiocy and Its Treatment by the Physiological Method*, a somewhat briefer version of *Traitement* and one that reflected both his deepening medical outlook on idiocy and the influence of American social policy. It was, incidentally, *Idiocy* that Maria Montessori would copy line for line as she began to develop her own system of education (Fynne 1924, 213–216).

In 1873 and 1876, he published on the subject of medical thermometry and, along with his son, was credited with introducing standard measures of assessing human temperature in relation to disease and illness to American medicine and to the general public (Dana 1924; Seguin 1873, 1876*b*, Wunderlich and Seguin 1871). He was also interested in and published on the use of the metric system as a standard measure in medicine (Seguin 1876*a*). In 1873, he was the US representative at the International Conference on Education in Vienna, and in 1876, 1877, and 1878 he represented the American Medical Association at conferences in Europe. As a result of trips to these conferences and visits made to British and continental institutions, he published two editions of *Report on Education* (Seguin 1875, 1880*c*; see also 1878*b*), both of which reviewed the status of common schools and special education in Europe and America, revealing much of Seguin's insights and biases in the last years of his career. In June 1876, he became the first president of the Association of Medical Officers of American Institutions for Idiotic and Feeble Minded Persons at its inaugural meeting at the Pennsylvania Training School. At meetings of that organization, in lectures in New York, and in publications, he developed the curious notion that the senses, especially touch, codetermined with the brain the starting point of human neurological activity. In January 1880, he officially opened a private school (informally begun in 1878) for the idiot children of wealthy New Yorkers, and, in May, he married Elsie Mead, a teacher at the school. In October 1880, after a brief illness, Seguin died. After his death, his widow expanded the Seguin Physiological School from three day students in 1880 to twenty-five residential students and additional day students. In 1894, she moved the school from Manhattan to the small town of Orange, New Jersey, where she operated the facility until her death in 1930 (American Association for the Study of the Feeble Minded 1930, 260; "Death of Elsie Seguin" 1930; *New York Times* 1880*a*; Seguin Physiological School 1894, 1896, 1905, 1906, 1911).

7. The omission of this passage from the *Appletons'* article suggests that Seguin intended to direct his criticism of larger schools for idiots to his American medical colleagues.

CHAPTER 3

✣

The Burden of the Feebleminded

I n 1857, an anonymous writer for the *Christian Advocate and Journal* published a description of a visit to the Pennsylvania Training School for Feeble-Minded Children, then at Germantown. After arriving at the facility, "situated in an elevated, healthy, and retired spot," the visitor met with the superintendent, who discussed the daily regimen of the pupils: up at half past five, light physical exercise at six, from eight to nine dumbbell exercises for the smaller children and "moderate out-door work, bed-making, etc.," for the larger. The writer next observed the children, "well combed, washed, and dressed," congregated in a classroom, where "they all sat in silence for a few moments with their hands clasped, and in concert . . . repeated the Lord's Prayer and the 23rd Psalm."

Although normally the group was afterward broken down into three classes, at the visitor's request the pupils remained together to demonstrate the range of "general exercises" conducted at the school and their capabilities at their lessons:

A geography class was first called up, and it would have put to shame many older and wiser heads, to have listened to the readiness with which they answered a multitude of questions, from an outline map of the United States. They are exceedingly fond of this study, and always consider it a recreation. It is taught by chorus, a mode by which alone they could arrive at such proficiency. Even the very little children seemed responsive to the larger ones, especially "Alice," who was an echo for every answer made. This child was admitted about a year ago, and from being a repulsive-looking semi-mute, is now as interesting a "chatter-box" as one would find anywhere. Geography finished, what is called "the quiet exercise" was introduced; by this is meant a phonetic exercise for the improvement of vocalization, which has been introduced among them with marked advantage. . . .

This concluded, a miscellaneous exercise in form and numeration was engaged in. "James," a most pitiable object, whose ponderous jaws, set with irregular teeth, were always wide open, his eyes fixed on vacancy or staring at the ceiling, and his gaunt body incessantly swaying from side to side; this apparently lowest and most unpromising case in the room, astonished me by naming several geometric figures, when made upon the board, in reading all the letters of the alphabet, and some half a dozen words, and in counting thirty understandingly. . . . "James" is now regarded a very promising case; apparently the most deplorable and obtuse when he entered, ten months ago, he is now found to possess a remarkably sensitive and reflecting mind, for this class of children. The poor boy, without advantages of any kind, has for long years remained under a cloud, which is dispelling before the kindly influences into which he is now thrown. . . . "Grubb," in February last, knew not a figure; he now adds and multiplies almost ad infinitum. "Alfred," an interesting semi-mute, by processes of his own, exhibits great natural talent for figures, adding, multiplying, and dividing. Some exhibit much taste in drawing.

After lessons, the children sat down to eat dinner "in perfect silence" at "a long table neatly furnished," a "sight unsurpassed in the best regulated family of juveniles. . . . At the signal from a bell, all took their forks properly in their fingers, and commenced eating as deliberately, in most instances, as ordinary children." After dinner, the afternoon was spent in light exercise and a variety of activities, from playing with blocks to sewing or grammar lessons, depending on the child's level of ability. The visitor was also impressed with the school's activities on Sundays:

> The Sabbath day is observed by appropriate exercises. Psalm recitation and singing, and what the children call a "sermon," are engaged in, in the morning. What is in effect an experience meeting is held after the sermon; the more advanced pupils, one after another, rise and narrate, first, what they have done that is bad, for the week past. They are very sensitive to gentle reproof, and their confessions are often accompanied with tears. The advantage of this attention to a form of worship and moral teaching has been very apparent in some instances. One boy, with strong thieving propensities, seems almost cured. He was a moral idiot; but after being taught the character of and his obligations to his heavenly Father; his clothes, his food, his friends as being supplied by him, and the return he should make for all these blessings in being good, he has become very correct in his life, and is one of the most devotional in the school. (cited in Kerlin 1858, 138–147; see also Experimental School 1866, 20–30)

The antebellum institution that the anonymous visitor described was a small facility in a small town. Made up of children, the facility was primarily a school. Although now including daily medical inspections and operated by physicians, the Pennsylvania Training School saw to it that its 1857 visitor observed *school* activities.[1] The next year, in some copies of his *The Mind Unveiled*, Kerlin (1858) included a group portrait of eight male imbeciles (Figure 3.1). In the photograph, each holds an object or objects of learning—a slate, blocks, a violin, dumbbells. Although Kerlin no doubt intended the portrait to demonstrate some of the boys' medical anomalies, the photograph also served to show their educational activities

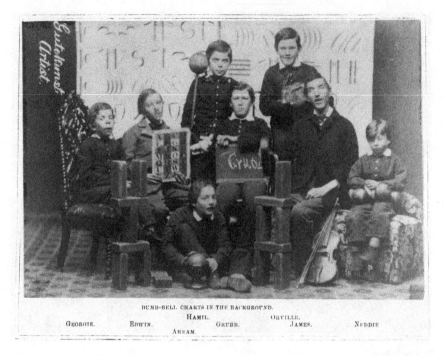

Figure 3.1:
Imbecile boys, inmates at the Pennsylvania Training School for Feeble-Minded Children, 1857. (From Isaac N. Kerlin's *The Mind Unveiled*, 1858)

and achievements. In 1858, the growing medical emphasis in the institution still maintained its important link to education.

Education was still on the minds of New Jersey commissioners who, in 1872–73, were charged with founding the state's first school for the feebleminded. In their report, they concluded, "[t]hat these institutions should not be asylums, or receptacles for the mere custody of their inmates, nor State alms-houses for the 'indigent poor' only; but that they should be schools for the education and training of our defectives for intelligent and self-supporting members of society, free to all, whether rich or poor" (New Jersey *Report* of 1873, 21). To arrive at this conclusion, they solicited information from the six superintendents of the nation's existing facilities. Responses came from Henry M. Knight of the Connecticut School for Imbeciles, Charles T. Wilbur of the Illinois Institution for Feeble-Minded Children, E. H. Black of the Kentucky Institution for the Education of Feeble-Minded Children and Idiots, Hervey B. Wilbur of the New York Asylum for Idiots, Gustavus A. Doren of the Ohio State Asylum for Imbecile and Feeble-Minded Youth, and Isaac Kerlin of the Pennsylvania Training School for Feeble-Minded Children. The superintendents answered seven questions posed by the New Jersey commissioners. What is most telling about the responses is the group's common perspective about issues ranging from the proper location of the institution to the minimum age for student admission. More than anything else, the superintendents agreed that the New Jersey facility should be a school.

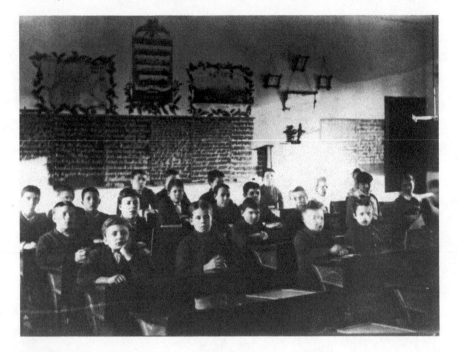

Figure 3.2:
Boys' classroom, Pennsylvania Training School for Feeble-Minded Children, 1886. (Courtesy of Southern Illinois University at Edwardsville, Lovejoy Library, Beverly Farm Records)

Twelve years later, in 1885, the year Kerlin published a handsome leather-bound collection of photographs of his facility, the image of feeblemindedness had changed. In 1858, the focus of the photograph (and the narrative accompanying the photograph) had been Grubb, Edwin, James, Georgie, Abram, Neddie, Hamil, and Orville—real people with real names. Now, the image of a large classroom with nameless people appeared. Likewise, the 1885 collection presented a picture of an institution. Located in a converted house in 1858, the Pennsylvania Training School (Figure 3.2, Figure 3.3) was now in a facility built specifically for its use. Now an asylum as much as a school, the 1885 facility's image was as much its buildings and its grounds as it was its nameless pupils, now called *inmates*. The collection proudly displayed three dozen photographs of buildings, supply rooms, a hospital, and landscaped grounds. There was a look of permanence about it all (Pennsylvania Institution for Feeble-Minded Children [ca. 1885]).

AFTER THE CIVIL WAR

The Civil War had conflicting impacts on idiot institutions. On the one hand, most facilities before the war had admitted private-paying pupils and depended on income from their families or wards. War left many Northern families strapped

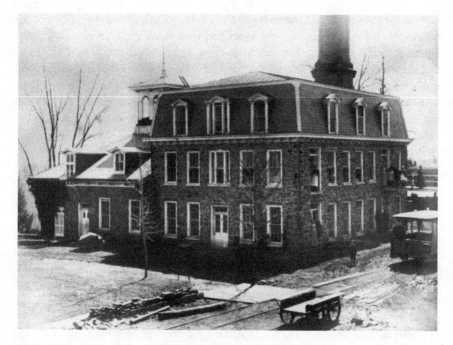

Figure 3.3:
The laundry, Pennsylvania Training School for Feeble-Minded Children, 1887. (Courtesy of Southern Illinois University at Edwardsville, Lovejoy Library, Beverly Farm Records)

for cash. Each asylum, too, had several pupils from the South, most of whom had been taught during and after the war years without reimbursement to the asylum. Kerlin, especially, nearer to Dixie than the others, had felt the loss of Southern payments. Inflation after the war added a further burden to the already stressed institutions as state reimbursements remained at prewar levels. On the other hand, family and general social disruption led to an even greater number of applications for admission. Thus, idiot institutions after the war found themselves without resources to meet new postwar demands (Pennsylvania Training School 1869).[2]

Limited resources, however, did not preclude some institutional expansion. Indeed, the populations of the institutions grew slowly but steadily in the decade after the war. The Pennsylvania asylum, for example, expanded from 175 in 1857 to 180 in 1868 and to 185 in 1871. Even five additional pupils after the war made for "an easier financial condition," Kerlin reported (Pennsylvania Training School 1869, 7). Having succeeded Parrish at the helm of the Pennsylvania facility in 1863, Kerlin soon saw that he could only meet postwar demand with public funds. In his annual reports, Kerlin (as did his cohorts at other institutions) began to emphasize more explicitly than before the war the need for dealing with two new groups of unserved idiots: the adult idiot educated in the asylum but still unable to find employment on the outside, and the low-functioning idiot, or "asylum grade," whose educational potential was low. The former consisted of lower-class inmates who, Kerlin claimed, could just as well remain at the institution where they would receive care more benevolent than they were likely to receive in almshouses or jails, and the latter included applicants whose parents had read about the marvelous successes reported in the popular press. Added to these groups were pupils who would be discharged either to their relatives or for work. Over the next decade, the group of *pupils* would be merged with the two new groups of *inmates*. Although most public institutions continued to operate on a nine-month school year (some even to the end of the century), they retooled for yearlong care and for education directed at skills used in the asylum, not on the outside.

When the Illinois Asylum opened in 1865, state lawmakers made provisions for well-to-do parents to contribute to their children's upkeep. Charles Wilbur soon discovered that almost all applicants came from families too poor to contribute more than the most basic support (Experimental School 1866, 15). By January 1868, without anticipated funds from parents, Wilbur found himself soliciting support from Civil War colleagues and friends in New England (Wilbur 1865–80, vol. 1, 34–35). By 1872, he had become increasingly concerned about pupils returning home for holidays and in the summer. Many communities, he claimed, were putting indigent pupils in almshouses, where the upright lessons of the asylum were soon lost. Even worse, female pupils from poor families often risked being "imposed upon" (Wilbur 1865–80, vol. 2, 132; Illinois Institution for the Education of Feebleminded Children 1873, 13). Although some well-to-do families still sent their idiot children to public asylums, after 1876, these facilities primarily housed poor children.

"What proportion of applicants are subjects for school education?" Kerlin asked rhetorically in his 1871 annual report (Pennsylvania Training School 1871). Three years earlier, in desperate need of additional legislative funding, he had boasted of the successes of discharged pupils to "the outside." With some in common schools, some in trades, and others doing domestic or farm labor, idiot pupils were still being regarded by superintendents like Kerlin as worthy of public support because of their potential for ordinary community life. Yet, by 1871, with financial stress relieved and demand as great as ever, the seeds of a new custodial arrangement planted before the war began to flourish. Kerlin wrote confidently:

> It is certain that of those who are sent out from the Institutions of this kind as "self-supporting," there are but few individuals who will not *always* need judicious and considerate guardianship; they lack the judgment or forecast which anticipates and provides for the needs of the future. . . . they fail of success, are bitterly imposed upon, or may become the easy dupes and facile tools of rascals and knaves." (Pennsylvania Training School 1871, 8–9)

In 1868, he had reported 57 of the 500 inmates who had been schooled at his asylum as "entirely dependent"; by 1871, the number of "hopelessly and totally dependent" had risen to 161 (Pennsylvania Training School 1869, 1871). Perception more than institutional demographics must account for this change. Postwar social stress added to major economic downturns between 1873 and 1879 and again between 1883 and 1885 allowed superintendents to make legislative appeals based not on success for productivity (the prewar appeal) but on either failure to be productive on the outside (in the case of trained adults) or failure to benefit from education (in the case of lower functioning adults and children).

Ironically, in Pennsylvania, the first custodial cases admitted were private-paying clientele. In 1871, when Kerlin responded to what he called the "spur of necessity," inadequate public support for indigent pupils had led him to advocate to his board of trustees for the admission of private-paying custodial clients (Pennsylvania Training School 1871). From Kerlin's perspective, these cases would help to subsidize the publicly supported educational cases. The arrangement, however, had its limitations. With increasing demands for the admission of public clientele, Kerlin, within the decade, had to begin searching for new ways to extend custodial care to the indigent. In part, demand shaped his search; in part, institutional survival. If state officials could be persuaded to pay for indigent custodial cases, local officials would have fewer people in their almshouses and the idiot institution would be on a sounder financial footing.

In Ohio, private pupils had never been important to the institution's survival. In 1869, a newly organized board of state charities had taken the step of recognizing three distinct classes of idiots, each worthy of admission to the state asylum at Columbus. Those classes included idiots capable of some schooling; "those so devoid of mind as to preclude the possibility of mental culture and yet possessing perfect physical organizations, susceptible of training, by mere force of habit to manual labor and cleanliness of persons"; and those who were totally helpless and in need of constant care (Pennsylvania Training School 1871, 13–15). To facilitate the differentiation of these distinct classes of what superintendents were increasingly apt to call *feebleminded* inmates was the plan by the Ohio board to authorize the construction of six one-story buildings. Known by the end of the 1870s as the "cottage plan" or "colony plan," these small buildings detached from the central (and usually large) educational building provided the physical structure for a newly emerging policy of differential custody (Pennsylvania Training School 1871, 13–15).

In 1868, before the development of this new architecture, the Ohio facility had housed 105 pupils, most of whom lived and received training in the multistoried educational building and returned to their homes after a course of schooling. By 1900, after the cottage plan was fully operating, the Columbus facility had more than one thousand inmates, many of whom were to spend their whole lives there. Even by 1879, the institution had acquired a reputation for its liberal admission policy. In that year, Charles Wilbur, superintendent of the Illinois Asylum for Feeble-Minded Children and younger brother of Hervey Wilbur, advised a Wheaton, Illinois, mother whose son was too old for the Illinois facility to move the young man to relatives in Ohio, where admission requirements were not so strict (C. Wilbur 1865–80, vol. 2, 91).

When fire destroyed the Ohio institution's large educational and housing structure in November 1881, Gustavus Doren, Patterson's successor at Columbus, had even greater freedom to expand the Ohio asylum to include several smaller buildings where "low grades," epileptics, and diseased inmates on the one hand, and child-bearing female imbeciles and able-bodied male imbeciles on the other, could be differentially housed. Indeed, the fires that plagued many institutions in the nineteenth century, despite their serious consequences, made policy shifts easier to accomplish ("Burned Asylum" 1881; Ohio Asylum 1868, 12, 1881, 5–7).

Supporting and even a bit envious of Ohio's expansion were Knight, Kerlin, and Charles Wilbur. Even Hervey Wilbur was not unsympathetic to Ohio's change of policy. Adamantly opposed to "institutional palaces," he nevertheless supported congregate cottages as an alternative. Pressed for greater openness in his institution's admission policy, he began calling for a place for unproductive and uneducable idiots, who seemed more prominent in postwar America.

The transition in Ohio occurred more quickly than in other states because of the Ohio institution's uniquely public character. The older facilities in Massachusetts, New York, Pennsylvania, and Connecticut had significant numbers of private pupils. Although parents at private schools like the one at Barre often arranged permanent custodial care for their children, parents and relatives of private-paying pupils at public facilities usually expected educational results and, at least prior to the 1880s, tended to have their children return home after a normal course of instruction. As noted earlier, they wrote of their children's amazing improvement.[3] Ohio, not as dependent as the other facilities on educating private-paying pupils whose improved condition would be demonstrated in the community but faced with the same demands, could make the shift to custodialism with greater ease. Likewise, neither Patterson nor Doren, unlike the Wilburs, Knight, Howe, and Parrish, had ever stressed extrainstitutional productivity as a central goal of education. Influenced from the beginning by his friend William Awl of the state insane asylum, Patterson had always envisioned the Ohio facility as a hospital, not an extension of the common school. When, in 1860, Doren, Patterson's successor, requested legislative appropriations for "a farm [that] would also provide for the permanent retention and profitable employment of a certain number of adult idiots who would otherwise be obliged to find homes in county infirmaries, jails or lunatic asylum," Ohio in practice and perspective was making itself ready for custody (Doren 1902 [1891]).

Equally important in Ohio's change of direction was the establishment in 1867 of the Ohio State Board of Charities. This centralized state board, unlike the quasi-public boards of trustees in other states, was able in the early part of the 1870s to initiate what would become a trend: the shift from an emphasis on education to custodial care. The change in institutional control from local trustees to state boards did not come without the superintendents' opposition. Most had operated with trustees whom they had handpicked, typically founders of the school or other citizens with personal and philanthropic commitments to it, and were at first suspicious of state control over their facilities. State boards usually consisted of political appointees made by governors who might or might not be supportive of the institution. But the growth of public funding and actions by greater numbers of states to establish centralized charity boards ensured that, by the 1890s, other states were following Ohio's lead (Craig et al. 1893).

The institutional changes anticipated before the war and begun in states like Pennsylvania and Ohio in the 1870s were the result of cognitive constructions and social factors that shaped new directions in policy and practice in the following decade. On the cognitive side were, among others, the writings of Ray (1838), Seguin (e.g., 1866), and later the British superintendents Down (1866, 1867) and Ireland (1877). Socially, as I will note later, the United States underwent unprecedented social and economic change. The shapers of services for feebleminded people—superintendents, charity workers, and philanthropists—were not unaffected by these cognitive and social influences. Their public writings of promise, their private correspondences of complaint, both showed a sensitivity to the implications of change in the American social fabric that affected their occasional moments of public prominence as well as the more routine activities of building larger and more specialized facilities. In the midst of change and routine, superintendents established their professional legitimacy and, more often than not, made themselves indispensable. What were these changes, and how did superintendents and their supporters respond in making new policy and setting new professional prerogatives?

CONSTRUCTING FEEBLEMINDEDNESS AS A SOCIAL PROBLEM

The Association of Medical Officers of American Institutions for Idiotic and Feeble-Minded Persons

When Kerlin called together in 1876 six fellow superintendents of institutions for feebleminded persons to meet at the Pennsylvania Training School in conjunction with the nation's centennial celebrations, his motives were more professional than patriotic. Previously snubbed by the Association of Medical Officers of American Institutions for the Insane, who insisted that only lunatic asylum superintendents could enjoy membership, Hervey Wilbur was glad to meet with Kerlin, who had also included Charles Wilbur, Doren, Knight, Brown, and Seguin, in forming an association for their own kind (Association of Medical Officers 1877; Grob 1973, 116–121; McGovern 1985, 156).

The Association of Medical Officers of American Institutions for Idiotic and Feeble-Minded Persons was an attempt to put these medical men on a footing equal with the lunatic-alienists or at least to give them an equivalent-sounding title. Arriving on the scene later than their colleagues heading insane asylums, the superintendents of idiots were, by 1876, feeling confident enough in their stability to join together but uncertain enough about maintaining that stability to appreciate the support of each other.

As a symbol of their growing unity, they elected Edward Seguin (né Edouard Séguin) their first president. Only four years from his death, Seguin represented the system that had brought hope for the education of idiots. In the decade following his 1866 *Idiocy*, he expanded his interests to mental thermometry, kindergartens, and parks. Like his friend Hervey Wilbur, he had distrusted mixing "simple idiots" with idiots having other disabilities. Yet, like Wilbur, he had begun to reconstruct his vision of idiocy to include the necessity of custody for idiots of families with little means to provide training and care. In the last year of his life, he launched in Manhattan a private school for idiot children from wealthy families where, unburdened by pressures for institutional development, he could practice his physiological methods of education. Such private facilities, he claimed, should continue an educational focus, a focus becoming less and less central to the public institution (Seguin 1870*b*, 1870*c*).

Isaac Kerlin was elected secretary-treasurer. He would hold this position until 1892, the year he was elected president of the Association of Medical Officers and the year before his death. As secretary, he launched and edited the association's *Proceedings,* sending a thousand copies of its first edition "for distribution in such States as may be now projecting State Institutions" (Association of Medical Officers 1877, 8). Letters to Doren show both his active interest and central place in shaping the content of these proceedings for the next fifteen years and his ongoing efforts to disseminate copies to public libraries, colleges, ancillary organizations, and the popular press. Indeed, as a propagandist in the cause of feeblemindedness, Kerlin was aggressive and tireless, cajoling members to attend meetings, give papers, bring with them elected public officials, and "get the word out." As the titular head of the Association of Medical Officers for sixteen years, he initiated the first paradigmatic focus on the subject of feeblemindedness. With Howe's death in 1876, Seguin's in 1880, and Hervey Wilbur's three years later, Kerlin became the senior spokesperson for the emerging group of institutional superintendents (Doren Manuscripts, Kerlin letters to Doren: August 8, 1884; November 17, 1884; February 12, 1885; May 14, 1885; February 12, 1886; March 26, 1886; May 20, 1886).

The formation of the association in 1876 was timely for what would become a new surge in institutional development. Illinois began a school in 1865, and the city of New York opened a facility as part of the Randall's Island House of Refuge in 1866 to relieve the demands made on the Syracuse school. The next public facility started in Iowa in 1876. In 1877, Illinois moved its modest school in Jacksonville to a large, newly built structure in Lincoln. In 1878, New York opened the nation's first explicitly custodial institution at Newark. In 1879, Minnesota and Indiana opened institutions, followed by Kansas in 1881, California in 1884, Nebraska in 1885, Maryland in 1888, New Jersey in 1889, Washington in 1892, New York in 1894 (a fourth facility at Rome), Michigan in 1895, and Wisconsin in 1896. Several private schools also opened, especially after 1890.

The growth in the number of public institutions paralleled a growth in the size of their facilities. In 1879, Charles Wilbur instructed J. M. W. Jones, a local engraver, to print a second register of pupils for the Illinois Asylum. His first register, now full, had room for five inmates per page. The new register, Wilbur urged, should have room for nine inmates per page and should hold a thousand names. Although his new facility at Lincoln had moved from its first Jacksonville location less than two years earlier, an abundance of admission requests had convinced the Illinois superintendent to plan for future growth (C. Wilbur, 1865–80, vol. 2, 54).

With the growth in number and size came the burgeoning of staff members in each of the institutions. In turn, the multiplication of institutions and staff resulted in the growth of the Association of Medical Officers. Meeting each year, usually in late spring at one of the members' institutions, superintendents, often accompanied by their spouses and one or two staff members, shared formal papers and informal gossip on topics ranging from the latest developments in craniectomy to casualties of recent state elections. During this time, the social matrix of the profession developed and crystallized.

Feeblemindedness, Philanthropists, and Fallen Women

Another organization, the National Conference of Charities and Correction, founded in 1874 by leaders of the emerging state charity boards, became a forum for extending the matrix to a wider social welfare community. Meeting annually in urban centers, it became the nation's leading association concerned with prison reform, pauperism, insanity, delinquency, immigration, and feeblemindedness. As its membership grew throughout the nineteenth century and into the twentieth, it attracted local, state, and national politicians; philanthropists of varying ideologies; charity organization societies; and social scientists, who were, in the last quarter of the century, beginning to establish themselves in American universities (Bruno 1957; Trattner 1979, 236–237).

The National Conference's initial interest in feeblemindedness came not from institutional superintendents but from philanthropists and social reformers. Hervey Wilbur had been a member since the earliest years of the organization, yet his conference activities had focused primarily on the problem of insanity.[4] Not until 1884, when Kerlin took over the chair of the Committee on Imbecility and Idiocy, did superintendents become actively involved in the conference. At the 1884 meeting in Saint Louis, as members of the newly named Committee on the Care and Training of the Feeble-Minded, they began issuing reports that reflected and anticipated major changes in social policy for feebleminded citizens.[5]

Kerlin, with his organizational know-how, became the major force keeping feeblemindedness on the conference's agenda. Wilbur had supported new custodial trends, but not with the enthusiasm mustered by Kerlin. Kerlin's skills, however, only nurtured a conference interest in feeblemindedness initiated neither by Wilbur nor Kerlin but by members interested in general topics of social reform and philanthropy. In 1877, Richard Dugdale presented his study on the heredity of degeneracy; in 1879, Josephine Shaw Lowell addressed the conference on "One Means of Preventing Pauperism"; and, in 1881, Frederick Wines reported the results of his census of "defective, dependent, and delinquent classes" (Dugdale 1877a; Lowell 1879; Wines 1881). More than the influence of the superintendents, these studies provided a context in the social welfare community for changes superintendents were only beginning to hope for.

Although interest in heredity was not new to the 1870s, the conference members now had a forum in which to address this issue. Howe, Knight, Hervey Wilbur, Kerlin, and Doren were each fascinated by what appeared to be the continuity of disabilities over generations. In the language of a post-Weismann perceptive (one, of course, not available to the superintendents of the period), adverse environmental factors affected the phenotypical cells, which resulted in degeneration of the individual. Degeneration of the individual added to the already adverse environment. Such a context ensured disability, usually even more severe, for the next generation. Genotypical changes, then, were the result of phenotypical damage caused by the environment from one generation to the next. Thus, for example, superintendents believed that phenotypical damage caused by alcoholism in one generation could be passed on; a disabled child was the result of the poor "genetic environment" of the parent compounded by the poor home environment into which the child was born.[6]

Richard Dugdale presented this argument before the conference in his speech in 1877 and in his book of the same year, *The Jukes* (Dugdale 1877a, 1877b). Dugdale departed from an earlier generation of hereditarians in the sophistication of his assessment of intergenerational degeneracy. For Howe and the others, degeneracy among generations could take on markedly different forms—a drunk in one generation, a prostitute in another, and an idiot in yet another (e.g., Fish 1879). While acknowledging the possibility of intergenerational disability, Dugdale, before Mendel and Weismann, began to see the relationship between heredity and environment as less capricious but more complex. Disability itself was not easily predicted across generations, but intergenerational patterns were more predictable than previously thought. When Dugdale talked about "undervitalization," he acknowledged that specific types of degeneracy affected different generations; yet, he began to recognize patterns. Thus, alcoholism in one generation would not normally lead to a whole host of degeneracies but to "backwardness" or low birth weight, for example, each contributing to poverty.

Dugdale never stated, however, that heredity alone, apart from its interrelationship with environmental influences, led to irreversible social problems. Instead, unhealthy Jukes, Dugdale claimed, were much more likely to be paupers than were healthy Jukes. "Health, self-support, self-respect, longevity flourish where disease is not, therefore pauperism and prostitution fail" (Dugdale 1877a, 89). Added to this hereditary-environmental interrelationship was Dugdale's cautious position on the linkage of heredity to feeblemindedness and social vice. "We have remarked," he told the conference participants, "that the law of heredity is much more firmly established in the domain of physiological and pathological conditions than it is as respects the transmission of intellectual and moral aptitudes. In proportion as we approach features which are moulded by education, they are less transmissible, and more completely governed by the laws of variation, which are largely referable to environment" (Dugdale 1877a, 84–85). In his book he added, "Men do not become moral by intuition, but by patient organization and training. . . . We must therefore distinctly accept as an established educational axiom, that the moral nature . . . is the last developed of the elements of the character, and, for this reason, is most modifiable by the nature of the environment" (Dugdale 1877b, 56–57). Thus, to deal with such "hereditary" matters as alcoholism and syphilis, society should educate people about the harmful effects of both.

Dugdale's paper aroused no greater interest than other papers given at the 1877 meeting. It was not until after his death in 1883 that his writings began to find an interested audience, albeit one that misrepresented his message.[7] No longer seen as responsive to environmental influences, the Jukes family members were portrayed as hopeless degenerates, victims of their self-generated vices and ignorance. In such a light, their fame spread even into the next century. In 1910, the sociologist Franklin Giddings stated, "*The Jukes* has long been known as one of these important books that exert an influence out of all proportion to their bulk. It is doubtful if any concrete study of moral forces is more widely known, or has provoked more discussion" (Giddings 1910, iii). Frequent references to the study began to appear at meetings of the Conference of Charities and Correction and the Association of Medical Officers after 1885.

Almost always emphasizing the depth of the Jukes' hereditary degeneracy, these references reflected a legitimacy given to an important new tool in the study of social problems in general and feeblemindedness in particular, the *pedigree study*. From Charles Brace's 1880 discussion of "Margaret, the mother of criminals" and Oscar McCulloch's 1888 study of the tribe of Ishmael to Arthur Estabrook and Ivan McDougle's *Mongrel Virginians* (1926), studies of the lineage of degeneracy were increasingly used to demonstrate the immutable effects of heredity on certain groups of American citizens. (I consider pedigree studies more fully in Chapter 5.) What Dugdale began as an exercise in measuring the effects of environmental deprivation on various social problems of his day soon became an exercise in measuring the effects of various social problems on what was considered an otherwise stable environment.

If Dugdale's study had its greatest impact after its presentation, Josephine Shaw Lowell's 1879 address to the conference, "One Means of Preventing Pauperism," had immediate effects. Dressed in mourning black since the death of her husband of one year at the battle of Cedar Creek in 1864, Lowell transferred her personal tragedies into postwar service. The quintessential friendly visitor, Lowell involved herself in virtually all causes popular among the enlightened old guard of the last quarter of the nineteenth century (Fredrickson 1965, 211–216; Rafter 1992a, 1997; W. Stewart 1911; Waugh 1998).[8]

An economic depression beginning in 1873 had created a new class of paupers. As the depression lingered, the plight of many Americans became even worse. In 1874, six thousand businesses failed; in 1875, eight thousand; and in 1876, nine thousand. By 1875, five hundred thousand workers were jobless, and others with jobs found their wages reduced. Breadlines were long, and strikes were frequent and well-organized (Bining and Cochran 1964, 410–414; Brands 2010, 81–105; Folsom 1991, 126–139). In addition, increased immigration aggravated the competition for jobs. As a result, there was a growing population of rural tramps and urban "deadbeats." Although some of these were veterans affected by traumas of war, most were merely unemployed workers looking for jobs. Elites became increasingly alarmed by this "army" of undeserving poor:

> The dead-beat will never reform. . . . A standing commission of vagrancy should be instituted in every large city, and every county in the land, and institutions of industry established for the purpose of making these men self-supporting, and

of curing them of their wretched disease. We have lunatic asylums, not only for
the benefit of the lunatics, but for the relief of the community, and among the
dead-beats and tramps we have an enormous number of men who are just as truly
diseased as the maddest man in Utica, or at the Bloomington Asylum. . . . It is only
last year that we heard of a force of 500 of them approaching a Western city, to
the universal alarm of the inhabitants. . . . These facts menace both our homes and
our liberties. It is not a tramp, here and there, such as we have at all times; but it
is an army of tramps that can be brought together on the slightest occasion, for
any deed of rascality and blood which it may please them to engage in. ("Topics of
the Time" 1877, 416)

By 1878, things seemed worse, not better. A new panic that year caused additional hardship and anxiety. Only in 1879 did economic conditions begin to look
better (Folsom 1991, 126–139).[9]

It was with a return to financial equilibrium in the midst of lingering social disruption that Lowell presented her 1879 address. As a member of the New York State
Board of Charities since 1876, she had come to know the ins and outs of the state's
welfare systems. Not long after her appointment, she visited Wilbur's facility in
Syracuse and soon began to take special interest in its operations (W. Stewart 1911,
48–61, 63).

Less than a year after her appointment to the state board, Lowell began a crusade
that, with varying degrees of intensity, would continue throughout her life. She
believed that one group of paupers—women "of delinquent and vagrant classes"—
had not received the attention they deserved (W. Stewart 1911, 88–89; see also
Rafter 1992a, 1997). The "pauper of paupers," she reported to the Board of Charities
in January 1878, the fallen woman was often feebleminded and idiotic, ending up
in almshouses or on the street. In the board's tenth annual report she continued her
campaign: "In order to grapple with the gigantic evil and to stop the increase of pauperism, crime and insanity in this community, a reformatory for women, under the
management of women, governed on the same principles as those which control the
management of the State Reformatory at Elmira is required" (cited in W. Stewart
1911, 88–92; on fallen women, see also Kunzel 1995; Rafter 1997).

The idea of the reformatory was increasingly taking hold among reformers of the
period. Zebulon Brockway's Elmira experiment and Enoch and Frederick Wines's
views on penology were finding their way into the wider social welfare community. Emphasizing indeterminate sentencing, the careful segregation of criminal
types, and the separation of children from adults and men from women, these
penal reformers were already influential in the National Conference. When Lowell
addressed the membership in 1879, she applied the new penal reforms to a group
that up to this point had received little attention: vagrant, often feebleminded, girls
and women:

The legislature of New York, by concurrent resolution of May 27–29, 1873, directed the State Board of Charities to examine into the causes of the increase of
crime, pauperism, and insanity in that State. In compliance with this resolution,

an examination ... was made into the antecedents of every inmate of the poor-houses of the State.... Even a casual perusal of that report will convince the reader that one of the most important and most dangerous causes of the increase of crime, pauperism, and insanity, is the restrained liberty allowed to vagrant and degraded women. (Lowell 1879, 189)

Poorhouses and jails, she continued, were not the proper places for either vagrant women or prostitutes. Those settings merely exposed their female victims to lust-ful men and to their own weak wills. The children of immoral women, too, were no better off. They began life as did their mothers and as their own children would likely begin life. Such women needed "self-protection" from their own "moral leprosy." "To rescue the unfortunate beings," she told the conferees, "and to save the indus-trious part of the community from the burdens of their support, 'Reformatories' should be established, to which all women under thirty, when arrested for misde-meanors, or upon the birth of a second illegitimate child, should be committed for a very long period ... and where they should be subject to such a physical, moral and intellectual training as would re-create them" (Lowell 1879, 197–199).

Lowell proposed an institutional structure more like that of the emerging in-stitutions for the feebleminded than that of the prisons. First, she insisted, the institution needed a large tract of land, between 250 and 500 acres, "to allow of free out-of-door life without any communication of the outer world." "A series of build-ings," would be built, "each to accommodate from fifteen to twenty-five women, and so arranged as to afford ample means of classification." In charge of the institu-tion would be women who would train inmates in "all household work to support themselves by honest industry." This labor, she added, would partially support the institution at a relief to all taxpayers. There would be a separate school for "mental and moral training," and a female physician would ensure good health. All inmates would be classified according to ability and attitude, and each woman could move either up or down the grades. A board of managers would have the power to place the higher grade inmates "in situations where their wages should belong to them-selves but where they would still be under guardianship and liable to recommit-ment to the Reformatory in case of ill conduct" (Lowell 1879, 198–199).

Lowell's address was immediately embraced by members of the conference. Convinced of the urgency of her cause and always mindful of good press, she wrote William Letchworth, then president of the New York Board of Charities, to have a thousand copies printed "for use in our next campaign." She added, "If it is not printed, I shall have it printed myself" (cited in W. Stewart 1911, 95).

Lowell believed that many so-called fallen women were actually feebleminded. At the December 1877 meeting of the State Board, she had noted the shocking number of mentally deficient males and females in the state's almshouses. The board had then appointed William Devereux, William Letchworth, and Lowell to a committee to consult with Wilbur and the trustees of the New York Asylum about custodial care for idiots (W. Stewart 1911, 115–121). Wilbur cooperated with the committee's efforts, supporting the need for custodial care but resisting such care at the Syracuse school. In March 1878, the trustees agreed to operate on an experimental basis a custodial facility for women between the ages of sixteen and forty-five and their children. In June, the State Board finished plans for the facility, and, in September 1878, it had opened in Newark, about sixty miles west of Syracuse. For the next five years, Wilbur supervised this explicitly custodial facility for feeble minds, the first of its kind in the nation (see also Rose 2008, 64–119).

In 1884, after Wilbur's death, the State Board sought to remove the Syracuse trustees' authority over the Newark institution, and a year-long struggle between the trustees and the board followed in the midst of the trustees' search for Wilbur's successor. Lowell and Letchworth advocated for a permanent and fully custodial facility controlled by the State Board. In her April 1884 memorial to the legislature, Lowell called for "the establishment of further and definite provision for the custodial care and sequestration of idiotic and feebleminded girls and women, for their protection and the protection of the State from hereditary increase of that class of dependents on public charity" (cited in W. Stewart 1911, 118–119). In the end, the State Board won, and the Newark facility was placed under its control.

Charles Wilbur applied for his brother's position, but the Syracuse trustees and some of his fellow state superintendents blocked his application (Doren Manuscripts, letter from B. K. Eastman to Doren, July 19, 1884; letter from Allen Moore to Doren, July 29, 1884 [includes Doren's reply]). Sharing his brother's insistence on a separation of educational and custodial services, Charles Wilbur represented a policy increasingly outdated and made questionable by Lowell's efforts. Relieved of their power over the Newark institution, the trustees soon began to see the necessity for a new type of leadership. In 1885, they appointed J. C. Carson to succeed the elder Wilbur. Reflecting on the growth of the Newark facility, Carson told the Association of Medical Officers at their 1889 annual meeting:

> There are at the present time over 200 of these feeble minded girls and women provided for in this institution, and appropriations have been made that will extend its guardianship over 100 more. Many of its inmates have borne children prior to their admission, and several of them more than one. There is no doubt that the propagation of idiocy, which was formerly carried on through the medium of this class of weak-minded girls among the homes and poor-houses of our State, will henceforth be materially lessened. (Carson 1891a, 78)

Carson had no difficulty accepting the winds of change. Even before 1890, the Newark facility for magdalens had become known locally as "The Custodial" (Hahn 1980).

Like Dugdale, Lowell believed that the "hereditary" linkage of feeblemindedness and other social problems found its roots in women, women as givers and nurturers of new life. With the growing interest in heredity among reformers, she took up the cause of backward and fallen women before the National Council on Charities and Correction. Although her personal leadership waned in the coming decades as she began new philanthropic activities, the message of the "pauper of paupers" remained and spread to other states. By the second half of the 1880s, Pennsylvania had added a "girls cottage" for eighty women of child-bearing age; Ohio had established separate facilities for women; and, in 1886, Illinois, under the leadership of William Fish, had built a new "cottage" for one hundred "girls" (Powell 1887).

The fear of unrestrained feebleminded women ultimately found its voice among educators and superintendents. George Knight, son of and successor to Henry Knight in Connecticut, in 1892 called for "a life time under restraint, oversight, and wise direction" for adult female imbeciles. They are "often bright and pleasing," he reminded his colleagues, but are apt to "become the victims of licentiousness" (Goodheart 2004; G. Knight 1892, 159; see also Sanborn 1892). Catharine Brown at Barre, a protégé of Hervey Wilbur and earlier an advocate of physiological education, small facilities, and community productivity told her colleagues in 1886:

> The feebleminded woman must be . . . securely hedged in, or she becomes the easy prey of man's lust and the mother of criminals, thus perpetuating the endless chain of human weakness and crime. Not long ago the wife of the superintendent of one of our largest institutions for this class said to me, "We have twenty girls fitted for domestic service." I knew the supply of kitchen-helpers was everywhere limited, yet could only reply, "What housekeeper will, or can, engage a servant who must be perpetually watched?" (C. Brown 1887, 404–405)

Thus, joining the classification of moral idiocy stressed by Kerlin before the war were vagrant women of childbearing years who, in what social reformers believed to be their moral lethargy, became threats to common decency and to the well-ordered family.

Feeble Minds and the 1880 Census

A third reformer, Frederick Wines, added another dimension to the newly emerging vision of feeblemindedness. Wines began his career in 1865 as the minister of the Springfield, Illinois, Presbyterian church once attended by Abraham Lincoln. His clergyman-educator father, Enoch Wines, who was well known in social welfare circles as a penologist, was secretary of the New York Prison Association and co-founder along with Zebulon Brockway of the National Prison Congress. Following his father's interest in social welfare, the younger Wines became the secretary of the Illinois Board of Public Charities newly organized in 1869. There he remained for thirty years, removed only between 1892 and 1896 during John P. Altgeld's Democratic administration. As secretary of the board, he took up many national and even international causes, becoming one of the nation's best-known postwar shapers of social reform (Bruno 1957; Givens 1986).

Wines's adopted state, Illinois, grew rapidly in the two decades after the Civil War. Social reformers feared that Chicago, the emerging center of Midwestern commerce and industry, was developing all the problems associated with postwar boomtown growth. In central and down-state Illinois, these same reformers saw crowded and unsanitary conditions in county poorhouses and jails, all of which contained outcasts of various sorts.

When Wines took over the leadership of the Illinois Board of Public Charities, social welfare had been (and would for several decades continue to be) the province of sectarian organizations. Although a devoted Christian, Wines advocated for greater public provision of social welfare services (Platt 1977, 101–136).

In 1878, appointed a commissioner to the International Penitentiary Congress in Stockholm, Wines visited several British and continental institutions, especially those for delinquent, insane, and feebleminded inmates. He was struck by the use of labor in British reformatories, which, he believed, was not a means of punishment but "training for future usefulness." Labor, he insisted, should become the new American model for dealing with juvenile offenders. In addition, he was equally taken by the small detached cottages in institutions for the insane and feebleminded. These facilities seemed to manage more easily the wide diversity of mentally disabled individuals. On his return to the United States, Wines began to advocate for the salubrious effects of both inmate labor and institutional differentiation through the cottage system (Illinois Board of State Commissioners 1879, 273).

This interest in mental disability coupled with his reputation for careful statistical analysis led to Wines's appointment in 1880 as special consultant to the Census Bureau. Although census officials had collected data on insane and feebleminded citizens since 1840, social reformers did not believe the findings were reliable. Wines insisted that an accurate count had to go beyond institutionalized people. Thus, he sent questionnaires to nearly one hundred thousand physicians throughout the nation, asking them for information about idiots and lunatics in their communities. That he sent his questionnaires to physicians demonstrated the penetration in the growing social welfare community of the medicalization of feeblemindedness. With an impressive response rate of 80 percent, Wines developed what he and others believed was the first accurate picture of the proportion of mental disability in the United States (Gorwitz 1974).

Although its interpretations were cautious, Wines's report, *The Defective, Dependent, and Delinquent Classes of the Population of the United States* (1881; also see Wines 1888) had a tremendous impact on social reformers. According to his data, the rate of feeblemindedness was 153.3 per 100,000 people, an increase of 2.5 times the 1870 rate. This high rate, he claimed, was especially astonishing since the rate reported in the previous census (in 1870) had actually been lower than the one reported in 1850 (Kerlin in the 1870s had estimated a 1:1,000 prevalence). By the end of the 1880s, Charles Wilbur and A. C. Rogers were estimating that one in five hundred Americans were feebleminded (Pennsylvania Training School 1871; Rogers 1891a; C. Wilbur 1888).

The new census data also confirmed Wines's and others' belief that vast numbers of the feebleminded were receiving no care at worst or ineffective care at best. William B. Fish of the Illinois institution admonished his colleagues in his 1888 presidential address to the Association of Medical Officers:

> There is yet "much land to be possessed." When we consider that the census of 1880 revealed the fact that less than three thousand of the seventy-six thousand idiots and imbeciles were being cared for in public and private institutions, there

must come to us a deep sense of our responsibility as an Association committed to the advancement of the interests of this class of defectives. How much of misfortune and suffering do these figures represent? How many saddened homes? How many worn and weary mothers? How many fathers, struggling to keep their families from want, weighted down by this burden of misfortune? (Fish 1889, 14–16)

A SOCIAL BURDEN

Organized in their professional ranks through the Association of Medical Officers of American Institutions for Idiotic and Feeble-Minded Persons and integrated into the major forum for social reform, the National Conference of Charities and Correction, the superintendents in the 1880s found receptive ears for their message. Dugdale's pedigree study and Lowell's investigations linked feeblemindedness with other social problems, and Wines's census enumerations suggested that feeblemindedness was rapidly increasing in the general population and the unserved feebleminded were consequently more numerous than ever. All these cognitive claims, of course, developed in the aftermath of an economic depression accompanied by severe social distress. Dugdale and Lowell had become suddenly interested in feeblemindedness as a social problem in the 1870s because feeblemindedness had begun to seem more a problem affecting economically vulnerable people, families, and communities. Wines, too, "discovered" greater numbers of feeble minds, not necessarily because America had more but because economic and social stress allowed for new parameters and definitions of feeblemindedness.

When he assumed the leadership of the National Conference on Charities and Correction's committee on idiocy in 1884, Kerlin, already a masterful propagandist, found growing support among social reformers for major changes in policies affecting feeble minds. Now, before ever-stingy and politically changing legislatures, superintendents became advocates not merely for provincial programs affecting their own small groups of pupils but also for solutions to wider and burdensome social problems. As legislators in the 1880s and 1890s became convinced of the truth of the superintendents' warnings in the midst of profound changes in the American social fabric, superintendents found new meaning in their message and new directions in the construction of social policy.

Their message was simple. Feeble minds were a burden to society. Without intervention, the burden would continue to increase and to exacerbate other social problems. To deal with this burden, public officials and private reformers must expand the parameters of institutional care to include all types and gradations of feeblemindedness. Such expansion required an institutional arrangement to differentiate care at a reasonable cost to taxpayers. Once such an arrangement had been demonstrated, the task ahead became the multiplication of institutional care facilities throughout the various states.

To gain legislative support for the expansion of their facilities, the superintendents turned to the colony system, and, to make that system work inexpensively, they turned to a new vision of education and productivity. The colony system put high grades and low grades, epileptics and mongoloids, moral imbeciles and spas-tics, troublemakers and "household pets," under one institutional roof. A new vision of education and productivity ensured that trained feeble minds would have a place in which to be productive: that is, the institution itself. Feeble minds would care for each other there, raising food in the fields, doing laundry, or caring for lower grades. No longer would society have to worry about their returning to the almshouse or becoming a renewed burden on their families or communities. In the institution, capable feeble minds would be transformed from community burdens and lawbreakers to self-supporting and upright caregivers, thereby reducing the cost of operating the institution. This model ensured the growth and perpetuation of the institution.

Feebleminded people had always been subject to systems of classification. In 1877, Kerlin identified three basic types of mental defectives: superior grades, who in five to ten years would be able to return to their communities; orphaned idiots and imbeciles; and lower grades, who needed "habit-training, amusements, [and] exercise, aided by appropriate medical treatment" (Kerlin 1877, 21–22). Even as late as 1877, Kerlin was relying on *social* as much as *medical* factors to differentiate inmates. Almost immediately after he presented this scheme, however, the criteria of differentiation changed. Superintendents began to use the *ability* to perform tasks at the institution as the fundamental criteria for classifying inmates. In an address to the Michigan legislature, Charles Wilbur, then superintendent of the Illinois Asylum, recommended the London Community Organization Society's 1877 classification scheme. Feeble minds were classified as the permanently im-proved (which Wilbur noted was a small proportion of the total); the moderately improved, who were good for institutional farm and trade work; and the unim-proved or retrograding idiots, epileptics, and other asylum cases. Although re-maining opposed to losing the educational focus of the institution to the custo-dial, Wilbur stressed the value of institutional employment for the moderately improved, noting the cost savings to the institution resulting from their labor (C. Wilbur 1877).

With a scheme developed for retaining various types of feeble minds, super-intendents were only a step away from calling for open institutional admissions. Indeed, soon most of them were championing the admission of epileptics, the crip-pled, and so-called low-grade cases (e.g., A. Rogers 1888; G. Knight 1889, 1892; C. Wilbur 1877) (Figure 3.4, Figure 3.5). Open admissions, therefore, allowed su-perintendents to retain the two groups of clientele—custodial cases and trained high-grade adults—previously prohibited by most state legislation. The retention of one, of course, was necessary for the retention of the other. Without custodial cases, there was no need for long-term, labor-intensive care; without high grades there were not enough caregivers. J. C. Carson summed up the symbiotic relation-ship implied in the new classification scheme:

> The first efforts made for them, as we know, were all on the educational basis, and experience has shown that by far the majority of feebleminded children are teach-able, and that by a proper course of training quite a considerable number of them,

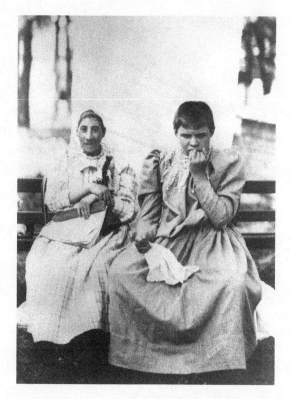

Figure 3.4:
Custodial cases: "low grades" ca. 1890. Inmates probably of the Illinois Asylum for Feeble-Minded Children. (Courtesy of Southern Illinois University at Edwardsville, Lovejoy Library, Beverly Farm Records)

by the time adult life is reached, become able, under well-selected surroundings, to care for and support themselves. Another large portion become useful in various ways about the institutions, at farming, at trades, at common labor, with the needle, in the laundry and kitchen, or in the care of others of their more helpless kind. Still another large number, although capable of a certain degree of improvement under proper training, require, by reason of markedly deficient mental capacity or physical infirmities, constant care and custody throughout their lives. These, then, are the results that may be expected from the school training of educable feebleminded. There are, however, others who are practically unteachable, and for whom no such results can be obtained, such as the excitable, the vicious, the epileptic and the paralytic. Such cases ought not to be associated in the schoolroom with the well behaved and more intelligent or teachable class, but require separate provision and custody.

He went on to note that "the adult female portion . . . should be kept under the careful custody of the State unless they can be released under exceptionally favorable and well-guarded surroundings" (Carson 1891a, 14–15).

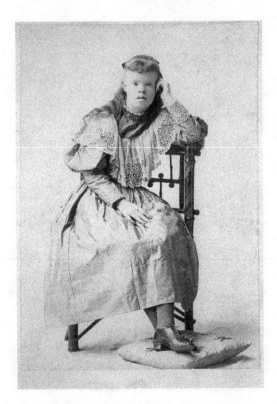

Figure 3.5:
Custodial case: "mongoloid idiot" ca. 1890. An inmate probably of the Illinois Asylum for Feeble-Minded Children. (Courtesy of Southern Illinois University at Edwardsville, Lovejoy Library, Beverly Farm Records)

Feebleminded women were thus especially singled out as candidates for custodial care. State after state in the 1880s followed New York's example of establishing facilities to keep feebleminded women of childbearing age from harm's way, although they generally established female custodial departments within existing institutions (e.g., National Conference of Charities and Correction 1889, 327). Superintendents, convinced that women worked best with custodial inmates, were quick to utilize female inmates in caregiving roles. Sometimes arriving at the institution pregnant or with infants, many women learned caregiving skills as they gave care. After gaining experience, many were given responsibilities in the institution similar to those of paid employees (Bragar 1977).

For this new policy of differential institutional care to gain a foothold, a new vision of education became necessary. Begun as "experimental schools" before the war, institutions had long ago demonstrated their ability to educate feeble minds. On a "permanent" basis by the 1850s, these educational facilities had thrived on their successes and continued to grow after the war. With the unwillingness of communities to reintegrate educated idiots and greater demand for the admission of lower functioning idiots (both exacerbated by economic stress and rapid social change), superintendents began in the late 1870s to reconceptualize the role of education in their facilities. "What per cent of persons can be expected to become self-supporting?" A. C. Rogers asked in 1888:

> Scores of feebleminded persons are today performing the work of regular employees in public institutions, and might under favorable circumstances earn a livelihood outside. But this is a busy, practical, money-getting age, when the satisfactory placing of children of normal faculties is no easy task, and only under favorable circumstances to be advised. This being true of normal persons, how small the field for those lacking in judgment and the higher qualifications for success! (A. Rogers 1888, 102)

In previous decades, superintendents had claimed that many, if not most, feeble minds were capable of providing for themselves after proper training. By 1889, however, Alexander Johnson, then secretary of the Indiana Board of State Charities, stated that only 10 to 15 percent would be "safe to send out." But he added: "to train to self-support is a very different thing. We hope to train sixty-five or seventy-five per cent to support themselves in the institution. What we need now is to adopt the principle of custodial care" (National Conference on Charities and Correction 1889, 318). George Knight at the Connecticut facility stated: "our highest grade . . . are [sic] capable of acquiring almost everything but that indispensable something known in the world as good, plain common sense. The greater proportion of this class can become self-supporting if the institution is large enough to find occupation for them within its own walls" (G. Knight 1892, 158).

To suggest, as the superintendents did, that few educated feeble minds could successfully return to their communities was not to deny the possibility of their education. Inability to meet the demands of the world did not mean that improvement under the direction of the institution was not possible. For improvement to occur, however, superintendents insisted that parents and educators had to view education not as an academic enterprise but as a vocational one. Although not entirely eliminating the three R's from their educational programs, the superintendents began to stress on-the-job training. J. Q. A. Stewart (1889) of the Kentucky Asylum reminded his colleagues that academic work provoked emotional stress in most feeble minds. Industrial work, however, provided an antidote to academic stress on the one hand and to idleness on the other. "It is hard to convince parents," Kerlin (1887a, 495) told the 1884 meeting of the National Conference,

> that the old forms of letters and numbers do not constitute an education for an imbecile child, even when they may be acquired. The best end attained in his training is, in reality, to induce in him the simplest conformity to the habits and actions of normal people—that he speak seldom, that he repress his emotion, that he move willingly and easily—so that he shall become an unobserved number of the common population, if thrown into it, or if retained under institution regulations, that his cost and care shall be as moderate as possible.

Just as academic training for *extrainstitutional* productivity began to shift to vocational training for *institutional* productivity, so too did gymnastic training, a central component in Seguin's physiological method and an important part of the curricula of all the institutions, begin to change. In the 1892 minutes of the *Proceedings of* the Association of Medical Officers, both Kerlin and A. E. Osborne, superintendent of the newly opened California institution, reported the establishment of military drills at their facilities (Figure 3.6). Both acknowledged that drills helped build self-control and discipline in male inmates. Pleased with the results, Kerlin, despite the reservations of his Quaker trustees, had even extended drills "to the little children." Seguin had used gymnastics to "excit[e] the will," to stimulate pupils out of their indifference and lethargy, but Kerlin and Osborne, and eventually many other superintendents, began to use physical training as a tool for inmate control (Association of Medical Officers 1892, 367–369, 382).

The shift to control, of course, was in part the result of institutional growth. Superintendents like Hervey Wilbur, Howe, and Richards had worked individually with pupils whose success had depended on the personality and intimate engagement of the superintendent and his staff. As their schools grew, superintendents became administrators, concerned more with the efficient operation of their institutions than with the educational needs of individual pupils.

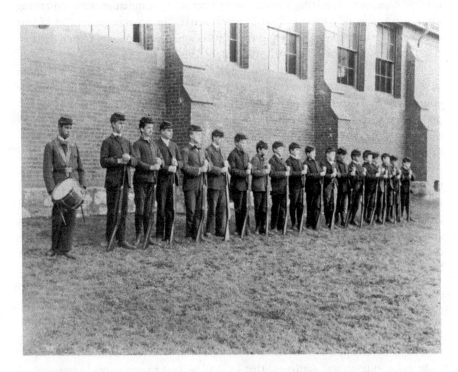

Figure 3.6:
Military drills, inmates at the Massachusetts School for the Feeble-Minded, ca. 1890. (From the author's collection)

An educational emphasis on *resocialization* thus shifted to an emphasis on *prevention*; that is, the prevention of crime, pauperism, and additional generations of feeble minds. For Catharine Brown in 1886, education no longer provided the sanguine possibilities she had hoped for as a young teacher in Barre. Joining her colleagues, she insisted:

> Although the feeble body has been invigorated by gymnastic exercises and labor teaching, the useless hand trained to dexterity, and the intellect quickened to perceive and comprehend simple details, we have not yet been able to strengthen the will nor develop the moral nature to a degree that can enable the great majority of the feebleminded as they pass from our schools, to cope single-handed with the evil there is in the world. The man of weak intellect . . . will deteriorate till his last state be worse than the first. Because he has been lifted up a little way he has more temptation, is the better fitted to become the tool of the designing, the cat's-paw of the criminal. (C. Brown 1887, 404)

To educate a feeble mind was to improve the efficiency of the institution while also preventing vice. The prevention of crime, pauperism, and future generations of feeble minds, then, became the new goal of institutional care. Institutional authorities directed education for inmate productivity away from the needs of the community and back to the needs of the institution itself. Educated feeble minds became productive feeble minds—productive within the confines of the institution, where they learned "lowerclass skills and middle-class values" and were secure from a stressful, cruel, and temptation-filled world (Platt 1977, 69). "We have a few who are bright," Alexander Johnson told the conferees, "and many who are very sweet and nice. Still, they have weak wills and feeble minds. They would be unsafe in the outer world. They must be kept quietly, safely, away from the world, living like the angels in heaven, neither marrying nor given in marriage" (National Conference of Charities and Correction 1889, 319).

Moral Imbecility

Superintendents also renewed a concern for the prevention of what they began to call *moral imbecility*. What Kerlin had identified in 1858 as moral idiocy took on new relevance in the 1880s. The change in terminology marked a change in meaning given to the condition. Like Dugdale's Jukes family, Kerlin's moral idiots in 1858 were diseased because of "a want of nurture" (Kerlin 1858, 101). Although ruthless criminals, he claimed, they were amenable to correction and change and, in turn, capable of returning to their communities where, under proper supervision, they could live out their lives. This message was clearly the one made in the story and photograph of Grubb (see Chapter 1). As late as 1875, Hervey Wilbur (New York Asylum for Idiots. 1875, 14) agreed with Kerlin that feeble minds were frequently involved in crime but with proper training could be reformed or, better yet, prevented from being lured into crime.

By 1879, Kerlin had begun to refer to moral idiocy as "juvenile insanity." In a paper by that name, he claimed that "juvenile affective insanity" was more common than previously believed. Indeed, much of what passed for juvenile delinquency, he suggested, was the result of juvenile insanity and imbecility. Such conditions, he added, had a definite and predictable relationship with crime and tended to reoccur in later generations. Although he claimed a close relationship between heredity and vice, Kerlin remained optimistic about breaking the relationship:

> The theory that once an idiot, or once an imbecile, therefore always so, is neither scientific nor sustained in facts.... [P]hysiological education and hygienic treatment early applied to congenital imbecility and child insanity, will, in the great majority of cases, result in as favorable changes, indeed in a marked rising of the individual towards the normal scale, as is accomplished in treatment of the adult insane. (Kerlin 1879, 93–94)

In less than a decade, however, Kerlin changed his views. In his annual reports of 1884 and 1886, he began to speak of moral imbecility as a distinct category and, in 1887 and 1890, delivered papers addressing the topic. In 1891, reflecting on his 1879 work on juvenile insanity, Kerlin stated, "With further reading and observation, I would today class four of the five cases as moral imbeciles, and but one as really an illustration of juvenile insanity." He added, "I have described moral imbeciles as a class of children whose perversion or aberration is in the so-called moral sense; with either no deterioration of the intellect, or if slight, such as is secondary only. More of these abnormal children are to be found in reformatories than with us, probably to the extent of twenty-five per cent. The condition is radically incurable" (Kerlin 1892a, 191).

No doubt the influence of other reformers accounted in great part for Kerlin's change of perception. His 1879 paper had reflected the sentiments of the time. For example, Charles Brace's 1872 book, *The Dangerous Classes of New York*, reprinted in several editions in the 1880s, claimed the salubrious effects of hard work in "industrial schools" as an alternative to prison, especially for juvenile offenders. The juvenile prostitute, the waif, and the street child could all, under proper environmental conditions, learn to live moral and useful lives. Dugdale's *Jukes Family* in 1877 had also stressed the link between the environment and a variety of social and personal vices, and Enoch and Frederick Wines as well as Zebulon Brockway advocated throughout the 1870s for indeterminate sentencing for juveniles in facilities segregated from hardened criminals.

Kerlin's thinking, as reflected in his paper of 1887, however, was the product of a new era. In July 1881, Charles J. Guiteau, a disappointed office seeker and (to fascinated alienists like Kerlin) a mentally deranged criminal, shot President James A. Garfield, who died eleven weeks later. In the same year in Russia, a terrorist linked with one of the several populist movements of the period assassinated Alexander II. Pogroms soon followed, and, by the end of the year, Russian Jews, the predictable scapegoats, began arriving in the United States thus beginning the "new immigration" of Eastern Europeans. Against the background of these events,

Congress in 1882 passed the "Undesirables Act," which excluded convicts, paupers, the insane, and idiots from entering the country. During the same year, Herbert Spencer, the father of social Darwinism and at the peak of his popularity, lectured in the United States; the next year, Francis Galton published *Inquiries into Human Faculty and Its Development* (1883), introducing the terms *psychometrics* and *eugenics*, both of which would soon become important in the field of intellectual disability. In 1883, the nation began to go into another economic depression (Folsom 1991, 148–154), leading to a rise in labor disturbances. Although trade unionists formed the moderate American Federation of Labor in 1886, less respectable unionists were killed the same year in Chicago's Haymarket Square. In the mid-1880s, Cesare Lombroso's *L'uomo Delinquente* [*The Criminal Man*] (1876, see also Lombroso 1911), with its claims for a criminology based on the physically inherited characteristics of criminals, began to be known and discussed in the United States (Rafter 2010). It was in this context of political and economic unrest, coupled with a growing interest in heredity fueled by purveyors of social Darwinism, that reformers in the 1880s began to reassess their optimistic assumptions of earlier decades.

The first example of this reassessment in social welfare circles was Charles L. Brace's discussion of "Margaret, mother of criminals," in a paper read to the 1880 meeting of the National Conference of Charities and Correction (Brace 1880). Following Lowell, Brace acknowledged heredity as a much greater determining factor in the perpetuation of crime. With Wines's linkage of defective classes with dependent and delinquent classes the next year, the stage was set before the Association of Medical Officers and the National Conference for a reconceptualization of the linkage of crime, feeblemindedness, and heredity.

Kerlin, whose interest in that linkage went back to the 1850s and whose professional leadership in the 1880s was unchallenged, was a perfect advocate for the new view. There were two types of physicians, he claimed in his 1887 paper (Kerlin 1889). One type was conservative and held that vice was the work of the devil; the other was progressive and scientific and held that vice was "the result of physical infirmity." Placing himself in the latter group, Kerlin regarded his view of moral imbecility as one that went beyond the conservative view embodied in the law and theology: namely, that people are always responsible for their actions. Following the perspective initiated in America by Isaac Ray (1838), Kerlin held that vice was often beyond the control of the will. Traditional morality and jurisprudence, which held that the will shaped human action, failed to take into account the evolution of the moral faculty, which, like any other human faculty, could be damaged—indeed, permanently damaged. Kerlin insisted:

> Moral sense is a primary feeling, resulting from the long experience of the race, and … its perceptions are of the same kind, engendered in the same way, and possessed of receptive and volitional centres, perhaps less localized, but common to large areas of the nervous system.… Hence, as there are persons in whom we discover a partial or entire absence of color perception … or of any other special faculty—*nor can the absence be supplied by education* [Kerlin's emphasis]—so we have individuals who, from some inherent fault in, or some radical defect of, the

receptive centers, are destitute in . . . the so-called moral sense, and no environment and no education will supply the deficiency. (Kerlin 1889, 34)

If a flaw existed, then, it was centered not in the will but in the brain. Unable to
control the moral faculty, individuals might do wrong even when their intellectual
faculty knew their error:

> Coupled with the condition [a hereditary disrespect for "the virtues of civilized
> society"] is a singular apathy to the consequences of wrongdoing: the dock and
> prison excite no apprehension; the gallows has no terror; and death and eternity
> are faced with sensational stoicism; indeed, it is a frequently expressed doubt
> whether the impressions gained by this class from the punishable sequences of
> crime, as published in our daily press, are not outweighed by excitation to crime-
> doing; for these people are egoists, who will play their role on any stage which
> elevates them into notice. (Kerlin 1889, 37)

Thus, the imbecility of most moral imbeciles appeared to be *moral* rather than *intellectual*. Within the population of feeble minds, then, most moral imbeciles were
bright enough to get into trouble, but not bright enough to stay out of it. They were
not stupid; their moral faculty was merely underdeveloped. Unfortunately, their lot
was one of hopeless degeneracy.

The condition of moral imbecility, Kerlin felt, was best explained in evolutionary terms. "The moral sense being the latest and highest attribute of our rising
humanity, it is the first and most to suffer from the law of reversion to lower type,
when from any cause the progressive development of a family is broken in the birth
of a defective child" (Kerlin 1889, 37). Acknowledging Dugdale's and Brockway's
contributions, along with recent observations on "fallen women," Kerlin developed
a picture of hereditary vice that retained its earlier polymorphism but that also
emphasized the intractability of inherited conditions, a departure from Dugdale
and Brockway (at least the latter's early work). Kerlin identified four types of moral
imbeciles: alcoholic inebriates, tramps, prostitutes, and habitual criminals. These
types, however, manifested themselves differently over generations. Thus, one
form of degeneracy might appear in one generation, but another form in the next.
The third generation might, in turn, receive the degeneracy of either the parent
or grandparent or a new form altogether (Kerlin 1889, 32–35). Commenting on
Dugdale's work, he wrote, "Carefully examined, I believe the history of the Jukes
Family will be found repeated in thousands of the lives of these four classes of
mental defectives. Of them all it is said that crime life is less likely to take its origin
in heredity, and yet there is much to sustain an opposite view" (Kerlin 1889, 36).
By 1891, Kerlin was boldly referring to moral imbecility as "radically incurable"
(Kerlin 1892*a*, 197).

Kerlin championed his ideas before his fellow superintendents at annual
meetings of the Association of Medical Officers and to child savers at meetings
of the National Conference of Charities and Correction until his death in 1893.[10]
Kerlin's legacy was the attention he brought to "how to protect society from [moral

imbeciles] and at the same time secure to them a maximum degree of happiness within the bounds of their forced and necessary restrictions" (Rogers 1892, 324).

In the year following Kerlin's death, Martha Louise Clark, who identified herself as a teacher of imbeciles, extended the latest incarnation of the moral imbecile to the general public. In the November issue of *The Arena*, Clark contributed an article entitled "The Relation of Imbecility to Pauperism and Crime." From her perspective as an institutional teacher of the feebleminded, Clark told her readers that no imbecile, especially of the "higher grade," could successfully negotiate adult citizenship outside of the confines of the institution. Their moral and intellectual frailty, improved but ultimately unaffected by education, made them prone to poverty and crime. "Of all the streams of evil which flow into the national blood no one is more productive of mischief than that of imbecility." Restricting immigration might be necessary, but it was not sufficient to rid the nation of this breed of dependent criminals. As "either a human parasite or a beast of prey" with no conscience and no ability to avoid wrongdoing, but also not responsible for his own fate, the moral imbecile had best be confined in public facility for her own protection (Clark 1894, 788–792).

Low Grades, Epileptics, and the Cottage Plan

Moral imbeciles, fallen "girls," epileptics, low-grade idiots—all became part of a classification system in which their educability or potential for extrainstitutional productivity was not particularly relevant. By the new century, Martin Barr, Kerlin's successor at the Pennsylvania school, was convinced that he or any well-trained physician could differentiate feebleminded types merely through observation. Thus, Barr claimed, physicians could spot and classify types of feeblemindedness in the same way they could identify types of pox or types of insanity (Elks 2004). Nevertheless, discriminations based on ability were made more often than not to accommodate the needs of the institution. Thus, "high" grades were likely to be classified as such because of their abilities to perform complex tasks needed in the institution. An inmate who could set type for the institution's printing press, for example, was considered of a higher grade than another who could only plow a row or make a bed.

Institutional classification reflected other changes occurring in the institution— in its goals, its architecture, and its daily operations. For example, New York began to use its institutions to house specific types of classified clientele. Syracuse remained the education facility for higher functioning feeble minds. Newark served fallen or potentially fallen feebleminded women. A strictly custodial facility opened in Rome in 1894, and, at the Shaker community at Sonyea in 1896, the state began an institution for epileptics.

Most states, however, did not follow the New York pattern. By the end of the 1880s, the cottage or colony plan became the dominant structural and operational model of most American institutions. New facilities, although adopting some traditional features such as large tracts of land, segregated facilities for the sick, and physiological education for those who could benefit, discarded the large centralized structures where pupils were housed and educated and where staff living quarters were located. Instead, they were made up of many smaller, separate buildings that reflected the new emphasis on specialization by function, age, sex, and even type of disability. Probably the first cottage plan for feeble minds was Brown's private school at Barre, Massachusetts. As early as 1870, he had separated pupils by educational ability and medical condition, and also by family wealth (Seguin 1870b). In 1878, the Ohio Asylum became the first public facility to experiment with detached cottages for feeble minds (Ohio Asylum 1878, 5).

In this new environment, institutional officials segregated higher functioning inmates from the lower functioning ones. The institutional hospital, which had previously treated only sick residents, expanded care to include many custodial or asylum-grade cases who, not expected "to recover," were treated as perpetually sick. In such a framework, cleanliness, routine, and order easily replaced individual treatment and spontaneity. Although asylum cases were thought to be best cared for in hospital settings where they could be kept clean, fed, and not abused, such intensified custodial care brought new problems (Fernald 1893). Not unexpectedly, custodial care became a more frequent topic at meetings of institutional leaders (e.g., Powell 1887). In 1894, Walter Fernald, superintendent of the Massachusetts facility, now much expanded since the days of Howe, spoke of the need to avoid the bad smells inherent in the care of custodial cases. However, the care of low grades also offered an "educational opportunity" for other inmates. The custodial department provided a setting for the training of higher functioning inmates in caregiving skills. Well-trained higher grades became instrumental in controlling the foul odors about which Fernald and others had written (e.g., G. Knight 1889, 67).

Epileptics were considered another distinct class of clientele. Usually excluded from institutions before the Civil War, epileptics were more routinely added to institutional rolls beginning in the 1870s (Wines 1888, 255). Within the next two decades, many institutions began adding separate facilities for their care. Kerlin opened a building for epileptic males in 1890 and one for females in 1892 (Kerlin 1891b, 1892d). Doren had opened the doors of the Columbus institution to some epileptics after the Civil War, and, in 1889, he requested legislative funds for an "epileptic department" (Doren 1887; Ohio Asylum 1889, 12). Even Hervey Wilbur acknowledged keeping "four or five epileptics" from the earliest years of the New York school (New York Asylum for Idiots 1874, "Note" [no page number after page 16]). In 1887, A. E. Osborne of the California Home for the Care and Training of Feeble-Minded Children received state funding for a separate cottage for seventy-five epileptics. By the early 1890s, Michigan, Minnesota, and Maryland had begun making provisions for the care of epileptics within their institutions; by 1900, Nebraska, Kansas, Iowa, and Wisconsin had also opened separate cottages (Letchworth 1894, 1900; Powell 1900).

Epilepsy had always created an institutional as well as a medical problem for the superintendents (what constituted an epileptic condition itself was not well-defined). A large number (some suspected a majority) of feebleminded inmates suffered from epileptic seizures, although with widely varying frequency and intensity.

Some seizures had clear neurological origins, but others appeared to be associated with various forms of lunacy. Intelligent people also had seizures (although there was some debate over whether their seizures were "real"). Some individuals seemed to become feebleminded as a result of their seizures (Barr 1904*a*, 21–27, 309–313).

The newfound willingness of superintendents to deal with epileptics came about not only from the general expansion of services to different grades of feeble minds but also because of advances in the medical understanding of epilepsy. By the 1880s, autopsies had associated brain lesions with epilepsy, and some epileptics benefited from bromide (W. Wilson 1892). Mysteries remained; yet, in their ability to control epilepsy, superintendents added to their institutional authority and professional legitimacy. A. W. Wilmarth, colleague of Kerlin and later the superintendent of the Wisconsin Home for the Feeble-Minded, advocated the segregation of epileptics who, past puberty, had shown no improvement because they were apt to cause seizures in other inmates. Wilmarth, like most of his colleagues, believed that feebleminded people were susceptible to epilepsy by their mere association with confirmed epileptics. He also advised that epileptics should not be overworked or fed "nuts, unripe fruit, and abominations" (Wilmarth 1892). Osborne of California, however, thought work was beneficial to epileptics. "We are forcing the epileptic boys," he told the Association of Medical Officers, "to [do] this out-door work in fruit harvest with first-class moral as well as medical results. They take an interest in the work, do it quite well, and have fewer spasms while thus engaged" (Osborne 1892, 368–369).[11]

All this specialization—for moral imbeciles, wayward females, low grades, and epileptics, among others—was dependent on the cottage or colony system. Most superintendents, however, acknowledged that the colony system developed as a result of the great debate in the postwar period over how to cope with the growing number of chronically insane. Thomas Kirkbride's *On the Construction, Organization, and General Arrangements of Hospitals for the Insane*, published in 1854, had been the bible of asylum construction in the United States. Before 1880, Kirkbride's suggestions had influenced all American idiot institutions. Emphasizing a large central structure with winged corridors connecting several wards, the Kirkbride arrangement called for private and spacious rooms for patients, with small day-rooms and other wards for around twenty-five residents, and total patient capacity of no more than two hundred and fifty. All patients, officials assumed, were newly insane, hence not chronically disabled and thus unlikely to be poor or working class. Indeed, in most of the ensuing debate, all parties, despite their differences, agreed that chronic insanity was highly related to membership in the lower classes (Dowling and Towlinson 1974; T. Kirkbride 1854).

As the debate intensified in the 1870s and 1880s, the Kirkbride, or congregate, model became increasingly unpopular. It was becoming unworkable as the demand burgeoned for admissions of chronically disabled people. Pressure from poorhouses, jails, families, and employers, who saw their able workers caring for chronically disabled family members, led to a rethinking of the costly, cure-oriented older model. Would it not be better, the reasoning went, to house chronic patients at lower per capita costs?

New York was the first state to attempt to reduce patient costs. In 1865, it adopted what became known as the Willard plan, which called for separate facilities for chronic cases, to deal with the rapid increase in the chronically insane population in the state's poorhouses after the war. By emphasizing that the facilities were *asylums* and not true hospitals, proponents of the plan argued that more inmates could be accommodated in less expensive structures. After all, they reasoned, chronic and usually indigent cases needed care, not treatment. Not surprisingly, hospital superintendents were quick to object. They claimed quite vigorously that the proposed facilities would only commit custodial inmates to public indifference and bureaucratic neglect. Although the Willard plan had strong support, only four institutions were ever built following its model (Illinois Board of State Commissioners 1885, 71–80).

As Frederick Wines acknowledged in 1883, the debate, which had continued to rage into the late 1860s and the next decade, was essentially over money (Illinois Board of State Commissioners 1885, 77). Faced with growing demands for the care of large groups of unproductive citizenry, state legislators in the midst of economic downturns were receptive to calls for cheaper facilities that could house more inmates who were also increasingly from the lower classes.[12]

Throughout the 1870s and into the 1880s, the debate between the older generation of hospital alienists and the younger progressives continued, with the latter winning over social welfare reformers and philanthropists first and state legislators next. Some of the older generation came over, but most maintained control of the professional apparatus until, one by one, they died off in the 1880s. It was in this period, too, that Hervey Wilbur began his attacks on the Kirkbride model and on the alienists' exclusive claim to dictate treatment for the insane (H. Wilbur 1872, 1877).

In the midst of these professional debates, the Illinois General Assembly in January 1878, under Frederick Wines's prodding, enacted legislation leading to the first American institution for the chronically insane based entirely on the colony plan. Constructed as a facility with several two-storied buildings, with multibed dormitories on the second floor and a large dayroom on the first, the Kankakee model attracted reformers looking for a way to secure large numbers of people more cheaply (Figure 3.7, Figure 3.8). Wines estimated that the Kankakee system could be constructed at one-half the cost of the traditional Kirkbride hospital and operated with inmate labor at perhaps even less than one-half the cost. Higher functioning chronic inmates in the cottages were assumed to have free time—which in a hospital would have been absorbed in their own treatment—to provide care to the even more disabled. With proper administration and the use of labor-saving devices like the telephone, the superintendent in a large colony-planned institution could govern with no less care than his hospital counterpart. Although acknowledging the impersonal nature of institutions like Kankakee, where the inmate population might well reach one thousand, Wines saw the alternative of the almshouse or jail as a greater evil (Illinois Board of State Commissioners 1885, 65–92).

It would take another decade to put the colony system on the agenda of superintendents of institutions for feeble minds. Some, like J. C. Carson in New York,

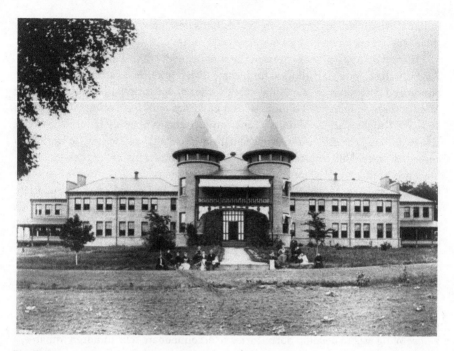

Figure 3.7:
Custodial building of the Illinois Asylum for Feeble-Minded Children at Lincoln, ca. 1885. (Courtesy of Southern Illinois University at Edwardsville, Lovejoy Library, Beverly Farm Records)

preferred the Willard plan; however, most, like A. C. Rogers and William B. Fish, successor in 1883 to Charles Wilbur, adopted some variation of the Kankakee model (Carson 1891*b*; Fish 1892; A. Rogers 1891*b*). Even Kerlin, whose original board of directors had included Kirkbride, began to adapt to the new model. In California,

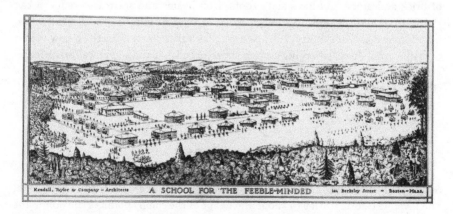

Figure 3.8:
Wrentham School for the Feeble-Minded in Massachusetts. (From the Proceedings of the American Association for the Study of the Feeble-Minded, 1924)

Indiana, Wisconsin, and Michigan, institutions developed in the 1880s and 1890s that were not encumbered by a large central edifice.

Fish and George Knight expressed the superintendents' enthusiasm for colonies. For Fish, the colony plan allowed for inmate differentiation: a "school; . . . separate buildings for the care of custodial cases . . . [and] epileptics; a hospital for acute cases of disease; industrial buildings; and buildings for a farm colony" (Fish 1892, 163). For Knight, the use of higher functioning inmates not only reduced costs but also eliminated the difficult task of securing and keeping staff willing to work with custodial cases. This unpleasant task, Knight reminded his colleagues, was willingly accepted by well-placed high grades: "none make tenderer care-takers, nor under supervision, more watchful ones. . . . The bright imbecile finds occupation, amusement, training, happiness, safety, both for himself and others, inside this usually to him happiest home he has ever known. . . . This is why the colony plan commends itself to us as superintendents" (G. Knight 1892, 159–160; see also L. Carlson 2001).

In 1889, the trustees of the Indiana State School for Feeble-Minded Children hired J. F. Wing of the Fort Wayne architectural firm Wing and Mahurin to design plans for the state's first facility for feeble minds. With the exterior of the administration building completed and with a state appropriation of $185,000, the task before Wing was to develop dormitories to accommodate four hundred inmates, a hospital, a chapel, a kitchen, a cold-storage building, a boiler room, a barn, and the interior of the administration building. After visiting the Ohio institution, where he received advice from Gustavus Doren, Wing decided on a plan that combined the overall institutional layout of the older Kirkbride model with living quarters based on the newer colony model. Thus, at the institution's center, facing south was a large administration building not unlike the type found at the Pennsylvania School, the Illinois and Ohio asylums, and at most other residential facilities of the period. Wing then added a two-storied L-shaped dormitory to both the east and west facades of the administration building. The hospital, chapel, kitchen, and so forth were in separate buildings. All the buildings were to be constructed of brick and stone and have slate roofs. Iron beams and staircases reduced the risk of fires, and tile floors in the halls and bathrooms reflected a concern for low maintenance and durability. Thus, Wing's plan for Indiana reflected a new vision of feeblemindedness emerging among superintendents and social welfare reformers, one of care and control based on differentiation, efficiency, and permanence (Doren Manuscripts, letter and drawing from J. F. Wing to G. A. Doren, March 18, 1889, box 5, folder 4).

CONCLUSION

Superintendents in the 1890s joined their associates in the state hospitals, prisons, and juvenile reformatories to adopt and adapt to the colony plan. As the dominant model for growing and specialized facilities, the colony system launched the field into a new century with a new vision of education and training, productivity, and control. Virtually all superintendents embraced the cottage system with its cottages housing different functional grades, sexes, and medical conditions. There were few detractors.

In 1893, Walter Fernald (1893), the young superintendent of the Massachusetts school, addressed the National Conference of Charities and Correction on the history of the care of the feebleminded. It was one of several summary addresses celebrating the twentieth anniversary of the conference. The depression of 1893 had not yet begun, and the conference approached its anniversary and recognized its growing prominence with confidence. Fernald's history, which became a much-quoted document over the next two decades, established an important myth about feeblemindedness, one that has been sustained even to the present.[13]

According to Fernald, institutions for feebleminded people began as experimental schools whose purpose was education. Having proved that feeble minds could be educated, these schools became permanent public facilities. As time went on, Fernald argued, early reformers began to see that they had expected too much from their pupils and had promised too much to anxious parents and public officials. To be sure, most feebleminded children could learn, but hardly enough to get along in the world. As adults, they could not learn to master the subtle complexities of nineteenth-century American life. Quickly seeing their errors, institutional officials began to envision a more realistic mission for their facilities: the protection of vulnerable people from a world that would take advantage of them and exploit their propensity for wrongdoing and vice.

As such, Fernald implied, superintendents had become victims not only of their own early optimism but also of a growing public demand to use state asylums to relieve communities of the burden of unprotected and vulnerable feeble minds. What Fernald failed to acknowledge (what as a participant he perhaps could not fully envision) was the participation of superintendents in these changes. No doubt, superintendents were hardly in control of factors that had placed new demands on state institutions. Yet to claim as he did that superintendents shifted their vision of the care of feebleminded people from the *school* to the *asylum* because of their doubts about the efficacy of education is to miss their reconstruction of the meaning of education. The asylum, like the school, continued to educate feeble minds. Seguin's methods and philosophy were followed well into the twentieth century.

What changed in the 1870s and 1880s had its origins, albeit faint origins, in the 1850s and 1860s. Faced with educated "simple" idiots who could not find jobs and multiply disabled idiots who were burdens to their families and communities, superintendents saw the potential of using the one to care for the other while also widening their own professional purview. Although they hardly controlled the events that precipitated the rapid growth of their facilities, they hardly responded to them as passive victims, burdened by new policies imposed on them by state officials. By the 1880s, the message they presented to state officials and social welfare authorities was one that made their institutions and their place in the institution increasingly indispensable.

Led by Kerlin and followed by a younger generation of superintendents like Fish, Rogers, Wilmarth, and Fernald was a group of medical men who saw in the public institution a place to establish and enlarge their personal and professional legitimacy. To be sure, some, like Fish in Illinois, would not survive state politics. Most, however, became quite successful in the politics of survival, exerting their influence on state legislatures and state executives and solidifying their nearly singular control over the operation of their institutions. As we shall see in Chapter 4, in spite of scandals and internal discord, superintendents found ways of expanding their influence and authority.

NOTES

1. On the topic of institutional visiting by the interested public in the nineteenth century, see Miron (2011). Miron recounts the common experience of visitors to asylums, prisons, and schools to observe the good work and accomplishments of the institutions. While touring the facility, they might buy an institutional souvenir, like a decorated teacup or plate, or, by the last decade of the century, a postcard.

2. In January 1868, at the newly opened Illinois Asylum, then in Jacksonville and a part of the State School for the Deaf and Dumb, Charles Wilbur wrote letters to New England acquaintances and Ohio Civil War friends asking them for money for books, journals, and school supplies. The legislature had appropriated $4,000 less than Wilbur thought was needed and had anticipated (Wilbur, 1865–80).

3. Occasionally, even former inmates acknowledged their own success. In 1884, Scott Strump, a former inmate at the Ohio institution, wrote G. A. Doren. At the time, Strump was living and working in Atlanta. "I am here doing business for this firm as foreman. I am married and settled down to a nice young lady of eighteen and have one nice little girl. I married well off. This is my second time, my first wife is dead" (Doren Manuscripts, letter from Scott Strump to J. D. Doorne [sic], February 20, 1884, box 3, folder 4).

4. In 1874, Wilbur visited British and continental insane asylums for the New York State Board of Charities. Attacking John Gray, the Utica superintendent who had always gotten bigger legislative allocations for the state lunatic asylum than Wilbur had for the idiot school, Wilbur criticized the American propensity for "extravagant, ornamental and palatial" asylums (McGovern 1985, 156; H. Wilbur 1876, 1877). The conference became an important forum over the next decade for this criticism of insane asylums. Oddly enough, Wilbur's interest in feeblemindedness went almost unmentioned in the proceedings of the conference during its earliest years. Other superintendents, too, showed little interest. In 1877, Wilbur was the only superintendent present at the annual meeting in Saratoga Springs. Not until 1880 was a committee on "imbecility and idiocy" formed at the conference's annual meeting held that year in Cleveland. Patterson, now the superintendent of the workhouse, home of refuge and correction in Cleveland, attended, but Doren of the idiot asylum was not present. At the 1881 meeting in Boston, "a report from the Committee on Idiocy and Imbecility was read by Dr. H. B. Wilbur of New York, but [was] withheld from publication" (National Conference of Charities and Correction 1881, xxxvi–xxxvii). Attending this meeting along with Wilbur were Doren and George Tarbell, Howe's successor at the idiot school in Massachusetts. In 1883, Wilbur died and the conference paid its respects. Although recognizing his abilities with even the most

disabled idiot, the conference eulogizers remembered Wilbur more for his work on insanity than for his work on feeblemindedness (National Conference of Charities and Correction 1884, xxx–xxxii).

5. Over its history, the committee had several names, sometimes changing annually.

6. For example, Wilbur wrote of degenerative heredity: "A majority may be classed as the result of hereditary neuroses in one or both families. That is to say, there may have been in the ancestral line insanity or idiocy, or some of the protean forms in which disease of the nervous system manifests itself. Not necessarily in the immediate progenitors, for physical traits, whether normal or abnormal, sometimes skip a generation or two, to appear again in remoter descendants" (New York Asylum for Idiots 1875; see also Sarason and Doris 1969, 214–218).

7. As E. Carlson (1980) has argued, *The Jukes* began to be misinterpreted even in Dugdale's *New York Times* (1883) obituary (also see Shepard 1884). Hahn (1980) claimed correctly that Dugdale began a long tradition of "cacogenic family studies" emphasizing a degenerative view of heredity. She fails, however, to note and explore Dugdale's faith in the ability of reformers to change the promiscuous female she so carefully depicts.

8. Nicole Rafter [Nicholas Hahn] (1992*a*), in this article sees Lowell's campaign to segregate feebleminded women as an early example of eugenics. My sense is that economic hard times more than proto-eugenics precipitated Lowell's activities at Newark, though the two, to be sure, reinforced each other.

9. Looking back on the time, Franklin Sanborn, whose philanthropic activities stretched back to his (and his mentor, Samuel G. Howe's) "Secret Six" support of John Brown, in 1881 reminded the conference in his presidential address:

Within the past three years we have seen our country recover from a severe and long-continued financial depression, during which many thousand working men and working women were thrown out of employment, and consequently became more or less dependent on charity for their support. This led to the formation of a large army of vagrants, who moved from place to place, sometimes in search of work, quite often from the mere restlessness and shiftlessness which enforced idleness produces, and then, in many instances, because the vagrant life was found to be a good disguise for various modes of depredation. Against an evil so great many measures were taken, and some laws were passed. (Sanborn 1881, 15)

10. Writing a decade after Kerlin's death, Martin Barr, his successor at the Pennsylvania Training School (by Barr's time, also called Elwyn Institute), noted Kerlin's tenacity:

The recognition of the moral imbecile, and the absolute necessity of a life-long guardianship, protection against temptation, and all the horrors of criminal procedure of which he must be but the innocent victim, were long and strenuously insisted upon by Dr. Kerlin in the name of science, of sociology, as a matter of political economy, of the protection of homes, and all that man holds dear. Through the press, on the platform, in his official reports as in private conversation, he did not cease to press home this truth, that a truly healthful status of the action depends upon eliminating from its arteries this most pernicious element and to point out this the only feasible plan; the gathering of these unfortunates into homes under the care of specialists, where trained to habits of self-support, protected from the world and the world from them, they might live out their brief day, unharmed by ignominy and the thousand ills the world would bring. (Barr 1904*a*, 68)

11. It would not be until 1912, with the introduction of phenobarbital, that physicians would successfully treat many cases of epilepsy and that superintendents would begin to rethink their pessimistic warnings about the condition (McGrew 1985).

12. Between February 1888 and December 1889, for example, the application form of the Illinois Asylum asked, "Are the parents able to furnish the child with clothing and pay expenses of transportation?" Of the 100 applications, 52 were able to meet these expenses, 40 were not, and 8 did not report (Illinois Asylum for Feeble-Minded Children 1865–1906, Applications 2101-2200; see also table 1).

13. On this myth, see Chapter 1, note 7.

CHAPTER 4

⌀⌿⌀

Living and Working in the Institution, 1890–1920

"If I live until a week from to-day (the 18th of May), I shall be 74 years of age," Charles T. Wilbur wrote William H. C. Smith, superintendent of Beverly Farm, a private facility near Alton, Illinois, in 1909. For nearly twenty years, Wilbur, the only living founder of the Association of Medical Officers of American Institutions for Idiotic and Feeble-Minded Persons and the first superintendent of the Illinois Asylum for Feeble-Minded Children, had operated the Wilbur Home and School, a private facility for "backward and mentally defective children and persons" in Kalamazoo, Michigan. Not participating in association activities after "some personal feelings between himself and his [Illinois Asylum] successor" at the 1884 meeting, Wilbur had recently renewed contact with the Association for the Study of the Feeble-Minded, the name since 1906 of the former Association of Medical Officers, and he planned to attend the 1910 meeting scheduled to be held at Lincoln (Figure 4.1).

The year was not a good one for the Illinois Asylum. Scandals and a rancorous state investigation left the young superintendent, Harry G. Hardt, in need of professional and moral support. Wilbur, who had witnessed seven different superintendents since his own departure from the Lincoln school in 1883, died in 1910, leaving his wife to attend the meeting that year as the last representative of the old era. Joining her were several second-generation stalwarts, A. W. Wilmarth of Wisconsin, A. C. Rogers of Minnesota, and Smith from Illinois, and some rising stars: E. R. Johnstone and Henry H. Goddard of New Jersey, George Mogridge of Iowa, J. K. Kutnewsky of South Dakota, and the association's president that year, Mattie Gundry of Virginia. All were present at least in part to support Hardt in what he believed had been an unfair and politically motivated state investigation. Several others, however, whose participation could usually be counted on, did not

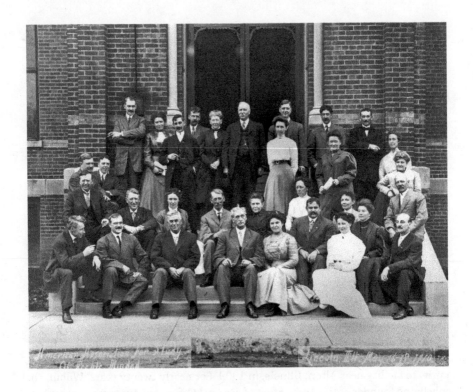

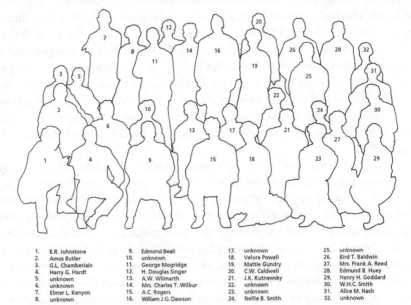

1.	E.R. Johnstone	9.	Edmond Beall	17.	unknown	25.	unknown
2.	Amos Butler	10.	unknown	18.	Velura Powell	26.	Bird T. Baldwin
3.	G.L. Chamberlain	11.	George Mogridge	19.	Mattie Gundry	27.	Mrs. Frank A. Reed
4.	Harry G. Hardt	12.	H. Douglas Singer	20.	C.W. Caldwell	28.	Edmund B. Huey
5.	unknown	13.	A.W. Wilmarth	21.	J.K. Kutnewsky	29.	Henry H. Goddard
6.	unknown	14.	Mrs. Charles T. Wilbur	22.	unknown	30.	W.H.C. Smith
7.	Elmer L. Kenyon	15.	A.C. Rogers	23.	unknown	31.	Alice M. Nash
8.	unknown	16.	William J.G. Dawson	24.	Nellie B. Smith	32.	unknown

Figure 4.1:
Participants at the annual meeting of the American Association for the Study of the Feeble-Minded, 1910. (Courtesy Southern Illinois University at Edwardsville, Lovejoy Library, Beverly Farm Records)

attend the meeting at Lincoln, preferring to avoid any taint of scandal (A. Rogers 1911; "Wilbur, Charles Toppan" 1900).

Wilbur's letter to Smith continued:

> The ideas concerning the aims and objects for the institutions for the Feeble minded are very different from what they formerly were. The whole aim of society is now to drive them into Colonies with very little effort as to their mental development.
>
> ... The developing or ennobling influences of the Public Institution with the inmates kept in large classes of their own kind or worse are not for their good. My views are decidedly changed since I learn that Society only desires to get rid of them and be protected from them when the older ideas were to uplift them by every means that could be used. Now when thus congregated in Droves like cattle it is about as much as we can accomplish to keep them comfortable and fed and clothed after a fashion, but without the affectionate influences most children get at homes. Shut up by themselves the large Asylum is no better than the County Poor house and in my judgement not as good for in the County Poor house they do get association with brighter individuals than themselves. With a large majority of the inmates Custodial cases I see [they] are now trying to take out the name of Asylum and substitute School. So with Insane Asylums which are very slightly curative in their influence but almost entirely custodial.

He concluded:

> Very few insane are cured or Feeble minded benefitted by the institutions, not because it is not possible but by the way they are managed by the Public. God help the Defectives of the land as man is failing to make much effort. (Beverly Farm Records, letter from Charles Wilbur to W. H. C. Smith, May 11, 1909)

Nearly forty years earlier, in 1870, Wilbur (1865–80, vol. 1, 172) had written all the important medical men in the field—Howe, Brown, Seguin, Knight, Kerlin, Doren—urging them to "note down briefly all the arguments" for "the direct and indirect usefulness and influence of idiot asylums upon the community." He would cite their opinions, he told the senior superintendents "in establishing our institution upon a permanent basis." Seven years later, he urged the Michigan legislature to expand state services to idiots, especially to those needing permanent, custodial care (C. Wilbur 1877). Thus, what Wilbur saw decades later and three months before his death was the maintenance of a cognitive and social construction of intellectual disability that he had helped to create but which had developed in directions he had neither anticipated nor advocated.

By 1910, the colony model had permeated virtually all public institutions for mental defectives. The scandal at Wilbur's beloved asylum in Illinois was the result, among other things, of the widespread acceptance of this model. The differential colony, with its emphasis on controlling various types of mental defectives, had become a place for people with all sorts of problems. By 1915, the population of

the Lincoln school had reached 1,888 inmates, with an annual state appropriation of $289,149. The total inmate population of noncriminal state institutions in
Illinois in 1915 was 20,934, housed in seventeen facilities, compared with 1,061 inmates in three facilities in 1869. Although institutional populations had increased
by 1,500 percent, state appropriations had increased by less than 1,000 percent
(Illinois General Assembly 1908, 144; Illinois State Charities Commission 1912,
68; Parsons 2011; US Department of Commerce 1919).

Such growth was further complicated by an increase in clientele with multiple
problems. In 1911, 16 percent of the population of the Illinois Asylum for Feeble-
Minded Children had epilepsy as a primary diagnosis (Illinois State Charities
Commission 1912, 68). Juvenile delinquents, most admitted as feebleminded but
many of whom superintendents believed were not, were also being added to the
institutions' rolls. These additions would become even more common after 1916,
when Illinois law for the first time allowed judges to commit people to most of the
state institutions. The "simple idiot" so preferred by Seguin and Hervey Wilbur
was becoming the exception rather than the rule in the institutional population,
although their low rate of admission primarily reflected a change in how "simple
idiocy" was defined.

If pressures to admit more and different types of inmates precipitated the growth
of public institutions between 1890 and 1920, schemes for adapting to those pressures through larger institutions and more complex institutional arrangements
marked their internal workings. Although the pressures were real and nearly every
annual report from every institution attested to them, most superintendents had
learned to use pressures to excite moribund legislators and what they believed was
an uninformed public. The task before them was different from the one faced by
the first generation of superintendents. Superintendents at the beginning of the
twentieth century did not have to demonstrate the productivity and educability of
their clientele. Rather, they had to show that their public facilities were orderly and
operated efficiently, without abuse or exploitation, and that they could expand as
demand required without undue burden on the internal consistency of the institution itself or on the taxpayer. Although superintendents had always had managerial and political roles to fulfill in the institution, these roles became increasingly
prominent yet more difficult to accomplish. As managers, superintendents had to
administer organizations that were growing in size and complexity. As politicians,
they had to cajole greater resources from skeptical legislators and unpredictable
governors.

Not unexpectedly, with these new roles came new relationships between the superintendent and the two other principals in the life of the institution: the inmates
and the staff. Because the latter left few written statements about their experiences
in the institution and the former left even fewer, the reconstruction of their experiences becomes inevitably difficult and tentative. The recollections of superintendents and their reports compiled for public audiences stressed the positive features
and accomplishments of the institution. Despite the bias implied in them, their accounts give a grounding for the experiences of the inmates and the staff. Although
the superintendents often omitted the disruptions and controversy that occurred,

they do show the many pleasurable and comforting aspects of daily life in the institution. Balancing their accounts are the reports of the scandals that shook several institutions during the period. Although not without their own hyperbole, these reports offer a critical, if not always unbiased, view of the underside of institutional life. Taken together, the personal recollections, official reports, and the scandals provide a picture of life in the institution.

THE INMATE

By the end of the first decade of the new century, just as many of the so-called boys and girls in public institutions for mental defectives were adults as were children. Many, perhaps most, were inmates who had reached maturity after training at the institution. A new group of adult inmates, however, joined this group. During the 1890s and early 1900s, institutions began to admit more inmates between the ages of fifteen and forty-five. These inmates, usually women of childbearing age and young men more often than not convicted of petty crimes, had not been institutionalized during childhood. Although classified by social welfare authorities and institutional officials as intellectually *slow* and *backward* but not viewed as classically feebleminded, their perceived superior capabilities ensured their less than smooth adjustment to institutional life.

Adjusting this group to institutional life became a growing concern for superintendents (e.g., Johnson 1923, 227; Wilmarth 1902). Newly admitted inmates were especially disruptive to routinized, institutionalized inmates. Most superintendents believed that organized work and play facilitated new inmates' adaptation. Undergirding both activities was the belief of the importance of routine. Routine meant predictable schedules, familiar sources of authority, and appropriate and dependable interpersonal relationships. Superintendents believed, and shared this belief among themselves, that when work and play deviated from prescribed routine, inmate adjustment in the institution was jeopardized. Given that the total institutionalization of mental defectives was an accepted, if not a fully explicit, policy by the end of the period, it is not surprising that superintendents went to great efforts to ensure that new inmates adjusted smoothly to the institution.

All American institutions of the period were in suburban or rural settings. Even at Syracuse and Columbus, where urban growth had begun to impinge upon the institution, the grounds of both facilities were large enough to convey at least a sense of the rural. All institutions had extensive gardens, and most had fully operating farms. In 1897, Walter Fernald, superintendent of the Massachusetts School for the Feeble-Minded, added a farm colony in Balwinville, a village about sixty miles from his Waltham institution and connected to it by a direct railroad line. This farm colony and others founded in the next decade by other institutions provided rural outlets for those institutions that could not acquire additional contiguous land for farming either because of its unavailability or its high cost. These outlets, not unexpectedly, became good places for adult inmates who had not adjusted well to the increasingly crowded institutions (Fernald 1902; A. Rogers 1903).

The rural setting, which had been so much a part of the curative apparatus of many groups served by American social welfare institutions, symbolized the rejection of urban society with its potential for vice, degeneracy, and abnormal behavior. The daily regimes in most institutions were typical of those of early twentieth-century rural life. At the Illinois Asylum, for example, inmates scheduled for work or school were awakened at 5:00 A.M. After washing and dressing, they did light chores around the cottage until 6:15, when breakfast was served in their cottage. For the "bigger boys and girls" at the Illinois Asylum, work began around 7:00 A.M. and continued to 5:00 P.M. with a half-hour rest for a simple lunch. The "younger boys and girls," those under fourteen years and considered "bright," began school around 7:30, with a comparable break for lunch (Illinois General Assembly 1908, 238–241; Johnson 1923, 232).[1]

After school and after work, institutions provided a variety of structured and routine recreation (Figure 4.2). On typical weekday evenings, especially in summer, inmates played baseball, threw horseshoes, or attended to personal needs. In winter, activities included skating, basketball, and playing musical instruments. Supper began around 6:00 P.M., after which inmates were also kept occupied. For example,

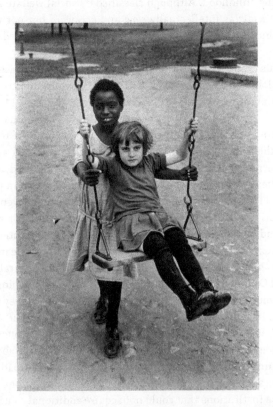

Figure 4.2:
Swinging, 1932. A photograph taken at Letchworth Village, New York, by Margaret Bourke-White. (Courtesy of Syracuse University Library, Special Collections Department, Margaret Bourke-White Papers)

at the Rome asylum in New York inmates might attend a Boy or Girl Scout troop meeting, or "boys" went to a meeting of the Royal Arch Sons of America, whose object was "to encourage good behaviour, stimulate each member to the saving of money and to promote the general welfare of each member and all with whom each and every one of them come in contact" (*Rome Custodial Herald,* August 1, 1916, 5).

The inmates' diet and the preparation of food were two important issues in the institution. A typical "country" breakfast consisted of fried or boiled beef, oatmeal, bread, and coffee. Younger children were given milk. On special occasions, eggs were served. Shortly after Alexander Johnson became superintendent of the Indiana School for the Feeble Minded in 1893, he insisted that inmates get eggs, if not often, at least more often than on Easter Sunday, the only day his predecessor had allowed such a delicacy. Lunches were simple, with soup, in-season vegetables, occasionally meat, and always bread and coffee. Supper consisted of items found in the other two meals of the day, plus an occasional sweet or seasonal fruit. The cost of providing all these meals was, of course, subject to scrutiny. Under the pressures of growing institutional populations, both Johnson in Indiana and Hardt in Illinois claimed the need to reduce the proportions of food given to each inmate (Illinois General Assembly 1908, 935; Johnson 1923, 235).

By 1900, superintendents were purchasing, as they had the resources to do so, modern kitchen equipment. In their professional journals, advertisements for the latest institutional stoves, utensils, and dishwashers were common. In a period when diet was still linked with the cause and prevention of mental defect and conditions associated with mental defect, it was not surprising that superintendents kept a watchful eye on the institution's kitchen. When Harry Hardt's new baker at the Illinois Asylum began to bake doughy bread, staff and later legislators were as concerned that Hardt failed to dismiss the baker as they were that inmates were being abused in other, usually more surreptitious, ways (Illinois General Assembly 1908, 935).

On weekends, most institutions had more extensive activities. Johnson began dances in the Indiana institution's chapel, insisting, however, that the sexes be strictly separated as they were in most other activities. The boys danced with "a detail of the women employees," and the girls danced with each other. Institutional leaders and staff usually planned special events for the holidays, with fireworks at the Fourth of July, pageants at Christmas, and renditions of the "Hallelujah Chorus" at Easter becoming the predictable fare. Hardt's wife reported that even her husband, not otherwise known for his camaraderie, received loud applause for his minstrel-show performance at the Illinois institution's 1909 Christmas program (Beverly Farm Records, letter from Mrs. H. H. Hardt to Dr. and Mrs. W. H. C. Smith, January 10, 1910). By the turn of the century, several institutions had even developed summer camps. Away from the institution for a week, inmates (usually the most capable and mobile and always segregated by sex) picnicked, went to the swimming hole, and did other activities that early twentieth-century American campers were learning and expected to do (Doll [ca. 1976], 15; *Herald,* March 1, 1923, 2; Johnson 1923, 188–191; *Rome Custodial Herald,* May 1, 1914, 6).

Most institutions had bands and orchestras and gave regular concerts open to the public (Figure 4.3). At the turn of the century, the Illinois Asylum boasted a senior band, a juvenile band, an orchestra, and an institutional chorus. Each of these groups practiced daily, including most Sundays (Beverly Farm Records, unsorted clippings, ca. 1880–1920; Hash 2010). In the summer of 1910, J. E. Wallace Wallin (1953) commented on his visit to Elwyn Institute (the new name for the Pennsylvania Training School): "An excellent band concert was presented by the inmates, one of whom had one of the largest hydrocephalic heads I have ever seen." Local townfolk visited the institutions, often on Sunday afternoons in warm weather and on Friday or Saturday evenings in cold weather. Sometimes poetry recitations and readings supplemented the musical concerts (see also Miron 2011).

Most institutional authorities allowed high-grade inmates to go freely about the institution. Wilmarth in Wisconsin noted that his "higher boys [had] free range of the institution grounds" with, of course, the exception of the girls' dormitories (Wilmarth 1902). Planners were so concerned about the possible commingling of the sexes at the newly announced Letchworth Village in New York (which opened in 1910) that they insisted that their (and the nation's most prestigious) landscape architect, Frederick Law Olmsted, use the Minnisceongo Creek running through the site to ensure the separation of males and females (Kirkbride 1909; Little 1912; Olmsted 1937).

The concern that female inmates might become pregnant made their safety a special source of concern for superintendents. Wilmarth acknowledged that they were given less freedom than their male counterparts. While noting that most female

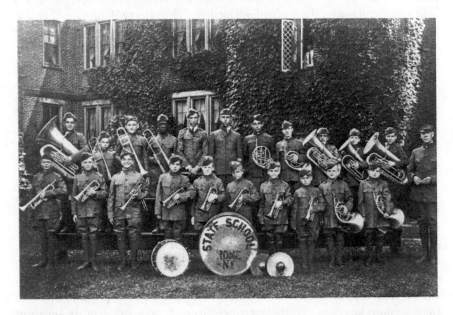

Figure 4.3:
Boys' band at the Rome State School in New York, 1925. (From James C. Riggs's *Hello Doctor: A Brief Biography of Charles Bernstein*, 1936)

imbeciles who "got themselves in trouble" were victims of the depravity of normal (as opposed to feebleminded) men, he took no chances. After all, many were in the institution because they had been, were, or might become pregnant (Wilmarth 1902). Some even brought children with them to the institution; others entered the institution pregnant, had their baby, and raised their child at the facility (e.g., *Herald*, January 1, 1922, 5). When he opened the Harper Cottage for 124 "fallen women" at the Indiana School in 1902, Johnson reminisced, "I dreamed of calling it [i.e., Harper Cottage] 'The Grange' and using as a motto a quotation from Tennyson's Marianna in the Moated Grange, 'He Cometh not, she said.' It was a place where no male comes; where there could be absolute freedom within the sacred enclosure" (Johnson 1923, 229). The institution as a place to rescue women from becoming victims of men's lust and their own "weakness of self-control" and at the same time to protect society from "the next generation of mental defectives" became not only social policy but also part of institutional practice and procedure. To prove that institutions could be havens for such women, superintendents had to ensure the chastity of their female inmates (Kunzel 1995; Odem 1995; Rembis 2011).

Inmate work at the institution was assigned on the basis of both sex and ability. Predictably, males labored on the farm; worked the heavy machinery in the laundry, print shop, or boiler room; and tended to the institution's assortment of animals. Females performed domestic chores, did the sewing and mending and the constantly needed hand laundry. Although higher functioning female inmates provided most of the care for custodial inmates, males also helped with some tasks (Bragar 1977; Johnson 1923, 223–229). Just as they were divided by predictable gender roles, work assignments were arranged according to predictable levels of perceived inmate capabilities; in some inmates, these capabilities appeared to be exceptional. When Martin Barr published his highly respected *Mental Defectives* in 1904, he thanked three "boys" for their help in the preparation of his book. One inmate had taken photographs for the book, another had done translations, and the third had typed the entire manuscript (Barr 1904a, vii). At the Illinois Asylum, Lizzie White, an inmate who entered the institution around 1900, taught music, along with the hired music teachers. They received $250 for ten months of service; she received $25 (Hash 2010).

Some inmates, especially those whom judges under newly enacted authority committed as incorrigibles to institutions for the feebleminded, were given tasks requiring only slightly less responsibility than those of regular employees. For example, Asa Carlin had been an inmate at the Illinois Asylum for eight years, placed there with his brother and sister after the death of their father. Carlin attended the institution's school and later worked as an inmate laborer. A bit rough and from a working-class background, he was nevertheless not stupid. Around 1905, after he had spent some time away from the institution, officials hired him back as an attendant at the Lincoln asylum to work with lower functioning clients. A few years later, he was fired and testified about his firing before an Illinois House Committee investigating the institution. His dismissal was not due to incompetence or cruelty to inmates, however, but rather to his objections to Superintendent Hardt's method of punishing his brother, also an inmate at the Lincoln school, by taking money from him (Illinois General Assembly 1908, 238–264). Obviously, Carlin's previous inmate status did not preclude his later employee status.

Another inmate at Lincoln, Walter Kaak, was one of the "bright boys" as he identified himself. At fourteen years and out of the institution's school program, Kaak was assigned to the laundry, where he ran the large electrical spinners that dried the large daily loads of clothing and bedding necessary at the institution. Kaak carried out functions indistinguishable from the hired help working alongside him. After a spinner shredded his left arm one afternoon in August 1907, lawmakers investigating the incident could not complain as much as they might have since they knew too well that inmate labor like Kaak's kept down institutional costs (Illinois General Assembly 1908, 238–241, 263).

A third inmate at Lincoln around the same time was Henry Darger. After the death of his mother, Darger's father, an infrequently employed and hard-drinking immigrant, placed him in a Chicago Catholic orphanage, but the placement did not work out. So, in 1904, social welfare authorities sent him to the Lincoln asylum where, like many other Illinoisan whose so-called feeblemindedness was the outcome of poverty, abandonment, and misbehavior, he would find himself abandoned and alone. As one of the "high grades" at the institution, then housing over 1,200 inmates, Darger received education in reading, writing, and cyphering, but spent most of his time working at one of the asylum's extensive farms. In his autobiography, Darger remembered the asylum as a place of camaraderie among his fellow early-teenage cottage mates, but also as a place of violence and strict discipline. He recalled with delight the boys sliding down the dormitory fire escape; yet, he also remembered the eruption of fights between staff members and among the inmates. He noted the practice used by the asylum authorities of giving an older adolescent inmate the power over groups of younger adolescents. From 1906 to 1908, Darger lived full-time on one of the asylum's farm, where through the summer and fall he worked ten hours a day for six days each week. Looking back fifty years later, Darger assessed his own intellectual ability, "I knew more than the whole shebang at that place" (Darger ca. 1960 [2014], 287–289). After several attempts to escape, Darger in 1908 ran away from Lincoln. He claimed to have walked the 170 miles between Lincoln and his godmother's home in North Chicago. Soon he found employment as a janitor at a Chicago Catholic hospital, where he would work until his retirement in 1963 (Biesenbach 2014; Darger ca. 1960 [2014], 288; M. Trent 2012; see also Chapter 8).

At most of the turn-of-the-century facilities, lower functioning male inmates also did simple but necessary tasks. Strong low-grade imbeciles, superintendents believed, were especially suited for construction. It was not uncommon to use them on new buildings that were being erected with some frequency during the period. The Massachusetts school employed inmate labor in the initial construction of its Waltham facility and continued their use into the new century (Fernald 1902). At the California Home for the Care and Training of Feeble-Minded Children relocated to Glen Ellen, inmates helped build several cottages (S. Cooper 1896). Other lower functioning inmates worked in the various institutional shops, fixing furniture, resoling shoes, doing minor building and roofing repairs, or cutting wood, or they attended to the institution's grounds. Lower functioning female inmates helped with the mending and hand laundry. These inmates performed much of the day-to-day work necessary for the maintenance of the institution.

The most common inmate activity, apart from work on the farm, was the care of custodial cases and small children. Basic to the cottage plan, this care allowed institutions to admit groups of mental defectives that in preceding decades had usually been excluded. At the Indiana School, the low-grade imbeciles and idiots were housed in Sunset Cottage. Segregated from other inmates, those with multiple and usually crippling conditions spent the day in bed while ambulatory cases stayed in the cottage dayroom. "Sunset Sisters," higher functioning female inmates, were assigned the care of one or more of these low-grade inmates. Seven days a week, every day of the year, the Sisters fed, changed, bathed, and attended to them. Not unexpectedly, many of them formed close attachments:

> Most appealing of all the touching sights in an institution, is to see the tenderness and patience exercised by a big over grown man-baby or woman-baby, towards a tiny child child-baby when put in their care. The maternal instinct is almost always present, and is often as strong in the males as in the females; fortunately for them and for us it is much stronger than the sex instinct. Here is a place which the imbecile can fill often as well as and certainly more willingly than a hired helper. (Johnson 1923, 224)

From the perspective of superintendents like Johnson, the care provided by high-grade feeble minds solved two perennial problems faced by most institutions: employee costs and employee retention. Inmate labor, of course, kept per capita inmate costs low. Fernald, Hardt, Johnson, and others boasted that their annual per capita costs were much lower than those of previous decades and of most other institutions in their respective states. None doubted that inmate caregivers made more inmate caregiving possible. One dependable hired employee could then supervise several inmate laborers. Also, inmate caregivers solved the problem of employee turnover. Superintendents complained of difficulties in retaining employees, claiming that many did not care for the long hours and the unpleasant monotony of caring for inmates whose conditions appeared to be unimprovable and who sometimes showed little concern or appreciation for their care. Others were unmarried young women and men whose greater concern, superintendents complained, was finding a mate. Higher functioning inmates, in contrast, not only tolerated the monotony and unpleasantries but, indeed, seemed to thrive on them:

> The Idio-Imbecile, but one removed from his weaker brother, to whose wants he may be trained to minister, finds here his fitting place, and the domestic service of these asylums may be largely drawn from this class, as also from that of his low-grade imbecile. Working as an aid, never alone, always under direction, he finds in a monotonous round of the simplest daily avocations his life happiness, his only safety from lapsing idiocy, and therefore his true home. (Barr 1904*a*, 137)

The institutional farm was the pride of several superintendents and where operated efficiently proved a source of savings and, in a few cases, income for the institution. But their benefits were more than just financial. According to Fernald, the farm colony at Balwinville provided an outlet for restless boys who had reached their classroom potential. Inmates there, often newly admitted to the institution as teenagers and young adults, were free, Fernald believed, to be themselves. Hard work and fresh air made them well-behaved and freed them from the sicknesses that disrupted institutional life. They were given a purpose suited to their abilities and temperament. Idleness and consequent bad behavior were unheard of. "They are very glad to go to bed at the end of a hard day's work," commented Fernald (1907). "Boys [who] have worked in the field all day require no night watchman. They go to bed and sleep. An attendant sleeps in an adjoining room, but we have little anxiety about the boys during the night. There are no locks on the doors, and the boys go and come as they please. We have had very few runaways from a class notorious for running away."

On the farm, inmates planted and tended the fields. Usually laid out for garden rather than cash crops, the farms became an important source of produce for the institution. As they purchased or rented more acreage, most institutions added cows and sometimes beef cattle to the farm. At the Illinois Asylum, institutional authorities even experimented with a herd of sheep. The sheep, state officials boasted, provided work for "boys of the school" and lamb for institutions throughout Illinois at "practically no expense for food or care" ("Lincoln State School and Colony" 1913, 129). Johnson at Indiana was especially proud of his superior breed of cattle, saving prize-winning bulls and cows for breeding and state fair contests and relegating inferior animals to the institution's tables. Other superintendents also encouraged inmates to work with farm animals in the belief that the feebleminded were fond of and had a special kinship with animals. Both the inmates and the animals seemed to thrive on the mutual affection they shared. In addition, animals, unlike crops, required the year-long attention of the inmates, thereby keeping them busy in the colder months of the year (Fernald 1902; Hornick 2012, 27–28, 49–53; Johnson 1923, 210–221).

By the beginning of the new century, several superintendents had negotiated working relationships with state agricultural colleges. Bernstein in New York, Johnstone in New Jersey, and Johnson in Indiana worked with their respective state colleges and agricultural authorities to test new crops and farming techniques and conduct experiments in animal breeding. The growing interest in heredity generated at the time was focused not only on inmates but also on the institutional farm (Johnson 1923, 211; "The Training School at Vineland" [ca. 1963]; Walsh and McCallion 1988, 2, 69–71).

The success of farm colonies was the result not only of their productivity but also of the relief they provided to growing and increasingly overcrowded institutions. Bernstein, who championed and extended the farm colony more than any other superintendent, frankly acknowledged: "As there is not enough beds to go round [the institution], and so many are sleeping on pads on the floor, any one who can make good in a colony should be in a colony, and not occupying a bed here" (*Herald*, November 1, 1925, 8).

By 1910, most institutions had farm colonies either contiguous to the main facilities or at some distance from them. Demonstrating the colonies' success, most institutions persuaded legislators to allow them to buy or rent additional farms. With farmland opening up because of urban migration, superintendents reclaimed land at bargain prices, with the hearty approval of public officials (Fernald 1907). Most institutions continued to acquire land until the Great Depression. By 1920, the colony farms had become an important linkage with another new trend, the parole system (discussed in Chapter 6). Important in the expansion of the institution and eventually in its extrainstitutional activities, the farm remained a source of pleasure and pride for superintendents in what were becoming increasingly bureaucratized facilities.

Work and play, issues of increasing concern in turn-of-the-century institutions, did not preclude an interest in education, the original, albeit now less crucial, focus of institutions. No longer the central function of growing facilities, the school continued, nevertheless, to be a feature of them.[2] Most institutions began to model their classroom and administrative structures after the public schools, ironically as those schools were beginning to emphasize vocational and "life-skill" curricula, which the institutional schools had stressed from the beginning. A teacher headed each classroom, and a principal, lead teacher, or school superintendent had administrative authority over the school. Most institutions had gymnasiums, and most had facilities for arts and crafts and vocational training. Specific vocational training began for inmates around their fourteenth year, although by 1920 most institutions had begun prevocational education for inmates even as young as five.

By 1900, most teachers either had normal-school degrees or had undergone apprenticeships, usually at the institution where they were teaching. Not infrequently, young women, and occasionally young men, began their teaching careers at the institution and remained there for a lifetime (Hornick 2012, 50–51). Marriage, a change in the administration of the institution, or the desire for a promotion might result in a resignation and possibly a search for a new position.

By the end of the nineteenth century, interinstitutional communication about job openings was common. Superintendents with junior teachers occasionally solicited senior positions for them in other institutions. If a teacher who had experience or training at another institution applied for a position, recommendations, often quite frank, were requested and given (e.g., Beverly Farm Records, letter from George Mogridge to W. H. C. Smith, March 23, 1917; Doren Manuscripts, letter from A. C. Rogers to Gustavus A. Doren, April 4, 1886, box 4, folder 5). When the staff of one institution visited another facility, it was customary for them to call on former employees (e.g., *Rome Custodial Herald*, July 1, 1914, 4). The network of superintendents, always strengthened by annual meetings of the American Association for the Study of the Feeble-Minded, provided an *invisible college* for the maintenance of a core of teachers in the institutions and, as I note in Chapter 5, for the establishment and maintenance of the field of special education.

Usually, teachers lived at the institution, often in small apartments in the same building as the school. Most, too, were engaged in extracurricular duties at the institution. Mary Douglass at the Rome asylum edited the institution's monthly newspaper. Nellie Blake taught during school hours at the Illinois Asylum and supervised a cottage during the evening. Other teachers helped with Sunday church services, writing and rehearsing Christmas plays, summer camps, summer courses for public school teachers, and the care of inmates during institutional epidemics. Usually from middle-class backgrounds, the teachers were almost always higher in the institutional hierarchy than either the attendant staff or the maintenance crew. At the Indiana School, they ate in a separate cafeteria (until Johnson stopped the practice). Usually, they had the authority (or sometimes they took the authority) to give orders to the attendants. If they married, as did Harriet Dix at the Pennsylvania Training School; Nellie Blake at the Illinois Asylum; Mary T. Douglass at the Rome, New York, asylum; and Alice Morrison at the Training School at Vineland, New Jersey, it was often to a physician or educator, not to an attendant or mainte- nance worker. With the advent of psychometric testing after 1910, some teachers began to shift their interests to psychology and social work and, as a result, began to identify with those professions (e.g., Beverly Farm Records, letter from Elizabeth Ross Shaw to W. H. C. Smith, January 18, 1911).

Typical institutional classrooms accommodated from ten to forty pupils. Most combined an ungraded structure with some attempt to divide students by age. Thus, pupils of dissimilar ages were apt to be together in a particular classroom, but preadolescents were not likely to be found with five-, six-, or seven-year-olds, for whom institutions began developing kindergartens. Seguin's physiological methods, especially those emphasizing preacademic learning, were used with the younger children.

Drawing on but modifying Seguin's system, several schools after 1900 began what they called "habit training." Although Seguin had seen physiological educa- tion moving pupils toward traditional academic skills, especially the three R's, most early twentieth-century educators either opposed the teaching of reading and writing to mental defectives or believed that the value of such education was merely the placating of those parents who insisted on having their chil- dren educated in reading and writing (American Association for the Study of the Feeble-Minded 1913; Johnson 1923, 183–186). Habit training of young children was directed at institutional adaptation, not skills needed on the outside. At the Training School at Vineland, New Jersey, kindergarten classes emphasized skills for institutional socialization—punctuality, obedience to authority, patience, teamwork, and respect for the rights of others. Students learned these skills in traditional settings—gymnastic play and exercises, nature study, musical ac- tivities, and object lessons. At Beverly Farm in Illinois, Superintendent Smith called his facility's educational activities "entirely individual [with] no classes" (Beverly Farm Records, New York State Commission to Investigate Provision for the Mentally Deficient, Questionnaire to Heads of Institutions of All Kinds in New York State and for Mental Defectives in All States, handwritten responses of W. H. C. Smith, December 10, 1914).

By 1920, most institutional schools had begun prevocational and even vocational training for kindergartners. Five-year-olds had several tools in the class toy chest that they were encouraged to handle and use in their play. By the age of six, young inmates were learning how to hammer a nail, punch holes in leather, or wash rags on a miniature washboard. All kindergartners also learned to tend a garden. Given the institutional emphasis on agriculture, planting seeds, weeding, and observing plant growth became an important part of the education of even the youngest children (Doll [ca. 1976] 13).

Older preadolescent children were taught practical life-skills—money recognition and simple reading and writing. Ironically, these practical skills were of little value in most institutions, where lifelong institutionalization was now stressed. At the Pennsylvania Training School, Martin Barr began to expand and refine a teaching method advocated by an earlier generation of superintendents. In the "object lesson," information about community life was conveyed through the use of miniatures. Barr, whose commitment to total, lifelong segregation of mental defectives was unequaled, insisted that feeble minds should have no intercourse with the outside world. His requirement that teachers use object lessons in classroom training added additional irony to life-skill education.

Other educational practices of the time lacked the irony of life-skill training; yet, they were a reflection of how liberal the view of what constituted education had become. At the Rome asylum, institutional officials called chores such as making beds, mopping floors, and changing the diapers of low grades "domestic training" (Douglass 1914). A photograph in the *Survey*, accompanying an article by Charles S. Little (1912), the superintendent of Letchworth Village, showed five "boys" shelling peas. The photograph's caption identified the activity as "home economics." Some parents complained about what they felt was a disregard for book learning. One Texas father wrote: "I feel greatly disappointed because of the fact that E— is doing no real school work." Other families hoped for the development of vocational skills. "I will appreciate hearing ... if in your opinion by a continuance at the school whether he can learn or be prepared so that he can keep himself employed and eventually earn a living," another father wrote. Most, however, had long since abandoned the hope of education to improve the lot of their children. Superintendents, seeing no need to resurrect lost hope, easily reformulated the meaning of education to fit institutional "community life" (Beverly Farm Records, letters to W. H. C. Smith, February 3, 1915, June 5, 1915).[3] A. E. Osborn, superintendent of the California Home for the Care and Training of Feeble-Minded Children, articulated most clearly this new purpose of institutional education when he wrote in 1891, "[W]e have the troublesome class, to whom, in very truth, 'a little learning is a dangerous thing.' Instead of books they need tools. Why supply them with the means of increasing their dangerous proclivities? Instead of school-room instruction, which too frequently sharpens their cunning and supplies means for the further elaboration of their vicious tendencies, it were better they were taught the alphabet of some simple handicraft" (*Institutional Bulletin* 1891, 9).

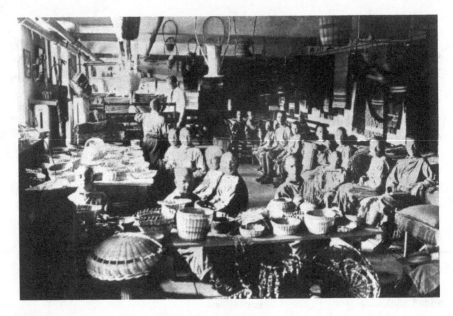

Figure 4.4:
Industrial training at the Rome State School in New York, ca. 1920. (From James C. Riggs's *Hello Doctor: A Brief Biography of Charles Bernstein*, 1936)

Many, probably most, inmates did not move beyond this institutionally focused domestic training. Some youngsters and teenagers, placed by relatives, social welfare authorities, or judges more for what the placers regarded as their misbehavior than for their feeble minds, however, progressed to more specialized vocational training (Figure 4.4). They were what Little (1912) called "finished workers" ("rough workers" were low grades). As noted earlier, some inmates assumed responsibilities in the institution hardly distinguishable from those of the salaried employees. Specialized training for male inmates included typesetting in the print shop, chair caning, brush and broom making, leather crafts, brick making, bricklaying, and carpentry (Figure 4.5). Female high grades learned weaving, basketry, sewing, and typing. At the Rome asylum, Bernstein began a nursing class (Figure 4.6). By 1925, thirty-eight female inmates had enrolled and twenty-one completed the course work (the others were dismissed or withdrew). In 1924, with the success of this program, Bernstein began a similar course for twelve "better boys." The graduates of these nursing programs found employment at their own institution, became nurses and nurses' aides at other county or state institutions in New York, and even took up private-duty nursing (*Herald*, May 1, 1923; August 1, 1924; March 1, 1925; September 1, 1926).

Problems, of course, occasionally arose during work, play, or school. When they did occur, they were usually settled immediately. Most responses to perceived misbehavior came from staff members closest to the inmate at the time of the wrongdoing. At work, this person was likely an attendant or maintenance worker who worked alongside the inmate. At play or in the cottage, attendants provided

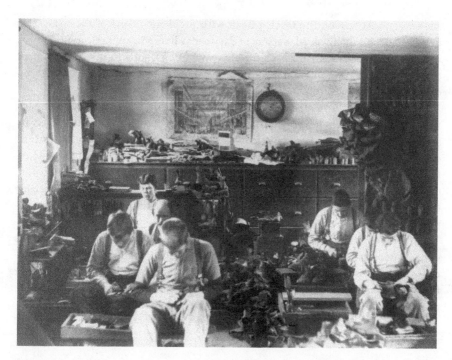

Figure 4.5:
Shoemaking shop at the Pennsylvania Training School for Feeble-Minded Children (Elwyn Institute), circa 1885. (Courtesy of Southern Illinois University at Edwardsville, Lovejoy Library, Beverly Farm Records)

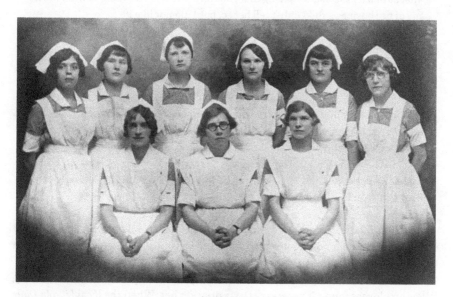

Figure 4.6:
Nurses' training class at the Rome State School in New York, 1928. (From James C. Riggs's *Hello Doctor: A Brief Biography of Charles Bernstein*, 1936)

supervision. At school, the teacher dealt with problems. Many of the issues that provoked problems involved matters of day-to-day living in an institution. Others, more serious, involved runaways or "elopements," as both Kerlin and Johnson called them. In one month alone (June 1880), Kerlin (1891*a*) reported sixteen escapes from the institution.

These matters were often exacerbated by overcrowded cottages; epidemics, which reduced the amount of staff time to devote to individual inmates; staff instability because of the frequent turnovers of attendants; classroom frustration, especially among older children; and the court-ordered placement of juvenile offenders with feeble minds. Added to these problems were the long hours of work expected of the attending staff, often under trying conditions. It is not surprising that tempers flared and that all actors in the life of the institution lost their composure from time to time.

An attendant at Beverly Farm protested to the superintendent that accusations of her immoral behavior at local dances were ill-founded: "They all know that I conducted myself well. If you have references to the dances that I went to why I got Miss Gaines's view on that before I went.... Who is it that made the charges I am not afraid to face him or her in any of them?" (Beverly Farm Records, letter to W. H. C. Smith, August 22, 1916). An inmate at the same facility wrote of her frustration with her attendants:

> When Cora brought me my breakfast this morning I told her I did not want it and I did not open the door for her and during the talk we had she told me that if I ate I would come back to the dining room the sooner or to that effect. I did not see what authority she had for saying that and think she was attending to what wasn't any of her business, tho I didn't tell her so, but I did not like it.

She continued in her letter:

> Yesterday I sent a note to Miss Curtis apologizing for giving way to my temper so on the occasion. I told you something of and also apologizing for the disturbance I made in the dining room Sunday but she has made no reply to it.... I think you told me Sunday I must mind the employees. I will tell you frankly I do not agree with you in this and I hope you'll withdraw it. I do not feel myself in duty bound to mind the young girls you have here tho' I trust you'll not repeat this. Of course I acknowledge your's and Mrs. Smith's and Miss Mattie's authority. (Beverly Farm Records, letter to W. H. C. Smith, ca. 1906)

In 1894, Melissa Ward, an attendant at the Lincoln asylum, became agitated while serving dinner to inmates under her supervision. Quite suddenly, she began to attack other attendants, making loud noises and cries and tearing her clothes. Opium and other narcotics did not seem to stop her unexpected behavior. Finally, fellow employees found it necessary to straitjacket her. When the local *Lincoln Daily News-Herald* reported the incident, what was most apparent was that it was recounted as if it was hardly unusual ("Commission in Insanity" 1894). Described as having a common-school education, fond of reading, "quiet and agreeable in disposition, no bad or vicious habits," Ward was portrayed as an otherwise normal person exhibiting the stress and "insanity" (the newspaper's conclusion) that must not have appeared so uncommon among institutional employees or to local newspapers.

FAMILIES AND THE INSTITUTION

Tensions also arose at the institutions from inmates' disappointing experiences with their families. Some after a visit home were eager to return to the institution, but others felt frustrated by parents and family who rarely took them home or visited them. Sometimes an unfulfilled promise from a family member sent an inmate into depression or, worse (from the institution's perspective), into several days of destructive behavior. In 1915, W. H. C. Smith wrote an inmate's aunt about the consequences of her sister's broken promise to her daughter:

> When Mrs. F— was here she evidently had planned to take V— home and told her so thinking she could go to Moody Institute. We have had a very unhappy time practically ever since with V— who when she found her mother was not going to take her demonstrated her instability by making threats to all but me, would take her hair down at the table, wash her face in [a] tumbler of water at dinner table and do so many things which in themselves were small but indicated an unsafe mentality and morale that after many evidences of insubordination and threats I at last had her brought to [my] office and blankly asked her if she was trying to make us send her to "Maplewood" again[.] [I]n a childlike manner she promptly admitted that was her plan and I of course told her she could not go again as they would not accept her. She broke down crying piteously and since then has been as nice a girl as you could wish but this will all be enacted over again and again. (Beverly Farm Records, letter from W. H. C. Smith, November 12, 1915)

The frustrations of inmates about their place in the institution and their absence from home and kin not surprisingly mirrored similar misgivings and uncertainties felt by parents and relatives. Many parents, especially in the first year of their child's institutional placement, felt great loss and concern. They worried about little things—things that, nevertheless, sustain intimate relationships—a warm coat for winter, comfortable shoes, properly fitted dentures, and countless other matters they had once taken care of themselves. The worries of many parents reflected the ambivalence they felt toward their now institutionalized children. Families with children at Beverly Farm, where parents paid for more individual care than they could expect from public facilities, looked forward to weekly letters from their children. Usually, these letters had to be written by attendants or teachers. The absence or sickness of one of these staff members usually meant a delay in letters home. Dozens of parents, some more sympathetically than others, wrote Superintendent Smith asking for more letters. Even when they rarely visited the facility, most parents wanted to be reassured that their child's day-to-day needs were being met. "Pardon dearie," wrote a mother to her daughter's teacher,

> how is little G— and doesn't she chill these morning[s?] [P]ut on little shirts with long sleeves if [it] continues cool and damp. I forgot to tell you [it] seems in trying to pick up pins, hair pins, needles and catching in threading needles that her fingers are dormant or so lifeless[.] [J]ust can't you lie a pin down and ask her to pick it up and you will readly [*sic*] see her condition. I have saw her work for 1 minute in trying to pick up even a hair pin . . . . [S]o pleas consider this when instructing her[.] [Y]ou see her fingernails are off almost into the quick from biting. [D]ress her warm dear and don't be too hard on her for she is mammas baby[.] [S]he is so constipated I have to give her something to move [her] bowels about once a week. So see this is done to prevent her from being sick. (Beverly Farm Records, letter to Instructor of the Girls' Department, September 21, 1917)

In similar fashion, a Chicago mother wrote:

> Dear teacher:
> Will you find out if S— is in need of anything and let me know. Also will you see if his shoes are big enough? His oxfords I know are but if his old shoes seem small wish you would throw them out. I don't want the child to suffer with his feet. If you will do that for me I will appreciate it very much. I miss him so, and often wonder if those little details are noticed. Wonder if he misses his mama. [H]e loved me so much it seems a pity to put him away. Is little S— learning to talk or is he just the same[?] Sometimes I still have hope for him although I know it is useless. (Beverly Farm Records, letter, July 13, 1914)

Other parents' worries went beyond the day-to-day. Several expressed concern about what they believed was their child's sexual vulnerability. A Chicago parent wrote W. H. C. Smith:

> A— is getting to be a big woman with a child's mind. I had her in a Academy up till now and her mind is not as it should be. We are afraid to trust her at home because she makes up with everyone and something might happen to her which would cause lots of trouble with us. Dr. have you an opening for her. She is strong and well and could do lots of work around the house. (Beverly Farm Records, letter to W. H. C. Smith, July 22, 1917)

Another parent wrote:

> When A— left Metropolis [Illinois] he worried us considerably talking about marrying and going with girls. Doctor, I am writing this in all confidence and beg you to see that no strange women try to influence him or take him away from Godfrey. Let no one take him from Godfrey but my sister Cora or I. Always see that he is in company with teachers or you. (Beverly Farm Records, letter to W. H. C. Smith, July 31, 1917)

Other relatives expressed mistrust of the institution's staff. One sister wrote her brother, an inmate at Beverly Farm:

Say—it makes us tired about your shoes. Don't you wear those that G— sent last everyday or don't the people there let you wear them. . . .

The reason papa doesn't send you any money is because they take it away from you—don't you see? You have a lot of money in someone's hand there and it is *awfully* provoking to us that they don't let you spend it your own way. I'll stick in a dime and you can surely put that in your pocket and get a little gum or something without anyone objecting. (Beverly Farm Records, letter, March 23, 1917)

Other parents and relatives came to terms with their anxieties, accepting their child or sibling as an institutional entity. When they had the means, they paid their monthly fees, and they visited on holidays. From time to time, they wrote letters or sent packages. But the break had been made. They now worried about time for summer visits, demands by their institutionalized relative to return home, and re-integrating the inmate into the family, if only briefly, at holidays. For some, reintegration was troublesome and awkward. Like loved but unwanted relatives, inmates often wore out their welcome. "I am inclosing check for $35.00 on D—'s account. How is he giting a long?" asked a father who lived only fifteen miles away from his son at Beverly Farm. He continued:

He is writing and calling me continually about coming home. Now Doctor, nothing would please me more than to let him do so if I was in a position to take care of him. But my being so situated that I am away from home every night, and no one at home but my wife and girls, and they are afraid to stay alone with him, it is next to impossible to me to comply with his wish. The last time he was home, he gave an awfull lot of trouble at nights, he would get up and wander all over the house, with out any clothes on and get lost and it kept some one up looking after him all night. He speaks of wanting to go [to the] Lodge. The last time we let him go to Lodge he had an attact, and disrupted the meeting, very sad to think about, but it shows you the position I am in. (Beverly Farm Records, letter to W. H. C. Smith, February 22, 1917)

Another well-to-do parent who had supported Beverly Farm through donations exceeding the tuition paid for his son's upkeep wrote Smith shortly after the Christmas season of 1913:

I am inclosing you a letter from S— [his son] and would like to know if these complaints originate from him or the mind of the writer. I am of the opinion the latter. . . . Is S—'s worrying about coming home [as] bad as this letter indicates? We have felt it best to keep him where he is, that coming home would only unsettle him. . . . The facts are his last trip home seemed to be very little appreciated by him. He saw very few people he knew, and they cared nothing for a poor afflicted Boy like him. He just sit[s] around the house . . . waiting [for] the time to go back.

I would not mind the expense if there was any thing to be gained but I fail to see the gain and think the money could be used by him to better advantage where he is in some kind of amusements like trips in summer for an outing. (Beverly Farm Records, letter to W. H. C. Smith, December 29, 1913)

The reluctance to have their children come home reflected the parents' coming to terms with the picture that the superintendents painted of their children's condition. At first, they might write to inquire about their relative's progress, but after a while that would usually stop. Most superintendents, of course, never believed that improvement was possible—certainly not the kind of improvement longed for by parents when they first put their children into the institution. When the New York State Commission to Investigate Provision for the Mentally Deficient in 1914 surveyed Smith about the "percentage that become self-supporting," he responded, "not 1 in 100" (Beverly Farm Records, New York State, Commission to Investigate Provision for the Mentally Deficient, Questionnaire to Heads of Institutions of All Kinds in New York State and for Mental Defectives in All States, handwritten copy signed by W. H. C. Smith, December 10, 1914). The prophesy fulfilled itself as parent after parent and sibling after sibling came to terms with the unimprovability of their loved one. In 1918, a middle manager in a well-known Chicago meat-packing corporation wrote an odd but revealing letter to Smith:

Am enclosing copy of letter I wish you would write me exactly as I have written it and send not later than Saturday 21st. This is a long story, however I'll not burden you with all the details but I am trying to induce a rich uncle to send D— back to school [i.e., Beverly Farm] as I haven't been able to finance it myself. He is a hard fisted old cuss and has to be shown and this letter from you will do the trick.

Whether Smith copied the letter as requested and sent it in his own hand back to the parent to use to trick the parent's rich uncle is unclear. What the letter provides, nevertheless, is a unique perspective on this parent's resolution of the fate of his daughter as prescribed by Beverly Farm:

Mr. T. L. C—

In reply to your recent letter in reference to your daughter D—, [I] beg to say that in my opinion she will always be a sub-normal child as far as her mentality is concerned. We found her quite backward in her school work and she made very little progress in that direction, however her nervous condition which was bad when she came here, was 50% improved when she left and I think the quiet healthful surroundings of our school was what helped her. She is a good dispositioned child, easy to control and if you care to send her back later on we would be very glad to have her. With kindest regards to Mrs. C— and yourself.

Very Truly,

Dr. W. H. C. Smith (Beverly Farm Records, Letters to W. H. C. Smith, July 19 [ca. 1918])

ORDER AND DISORDER IN THE INSTITUTION

Out of these issues and concerns emerged questions of how to deal with recurring inmate misbehavior, how to prevent the abuse and neglect of inmates, and how to cope with the concerns and misgivings of parents and relatives when they arose.[4] Responses to these questions were heightened by the scandals that occurred frequently in state hospitals for the insane and, to a lesser extent, in institutions for feeble minds throughout the last half of the nineteenth century. Responses were also shaped as superintendents shared among themselves their views on how they and their staff should deal with inmate misbehavior. In the *Manual of Elwyn*, shared with institutions across the nation, Isaac Kerlin (1891*a*) clarified for his employees precise requirements for discipline. Forbidding attendants to strike an inmate or even show their tempers, Kerlin laid out an elaborate and detailed set of instructions to regulate punishment and to maintain order.

From the institutions' beginnings in America, moral treatment had been a fundamental philosophy. According to the tenets of moral treatment, inmates were to be dealt with kindly, never abused, and restrained only to prevent harm to themselves or others. As institutions for feeble minds were transformed from schools to small institutions and then to larger facilities, commitment to moral treatment became more difficult as attendant staff grew in size and became less stable. By 1910, most superintendents had only limited direct contact with attendants who, unlike their predecessors of previous decades, might work at the institution only long enough to secure better-paying and less strenuous positions elsewhere. Julia Lathrop, a member of the Illinois State Board of Charities, complained in 1909 that better-educated upstate Illinoisans were difficult to attract to the Lincoln school because of the better-paying industrial jobs in Chicago (Illinois General Assembly 1908, 171).

Kerlin's warning, first made in 1879, showed that inmate discipline was already an institutional concern and that abuse of control occurred. A decade later, William Fish (1889) at the Illinois Asylum delivered a paper to the Association of Medical Officers on the issue of institutional discipline. Obviously sensitive about punishment, he advised its use only "until all else has failed." He added:

> Let the punishment, if needs be that it must be given, be given calmly, certainly without anger and never with any admixture of personality. I deem it the only safe rule to follow, to restrict the power of inflicting corporal punishment to the superintendent, or his assistant in case of his absence. It seems to me unwise to delegate the power to any one else, and I hold it wise precaution to place in a permanent form a record of the circumstances leading to the punishment, and to have it performed in the presence of a reliable witness.

Like Fish, Barr (1904*a*, 171–172) supported the use of corporal punishment only when all other forms of correction had failed. Barr advised that withholding a privilege was more appropriate than physical punishment. His views had not changed fourteen years later. In a letter to Daisy Denson, the secretary of the North

Carolina State Board of Charities and a leader in the founding of the first institution for mental defectives in that state, he wrote:

> For the high and middle grade children we occasionally use corporal punishment, but this is only administered after due consideration, and all other methods of punishment have failed. I am the one to decide and personally spank the boys, and either my chief matron or principal teacher attend to the girls. It is always administered in the presence of a witness, and an elaborate record is made of cause and effect. We find, however, that the best means of discipline is to deprive the children of some pleasure, and corporal punishment is resorted to only as an extreme measure.
>
> We also put the children to bed, and persistent runaways have a regular uniform of blue and scarlet, which they wear constantly.
>
> Under no circumstance do we deprive children of food. (North Carolina State Archives, State Board of Public Welfare, box 178, letter from Martin W. Barr to Daisy Denson, July 25, 1918)

When he took over the Indiana facility in 1893, Johnson (1923, 206) used corporal punishment for "exceptional offenders or grand offenses." By the end of the decade, however, he had stopped such punishment. He also insisted that the institution discontinue "search parties." His predecessor at the Indiana school had followed Kerlin's lead in organizing groups of attendants, trusted inmates, and sometimes local law officers to hunt down escapees from the institution. Johnson believed most inmates left the facility to gain attention, which the search party provided. Johnson shocked his staff by insisting that runaways be allowed to return to the institution on their own. By 1910, most other superintendents also opposed corporal punishment, although they did not follow Johnson's practice regarding escapees. When he took over the superintendency of the Rome asylum in 1903, Bernstein announced in his first annual report that no form of corporal punishment would be allowed (Riggs 1936, 22). Johnstone in New Jersey also forbade corporal punishment (Doll [ca. 1976], 15). His director of research, Henry H. Goddard, had insisted: "In this Institution the slightest approach to corporal punishment is followed by immediate dismissal" (North Carolina State Archives, State Board of Public Welfare, box 178, letter from Henry H. Goddard to Daisy Denson, July 23, 1918). The abandonment of corporal punishment reflected both the recognition of its potential abuse and the vulnerability of superintendents to charges of abuse by the public whose awareness had been heightened by well-publicized scandals at certain institutions.

The most prominent scandal of the period occurred in Illinois in 1907 and 1908. Drawing the attention of Chicago papers as well as the concern of superintendents in other states, accidents and claims of abuse and neglect at the Illinois Asylum led to a statewide legislative investigation of all public institutions in Illinois. The facts surrounding the incidents were complex and not entirely clear. Two days before Christmas in 1907, Frank Giroux, a sixteen-year-old inmate who had entered the asylum only nineteen days earlier, received a severe burn on his left ear, neck, and face (Figure 4.7). Probably as a result of an epileptic seizure (although, in the absence of a cottage attendant at the time of the occurrence, the circumstances of the accident were unclear), Giroux fell on an uncovered radiator, where he lay for several minutes. After an attendant found him, the institution's matron sent the injured boy to the infirmary, where two physicians who treated him claimed the burns were minor.

The next day, Christmas Eve, the boy's father appeared at Lincoln, having missed the telegram that Superintendent Hardt had sent him the evening before. Suspecting a cover-up, the senior Giroux, a Chicago theatrical agent, returned his son to Chicago. There, two prominent physicians examined the boy and expressed shock upon finding severe and improperly treated wounds. Incensed, Giroux reported the incident to John W. Hill, his state representative and a leader of a faction of the Republican Party at odds with the then Republican governor Charles Deneen. As a result of Hill's prodding, in January 1908, the Illinois House of Representatives authorized a special investigative committee with Hill as the chairman and five other members, both Republicans and Democrats, but none sympathetic to Deneen. Hardt, a Deneen appointee, had the backing of the

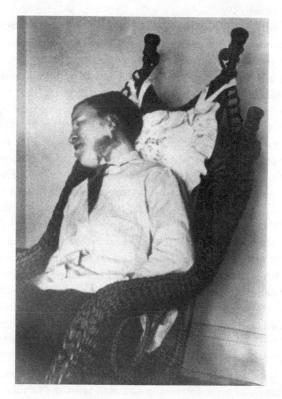

Figure 4.7:
Frank Giroux, an inmate burned at the Illinois Asylum for Feeble-Minded Children, 1908. (From the Illinois General Assembly's *Investigation of Illinois State Institutions: Testimony, Findings, and Debate*, 1908)

State Board of Charities. The board had considered both Deneen and Hardt as reformers who could reshape and bring humane treatment to the Lincoln asylum (and to other Illinois institutions), which, they believed, had become, to use Julia Lathrop's characterization, a "political football." Nineteen-eight was an election year, and Deneen was trying to be the first Illinois governor in nearly two decades to be re-elected. The investigation lasted from January to May of that year, the newspapers made much of it, Deneen survived the investigation and was re-elected, and, as a result of it all, Illinois replaced its seventeen institutional boards of trustees and its weak State Board of Charities with a five-member State Board of Administration having administrative authority over all Illinois public charitable institutions (Howard 1988, 211–217; Illinois General Assembly 1908; see also Willrich 1998).[5]

To superintendents in other states, the Illinois investigation represented a scandal of the sort more often associated with the insane asylums. Aside from the castration scandals involving F. Hoyt Pilcher in Kansas, publicized problems at asylums for feeble minds had been relatively minor. For example, Gustavus Doren and A. C. Rogers had received charges of incompetence and mismanagement, and Alexander Johnson had been accused of nepotism (Doren Manuscripts, box 1, folders 1 and 2; J. Holman 1966; Johnson 1923, 238–245; M. Thomson 1963, 29). And, in each of those cases, the superintendent had survived the accusations. While investigations of abuse and neglect had occurred in the facilities for feeble minds (see, e.g., "Discussions: Accidents" 1909), most had resulted in dropped charges. None had rivaled the attention shown the Illinois Asylum's scandal. It was so concerned with the national implications of the Illinois investigation that the Association for the Study of the Feeble-Minded showed its support for Hardt by making him president-elect of the association in 1909 and accepting his invitation to hold its annual meeting at Lincoln in 1910. Letters between William H. C. Smith, superintendent of the private Illinois institution, Beverly Farm and various state and national figures also attest to the importance of the scandal for leaders in the field and to the organized effort of some of the superintendents to support one of their own (Beverly Farm Records, unsorted letters, ca. 1908–10; see also "Dr. Smith Protests" 1908; Hardt 1909).

The investigation provides the contemporary researcher an unusual glimpse at the underside of institutional life. During several sessions at Lincoln, Springfield, and Chicago over the course of one month, the six-member investigating committee questioned a wide variety of people associated with the asylum. Shortly before the investigation was to begin, several inmates at the institution had come down with measles, four of whom died in the midst of the hearings. While the epidemic kept the committee at the Logan County Court House a few miles away from the asylum and prevented its firsthand inspection of the facility, it also added to the already tense situation. In Chicago and Springfield, the committee also interviewed several witnesses formerly associated with the facility, including the Giroux family. Under skillful and persistent questioning, especially by Chairman Hill and Walter I. Manny, a Democrat, witnesses painted the picture of a disjointed and disrupted facility.

Superintendent Hardt regarded the accident reports, which the committee required him to produce, as both a blessing and a problem. On the one hand, the reports seemed to support his and the Board of Charities' claim that Illinois needed a separate facility for epileptic inmates. Most accidents in the institution involved injuries occurring during a seizure. Some epileptics had daily, even hourly, attacks, making them susceptible to frequent injury. On the other hand, the reports opened to public scrutiny several cases of staff carelessness, neglect, abuse, insensitivity, and indiscretion.

The case of Minnie Steritz was especially damaging. In May 1907, Steritz was severely burned while left unattended in a bathtub and died a week later. One attendant was fired as a result of the incident. The attendant claimed her innocence, blaming the inattention on her supervisor, whom Hardt had recently hired. Under questioning, Hardt claimed:

> The child was of such a kind, that the pain, I don't believe would affect her very much; I know I have seen her dressed part of the time, and she showed no indication of pain, and I know it would have been painful to myself or any other normal being. She did not have the sense of pain developed to the extent of a normal individual. (Illinois General Assembly 1908, 45–46)

Later, John Wagner, a former trustee of the asylum appointed by Governor Deneen's predecessor, testified that Hardt had tolerated physical violence by staff members appointed by him and reduced the quantity and quality of the food served at the institution. He criticized Hardt also for his cold and distant manner with inmates and reported hearing that Hardt had also stolen money from them (Illinois General Assembly 1908, 76–90). During the hearings, newspapers reported that committee members had claimed that some of the physicians at the asylum were "dope fiends." Others testified on the case of John Morthland. Convinced that his recurring epileptic attacks were the result of sexual indiscretion, Morthland attempted almost successfully to castrate himself. When he died four days after his self-mutilation, few in the press or public were inclined to believe the attending physician's insistence that death was the result of his epilepsy. Another inmate, eight-year-old Virgene Jessop, received bites and scratches on her arms, face, and abdomen on the night of March 21, 1907. Several employees testified that the wounds were made by rats. The most damaging claim given by many of the same witnesses was that Superintendent Hardt had tried to cover up the incident.

Finally, the committee took the testimony of Walter Kaak and Asa Carlin. Kaak testified in Chicago not only about his own accident (in which he had lost an arm) but also about other examples of abuse and neglect at the Lincoln facility. He claimed that an attendant had kicked and slapped him. Soon after the incident, he had written Governor Deneen to complain. Kaak's testimony then revealed that the governor had merely sent the letter to Hardt, which made both the governor and the superintendent appear unconcerned about Kaak's complaint. His accident a few months later, of course, made their inaction look even more callous. Carlin, too, provided specific incidences of inmates being beaten by attendants.

Added to all this, reports surfaced that Harriet Hook, an assistant physician at the institution, had been keeping body parts of autopsied inmates. Most of these autopsies had been done without the permission of relatives. When more than one attendant testified that Dr. Hook, in anatomy lectures newly instituted for the attendants by Hardt, had casually referred to specific body parts as being those of deceased inmates well known to the attendants, the committee and newspapers throughout the state suggested ghoulish activities at Lincoln. As the public then still suspected hospitals of experimenting on the living and the dead, these careless activities hardly diminished concerns about the facility.

At the end of the investigation, the committee recommended major changes in the administration of Illinois state institutions. Although it urged a new facility for epileptics, most of its recommendations focused on centralizing authority for what, up to this time, had been decentralized administrative boards for the various institutions. Few acknowledged, however, that Illinois institutions had been perennially underfunded and had become political rewards for individuals backing successfully elected governors.[6]

Superintendent Hardt survived the investigation, although by 1913 he had moved on to a private medical practice. The informally sanctioned physical punishment of inmates was "officially" eliminated in favor of the administratively sanctioned use of secluding misbehavers. By 1913, inmates had begun to call the place of seclusion, "the jail." Located on the top floor of the main administration building at the Lincoln asylum, it was a low, dark room where iron bars covered a single small window. Hot in summer and without heat in winter, it became the postscandal alternative to beatings ("Lincoln State School and Colony" 1913).

THE ATTENDANT

The investigation revealed that rapidly growing public institutions, often underfunded by capricious politicians, were vulnerable to abuse, neglect, and accidents despite the best intentions of concerned and even vigilant superintendents. All institutions relied almost exclusively on the care of custodial inmates by salaried attendants and higher functioning inmates. Usually receiving their training through an unstructured apprenticeship, both groups were prone to the stress and carelessness that affect all untrained, overworked, and underpaid people. By 1910, most institutions initiated training programs for attendants. Most also tried to formulate hospital-like discipline, while also offering clubs, sporting events, and outings for the attending staff.

Life at the institutions was hardly easy for the attendants. Although many literally spent their lifetimes at the institution (even being buried there), good attendants, superintendents complained, were difficult to find and even harder to retain. By today's standards, work in the institution at the turn of the century required a commitment approaching monastic proportions. The Illinois Asylum, whose requirements were not atypical, had two attendant shifts. The night, or second, shift worked from 7:30 in the evening until 6:00 the next morning. It was a reduced shift, with usually only one attendant on duty in each unit. A night supervisor made rounds from building to building to assist the attendants and to make certain they refrained from sleeping on the job. Although most inmates slept during the shift, the night attendants were still usually kept busy. Inmates might soil themselves and need new bed clothes. Some might become sick in the night and need attention. Most cottages had at least one inmate who would "come alive at night." Some inmates were known for biting other inmates and had to be watched and sometimes restrained. Second-shift workers were expected to watch for and stop sexual indiscretions. In addition, if a lone attendant became preoccupied with a sick inmate or was preparing evening medicines, an inmate could easily slip out of the cottage. Evening escapes were especially troublesome because they usually required search parties at an inconvenient time.

The day shift's formal hours were 5:30 in the morning until 7:30 in the evening, when the second shift arrived. But, in fact, the day attendants were always on call and could be summoned at any hour. Usually, two to four attendants worked in each cottage, depending on the number and needs of its inmates. As a rule, young children and more severely impaired inmates required more attendant care than did older and more capable inmates. Female attendants cared for older "girls" and young children, male and female. Male attendants cared for older "boys." Care included basic maintenance of inmates and the cottages. Attendants might be watching after inmates in the dayroom, the bath, the dining room, or the sleeping room. If not dealing with an inmate, they were apt to be sweeping or mopping floors, preparing the medicine tray, or moving furniture. Laundry, too, was always a problem. At Beverly Farm in Illinois, attendants in 1911 petitioned Superintendent Smith for relief from the heavy demand of laundry duties (Beverly Farm Records, letter from Erma C. Bishop et al. to William and Nellie Smith, August 8, 1911). In addition to these duties, lower grades had to be fed, and great care had to be taken lest they choke. Many were not toilet trained, so cleaning was a constant activity. Attendants working with high grades had any number of behavioral problems to resolve.[7]

Attendants also had to deal with inmates' homesickness; concerns about approaching holidays, which usually meant ambiguity about returning home; and other anxieties. Issues of life and death were always magnified by distance from family. Personal sickness, family inattention, a death, the marriage of a sibling, and so forth could precipitate an inmate's anxiety, necessitating the attention and time of attendants. "My dear son, C—," began the letter from a father living in Chicago to his son at Beverly Farm:

> Well how are you any way [?] I suppose you will be surprised to hear from me. But you know how busy I am all the time, and that is reason I don't get to write. But I will try and do better after this. Now we got your letter this a.m. and sorry to hear that you want to come home. But C— you must not think of that because you would not be here a week till you would want to go back. There is nothing here C— for you to do and you know it. You must learn to like every body there and I am sure they would never say any thing to you only for your own good. You know it is terrible to

go through this world with out an education and you must make up your mind to be a striker. We never make anything by wanting to be changing around. Also your mother is in poor health and I want her to get well before you come home. I will come and see you in a few weeks and then we can have a big talk. . . . Now be a good boy and do as Dr. Smith wants you to and I am sure you will be well paid for it. You know we would like to have you home. But as I said before there is nothing for you to do. Now try C— and be Satisfied. (Beverly Farm Records, letter, March 17, 1913)

In 1906, an inmate from Chicago wrote a letter home that was never sent by institutional officials:

My Dear mamma and papa and aunt Carrie. I would not mind comming back home at once. I would like to come right now if all of you would let me come home at once. Would you please let your boy . . . come home right away. . . . If the three of you want to please me just tell me that I can come at once. And I would be tickled to death to think that I could come home once more. To think that I could come back to home sweet home once more. Just think how sad I am up here away from you three. I am awful sad up here away from you three. I believe that you three don't care for me any more or you would let me come home at once. I would help my dear papa on the wagon and my dear mama in the store. (Beverly Farm Records, letter [ca. 1906]).

By 1915, most public institutions were caring for inmate populations of more than one thousand children and adults. California, Illinois, Indiana, Iowa, Massachusetts, Michigan, Minnesota, New York (at Rome), Ohio, Pennsylvania, and Wisconsin all had institutional populations exceeding one thousand, and Illinois, Massachusetts, Ohio, and Pennsylvania had populations approaching two thousand. The age range of the inmates had also expanded, with institutions serving inmates as young as one month and as old as seventy years (US Department of Commerce 1919). As institutions became more populated and diverse, the hierarchy of attendant care became more complex. In some institutions, a "matron" supervised the care of all inmates; in others, she supervised the care of only female inmates and a "supervisor" oversaw the care of male inmates. In either case, supervision of the attendants was a twenty-four-hour-a-day job. Despite the heavy demands made of them, most matrons and supervisors were devoted to their institutions. Some, as Johnson (1923, 205) noted, were perhaps too devoted: "My first matron often boasted of her loyalty and would declare that if the superintendent ordered her to transfer the contents of the attic to the cellar and of the cellar to the attic, she would do it and ask no questions."

Beneath the matron and supervisor in the institutional hierarchy were "charges." These were essentially middle managers, who, as institutions grew larger, provided intermediate supervision to areas of cottages, each with several attendants. Most charges had progressed from the ranks of the attendant staff. With little formal training other than their on-the-job experience, they often found themselves supervising attendants who had been their peers. Sometimes this arrangement worked well and sometimes it did not.

Despite the efforts of some superintendents and some state civil service administrators, most attendant care was drawn from the population of residents living
near the institution. Since most institutions were in rural areas, the attendant caregivers tended to be a homogeneous group. They had often grown up knowing each
other and were not infrequently related by blood or marriage. Although this homogeneity may have been beneficial, at least to the attendants, it created problems,
especially for supervision and in times of institutional change.[8]

When Hardt arrived at the Illinois Asylum from Chicago in 1907, he found what
he believed to be a too informal, lax, and undisciplined attendant force. Often
supervised by kinfolk who, Hardt believed, tolerated immoral behavior among
staff members, cruelty to inmates, and disrespect for professionals (especially
physicians) at the institution, attendants had become unruly. By all accounts, his
predecessor had developed a good relationship with the attendants by tolerating
their need for informal arrangements among themselves and by tacitly accepting
their self-imposed limits on disciplining inmates. Visits from town folk and parties among on-duty staff members were allowed, and attendants were permitted to
spank, box the ears of, and paddle inmates who were disobedient (Illinois General
Assembly 1908, 76–90, 131–135). Henry Darger (ca. 1960 [2014]) wrote about experiencing all three methods of disciplining during his incarceration. When Hardt
tried to make what he believed were necessary changes to these informal arrangements, attendants resisted. First, he hired new supervisors and charges from outside of Lincoln. Next, he limited the already restricted extrainstitutional time off
of attendants and prohibited the free access of town people to the facility. Third, he
forbade the use of corporal punishment by attendants. Finally, he demanded that
attendants stand in the presence of a physician. This last change was too much for
attendants like T. B. Coates, a sixty-seven-year-old veteran of what he believed was
formerly a congenial place to live and work. He resigned and later testified before
the 1908 Illinois House investigating committee:

> Well, it seems to me that when a superior comes into the play room they complain
> of not making obeisance to them, arising to our feet.
>
> Well, I think we were not used as we ought to be used. We are not so much their
> inferiors that we have to be used like dogs, I don't think. I claimed that I was a
> man, and a white man. I want to be used right, and when they would come in there
> we got it into our heads always we would get what we call in common phrase a
> "jacking up." We looked for it. There was nothing good to be said for us.
>
> It was always fault finding, criticizing, or something of that kind, whenever
> they came into the room. We looked for it, and sometimes it was disagreeable.

When questioned further about these indignities, about being treated "like
dogs," Coates explained:

> Well, I could not name any particular that I think of. What I had reference to more
> particularly was allowing no privileges, being shut off entirely, taking our usual
> hours away from us, that we had for recreation, hours off, and placing us in the

work the whole time and allowing us only one permit a week to go out where we would get some fresh air here in town. (Illinois General Assembly 1908, 133)[9]

In rural, homogeneous environments, changes in the formal and informal arrangements within growing and more complex organizations were difficult to achieve. In the hands of an inexperienced and insensitive leader, such changes were even harder to accomplish. Some superintendents, for example, Johnson, Bernstein, and Barr, tried to avoid these difficulties by developing organizational relationships that they hoped would promote attendant solidarity without sacrificing order, discipline, and good care. To maintain order and discipline, Barr followed Kerlin's lead in using an employee handbook. *The Manual of Elwyn* (1891*a*), published less than two years before Kerlin's death, was a compendium of rules and regulations issued by Kerlin since the 1860s. A few years later, Barr added the manual to his *Acts of Incorporation with Amendments and By-Laws of the Pennsylvania School for Feeble Minded Children* (Pennsylvania Training School for Feeble-Minded Children. 1894). Around 1910, he began requiring all staff members to sign the "house copy" of this manual. The rules became the principal source for organizational solidarity at the Pennsylvania school. The continuity of perspectives between Kerlin and Barr, and later between Barr and his successor E. Arthur Whitney, also strengthened this solidarity. At Elwyn Institute, codified rules and continuity of leadership maintained institutional traditions, which proved able for the most part to overcome the extrainstitutional relationships so prevalent in other facilities. Added to this was the large labor pool available because of the school's proximity to a large urban center. Unlike most facilities, the Pennsylvania Training School had little trouble finding help. Thus, Barr (1904*a*, 135) could be more particular about the people he hired than some of his colleagues in other states:

> The character of attendants is of the first importance, as these are they who live with the children; it should combine that firmness, tenderness, and balance that constitutes an even temperament, capable of recognizing and meeting an occasion without loss of self-control. The duties include not only the care of the idiots, both unimprovable and improvable, but the training and direction of idio-imbeciles as aids; and this dealing with natures often wholly animal requires a certain refinement and dignity of character, at least an entire absence of coarseness, while a knowledge of the simple manual arts, and, if possible, of drawing and of music, will do much to soften and brighten these darkened natures.

If Barr by location and tradition could maintain attendant cohesion, Johnson in Indiana and Bernstein in upstate New York had to rely on more innovative, and less predictable, approaches to maintain order and stability. Johnson recalled his father's Chartist loyalties. He considered himself somewhat of a radical and insisted on the destruction of the barriers between classes of employees at the Indiana School. To facilitate this classless democracy, he closed separate cafeterias, instituted employee dances and socials, and personally took part in activities that placed him in close contact with attendants. As a social worker, Johnson was one of the few superintendents at the time who was not a physician. The gap between medical and other personnel at the institution that most superintendents maintained was thus probably less important to Johnson.

Bernstein in New York also went to unusual lengths to build employee solidarity. Around 1920, he formed the Rome State School Council made up of nonprofessional staff. The council considered their pension options, arranged dances and socials, set up employee reading and game rooms, and formed baseball and basketball teams (*Herald,* December 1, 1921, 5; January 1, 1922, 6; March 1, 1922, 6). As early as 1907, Bernstein had established a training program for attendants that provided two years of hands-on training supplemented by lectures. During the same year, he instituted paid vacation (two weeks) and "reasonable sick-time" for attendants (Bernstein 1907). In 1914, he provided a "passenger auto truck" to transport employees between Rome and the institution (*Herald,* April 1, 1914, 6).

Thus, compared with most facilities of the time, the Rome asylum was a humane place for attendants to work. Many, like Julia C. Cully, worked there their whole lives. When she retired as matron of the Rome asylum in 1935 after thirty-seven years of service, Cully even moved into a small house on the institution's grounds to "keep in touch with the hundreds of friends among patients and employees to whom she [was] so well known, and who wish[ed] for her a very happy future" (*Herald,* January 1, 1935, 5). In 1921, four attendants and one teacher were married at the institution (*Herald,* April 1, 1921, 3). In 1922, Mary O. Maxwell, an attendant, was hospitalized at the institution when she became ill. She died several days later, and although she was not buried at the institution, a funeral service for her was held there (*Herald,* March 1, 1922, 4). The hospitalizations and burials of employees at institutions were not uncommon, especially in rural areas or if employees did not have relatives to care for them.

CONCLUSION

Attendants who adapted and committed themselves to life and work in the institution (often for the duration of their lives) became part of an institutional community that had its own internal system of meaning and purpose. In short, attendants, like inmates, became institutionalized as their personal identities became subsumed by their near total involvement in the institution. Superintendents often joked among themselves about the frequent inability of visitors to distinguish among the inmates and the attendants: both groups had become institutional people.

This institutionalization, of course, did not ensure that all care was good care. Much of it was; some of it clearly was not. Six years after the scandal at the Illinois State School and Colony at Lincoln, Caroline Lutz wrote William H. C. Smith for advice on how to handle charges against a carpenter employed at the school. Lutz had been appointed to investigate the accusations. A female inmate had reported that the carpenter had put his arms around her. This charge was enough to elicit new reports of his past indiscretions with inmates. The superintendent at the time, Thomas Leonard, claimed that the word of inmates could not be believed and thus there was no proof for the charges against the carpenter. Feeling uneasy about the superintendent's claim, Lutz consulted with other authorities including Smith. All these authorities, Lutz noted to Smith, confirmed the unreliability of an inmate's word (Beverly Farm Records, letter from Caroline C. Lutz to W. H. C. Smith, February 1914).

Institutionalization itself did not ensure a community of caregivers and care receivers. The demands placed on institutions to take more inmates with more diverse and often complex problems inevitably found its consequences in increasing burdens for attendants. The attendant, not the educator or the physician, was, in fact if not in rhetoric, the most crucial actor in the lives of inmates after 1890. Care, not education or treatment, had become the central focus of institutions by the turn of the century, and attendants, not educators or physicians, were, along with their inmate assistants, the principal caregivers.

The frustration expressed by Charles Wilbur in his 1909 letter to William H. C. Smith, noted at the beginning of this chapter, is the frustration of a leader in the field of mental deficiency who began his career in one era and was ending it in another. The era of care had supplanted the era of education. And the idea of care, as Wilbur knew, was one based on a growing fear of feebleminded people. Even before his death, institutional officials were beginning to call mental defectives "burdensome" and "menacing."

Ironically, the institution was a place where feeble minds could be freed from their burdensome and menacing potential. Most members of the institution—the inmates, the attendants, the maintenance staff, and even some of the teachers— were not caught up in the extrainstitutional movement to convince public officials and private citizens that burdensome mental defectives had to have lifetime care, their freedom to marry and have children prohibited, and their impulse to indulge in social vices restrained. Most were there to care as best they could for people who, they believed, needed care either because of their inability to care for themselves, because no one else would care for them, or because their behavior or potential behavior made them threats to the social fabric. What caregivers between 1890 and 1920 became a part of was an institutional structure that, duplicated in state after state, would be familiar to attendants and inmates in 1960 and even 1970. Between 1920 and 1970, institutions would absorb popular images from American society; yet, the structure and patterns of institutions for mental defectives would, despite the absorption, change little between those years. Only the numbers would increase. As I shall hold in Chapters 5 and 6, although institutional populations would grow, the influence of the superintendent would begin to diminish after 1920 as the state began to centralize authority it had originally shared with the superintendent.

What would change after 1920 were factors more likely outside than inside the institution. Until the 1970s, institutions would languish in the routinization formed in the 1920s. What would occur in the decades between 1910 and 1970 would be a rhetorical flourish that would affect not the structure of the institution, but only its size and its continuity of purpose and meaning for five decades.

NOTES

1. In the Beverly Farm Records, there is a rare example of a description of an institution from the perspective of an inmate. The inmate had lived at Beverly Farm in Illinois, but his family moved him to Vineland in New Jersey. He wrote the Smiths of his impressions of Vineland, especially as they compared with his views of Beverly Farm (Beverly Farm Records, letter to W. H. C. Smith, August 4, 1919).

2. A. C. Rogers, for example, reported that out of 1,113 inmates at the Minnesota School for Feeble-Minded and Colony for Epileptics, 507, fewer than one-half, attended the institution's school (Beverly Farm Records, letter from A. C. Rogers to W. H. C. Smith, June 3, 1908).

3. In 1908, A. C. Rogers noted that 489 of the 1,113 inmates at the Minnesota School for Feeble-Minded and Colony for Epileptics were "low-grade imbeciles not in school" (Beverly Farm Records, letter from A. C Rogers to W. H. C. Smith, June 3, 1908). Interestingly, however, Rogers was never reluctant to use these "low-grades" for institutional maintenance and upkeep. Indeed, even "low-grades" became a part of the institution's efforts for cost containment, which, in turn, became an important part of the superintendent's quest for legitimacy with the legislature.

4. For a collection of letters between parents, children, and officials at the Albany, New York Orphan Asylum from the 1880s and 1890s, see Dulberger 1996. As this collection shows, there are similar concerns between parents who have children in the feebleminded institutions and parents with children in the orphan asylum.

5. On the situation of child welfare and institutional services for children in Illinois at the time, see Gittens (1994).

6. Ironically, after the scandal at Lincoln, per capita costs went down, not up. In 1908, the year of the scandal, the per capita cost was $201. By 1916, it had dropped to $165. Most of the decrease was the result of a population increase from 1,153 in 1908 to 1,922 in 1916 (Moore 1928, 102).

7. Some of the most revealing observations by an attendant are in the letters of Grace H. Kent. A Vermonter, Kent was hired in 1920 as a psychologist at the newly opened South Carolina Training School. Soon after her arrival in South Carolina, however, she found that she had to become an attendant, cook, and secretary and was only occasionally a psychologist. Between September 1920 and March 1921, she wrote twenty-one letters home. They make up the third chapter of Whitten's history of the South Carolina school (Whitten 1967). Her letters not only offer a unique perspective on a newly opened facility but also show the tenuous and often complex relationships among staff, inmates, and the community.

8. Seymour B. Sarason (1988, 145) remembered his first position in 1942 as a young psychologist at the Southbury Training School in Connecticut. Although two decades beyond the purview of this chapter, Sarason's experience speaks to this institutional homogeneity. Sarason remembered: "And that was the dark side of life at Southbury: the seemingly endless number of interpersonal, interdepartmental, intradepartmental, sexual, and professional sources of friction. It was one big soap opera. I was not viewing it, I was part of it."

9. I have never found a diary or other detailed remembrances of attendants at institutions for feeble minds. Carrie White Lively's account of her experiences at Central State Hospital in Indiana around 1899 probably comes close to conveying what it must have been like for an attendant at the nearby Indiana State School for Feeble-Minded Youth (Lively 1983). For the perspective of attendants in the early 1970s, see Bogdan, Taylor, de Grandpre, and Haynes (1974) and Hornick (2012).

CHAPTER 5

༄

The Menace of the Feebleminded

At Century's End: Human Weal or Human Woe?

Horatio Alger's death in 1899 hardly marked the end of what Merle Curti (1951, 644–648) called the "cult of the self-made man." Over a period of thirty years, beginning with *Ragged Dick, or Street Life in New York*, published in 1867, Alger wrote 119 popular, much-read books. Discharged from his Massachusetts pulpit in 1866 for the "revolting crime of unnatural familiarity with boys," he transferred his sexual frustration and professional failures into writing potboilers about working-class boys who achieved worldly success (D'Emilio and Freedman 1988, 123). Crucial to their ascendancy in novel after novel were the boys' perseverance, courage, and—above all—their intelligence. Intelligence, although usually linked to other virtues associated with success, was a necessary, if ambiguous, requirement for self-made boys. Most were poor, unpolished, and uneducated. Many were newly arrived immigrants. Yet, besides their pluck and gumption and ability to work hard, the rags-to-riches boys were always intelligent, especially in the ways of commerce and day-to-day survival. Not an effete, academic intelligence, nor a deceitful, dishonest one, the smarts of self-made boys were get-ahead and worldly, but also moral, honest, and fair. Stupid, immoral boys did not become self-made men.

The linkage of intelligence, morality, and success was reproduced not only in Alger's predictable plots but also in "thousands of tons of books based on the very acceptable theme of the individual rising above his surroundings to a triumphant material success" (Curti 1951, 648). Adult literature had its parallel, if less singular, spokespersons. Before World War I, self-help authors like Russell Conwell and Orison Swett Marden and novelists like Owen Wister, Frank Norris, Hamlin Garland, and Edgar Rice Burroughs extolled the virtues of strong, successful men.

Even the poor and the uncouth could be successful. By relying on their own abilities, skills, and know-how, little men could become big men.

Marden published 250 editions of *Pushing the Front; or, Success under Difficulties, a Book of Inspiration and Encouragement to All Who Are Struggling for Self-Respect along the Paths of Knowledge and of Duty* (1894). By 1920, three million Americans had purchased his books. Working his way through Boston University and later making a fortune in advertising and resorts, Marden was broke after the panic of 1893. Indeed, his first book was an attempt to come back from financial ruin. Preaching a gospel of success through positive thinking and self-confidence even in the midst of a national depression, Marden represented the popular outcome of an optimistic undercurrent at the *fin de siècle* (Connolly 1925; Curti 1951, 649–650).

Women, too, began to develop their own cult of success. More than ever before, the measure of success for the modern woman was her success as a wife and mother. At the same time, the roles of wife and mother were crucial to newly emerging concerns: child development on the one hand and marital success on the other. As reproduction replaced production as the principal function of the family, women's sexuality became more obvious and more problematic. The Gibson Girl became a new ideal for unmarried and even married middle-class women at the turn of the century. Tall and beautiful, strong and even a bit athletic, she reflected a new, although still ambivalent, sexuality. Like her male counterpart, the modern young woman could take chances. Indeed, her success depended on her ability to take risks and experience new freedom, avoiding the slavery of early marriage and unwanted children.

Once marriage and child-rearing began, however, the successful woman, freed from the drudgery of endless chores in the modern household, had time to pass on risk-taking to her children, to use her skills to promote her husband's rising social prominence, and even develop her own civic interests and responsibilities. Women's magazines of the period, such as the *Ladies' Home Journal* and *Woman's Home Companion*, provided in issue after issue advice on becoming more successful as a mother and wife. Although the measure of her success was quite different from that of either her husband or her brother, the successful woman in 1900 shared with them two attributes: she was intelligent, and she was moral. To be sure, as physicians and popular writers of the period warned her, the overuse of her brain might make her ill. Nevertheless, the modern, successful woman required intelligence and propriety to develop her children's "self-made" self-image, promote her husband's social affairs, and also keep herself active in the various "self-made" social commitments expected of her (S. Rothman 1978; M. Ryan 2006, 201–244).

Interestingly enough, this cult of success for both men and women allowed for the success not only of members of poor and working classes but also of people with disabling physical and mental conditions. Helen Keller's story was well known to Americans at the turn of the century (e.g., Keller 1903, 1905). Because of her superior intelligence, she had even surpassed Laura Bridgman, Samuel G. Howe's blind and deaf student of the previous generation, succeeding not only at Perkins

Institute but also at Radcliffe. Keller raised herself to prominent success through hard work, courage, and brains. In 1897, Charles Steinmetz, a hunchbacked, nearsighted immigrant, published *Theory and Calculation of Alternating Current Phenomena.* Few people understood it, but Steinmetz's fame soon followed. Popular magazines made Steinmetz an American hero. His disability seemed to magnify, not diminish, his popularity. Thomas Edison, another man interested in electricity, was deaf. Popular literature for children and adults marveled at his achievements despite his handicap. In 1908, Clifford Beers published *A Mind That Found Itself.* Beers, the scion of well-to-do New Englanders, had been hospitalized after a suicidal attempt brought on by a delusional belief that he was about to become epileptic. After three years in various psychiatric hospitals, he wrote about his experiences, describing them as brutal and cruel. With the backing of prominent psychiatrists, academics, and philanthropists, he later launched what would become the influential mental hygiene movement. Demonstrating that even a crazy man could pull himself out of the mire of insanity, Beers in the first and second decades of the new century extended the cult of success to mentally handicapped people (A. Deutsch 1937, 302–310). Despite their afflictions, physical or mental, with persistence, courage, intelligence, and good living, some disabled Americans succeeded and went on, especially in popular literature, to become examples for others. Again, intelligence and morality were important elements of their rags-to-riches (or disability-to-overcoming-disability) stories.

The effect of this cult of success on feebleminded people and their families at the turn of the century is nearly impossible to document and assess. Cultural effects, though powerful, are not easy to measure in people, even in those who leave written reminders. What is reasonably certain is that the success motif, with all its accompanying aspirations and mythology, affected American citizens during this period of rapid national growth and change. Feeble minds and their families could not have remained unaffected. That feeble minds were the embodied antithesis of late nineteenth-century success must have been felt, sometimes painfully so. At the turn of the century, Charles Eliot Norton, professor and former president of Harvard University and editor of the *North American Review*, advocated for "the painless destruction" of insane and deficient minds. Newspapers throughout the nation printed stories about Norton's position, for example, "Dr. Charles Eliot Norton, Who Favors Death for Hopelessly Incurable Persons" ([ca. 1896]; see also Norton 1896; Lavi 2005).

Letters from parents in the Beverly Farm records suggest that they absorbed these constructions. "I have hoped that you could teach the boy to eat things that he ought to eat and in a decent manner," wrote a Texas aunt, "to tie his shoes and such little things, and to read and write a little of course his father hopes for more than that, but it seems to me it will be a long time before he can do much more" (Beverly Farm Records, letter to W. H. C. Smith, December 6, 1913). A father from Chicago wondered "whether our little girl is beginning to find herself, or show indications of substantial improvement. I should dislike to be informed to the contrary, and we are hoping and praying that through the instrumentality of your direction and service she may be restored to normal condition" (Beverly Farm Records, letter to W. H. C. Smith, March 23, 1917). An attorney from Oklahoma wrote Smith about his daughter:

> We hope to have a letter from you any day now, telling us how our little one is getting on in her new home. The little details, such of them as you can give, will be appreciated. The crumbs, even, will feed graciously our hungry hearts. And also, as soon as you have made up your mind, or formulated your judgment about her case, we shall hope to hear about that, and will not ask you to conceal or withhold, but will submit to, and prefer, perfect frankness, in so far as your conclusions enable you to announce a clear judgment. (Beverly Farm Records, letter to W. H. C. Smith, October 7, 1913)

Superintendents, who of course left more records than did the parents and relatives of feeble minds, were quick to talk about their age as a time of hustle and bustle in which feeble minds were always left behind. Especially in cities, where success or failure became not only a cultural preoccupation but indeed a fundamental norm, being feebleminded or having a feebleminded child or feebleminded sibling threatened to violate the preoccupation and defy the norm.[1] Without a head, one could not get ahead. Having a child or brother or sister without a head also made getting ahead a more difficult proposition. If this powerful, yet subtle cultural development affected the popular image of success and—by implication—failure, it was also reflected in scientific, literary, religious, and sociopolitical movements of the period. Being not the rationalistic optimism of a century earlier nor the romantic optimism of the 1840s, faith in progress at the end of the century combined elements of social Darwinism and a better understanding of heredity with a concern for race purification and perfection.

Herbert Spencer and his American disciple, William Graham Sumner, were optimistic about the improvement of human beings in the modern age. They believed that the relationships between human beings at all levels of interaction could be reduced to scientific principles. Reinforced by Darwin's observations on the natural order of plants and animals, the social Darwinists were confident of their understanding of the relationship of people in the social order. That order was governed by what Spencer called "the survival of the fittest." The social order bound by this survival principle was as fixed and as "natural" as those principles governing the natural order. To tamper with the natural order risked jeopardizing the operation of nature itself. Social relations, not unlike animal migratory behavior or gravity, had their grounding in the natural order of things. Not surprisingly, Spencer and Sumner emphasized a laissez-faire opposition to governmental involvement in the social order. What nature dictated, people in their collective activities should modify only with great caution and then only during unusual circumstances. Knowledge of these principles and proper application of them ensured social progress. Although unsure that leaders would have the resolve to act on them, the social Darwinists were confident of the principles of social relations and of the potential of those principles to free people from the mistakes of their former ignorance.

Linked with social Darwinism was a growing interest in heredity. Darwin and his generation had remained puzzled by the mechanics of heredity. But later theorists began to illuminate its mysteries. Francis Galton, influenced by his cousin, Charles Darwin, and Spencer, used the idle time created by the same fortune that sustained Darwin to speculate throughout his long life on the characteristics of human variation. For Galton, and later for his pupil, Karl Pearson, aggregate differences among people showed two fundamental attributes. First, aggregate differences tended to take mathematical shapes allowing interested parties like Galton and Pearson to predict over a given population the variation of a given variable such as height, weight, or intelligence. Second, although wide differences existed among aggregate groups of people on many dimensions, differences among generations of people did not show such variations. Thus, human characteristics appeared to distribute themselves randomly in the population with wide variation; yet, within families, they appeared to remain fairly stable (J. Brown 1992; Chase 1977; Gillham 2001; Gould 1981; J. Haller 1971).

At the turn of the century, Hugo de Vries, William Bateson, and others were drawing on the work of Gregor Mendel to develop new understandings of heredity. Their ideas at first challenged Galton and Pearson but were eventually integrated into their mathematically grounded theories of heredity. By 1930, this integration would lead to a view of heredity that recognized its aggregate regularity but also acknowledged individual variation caused by random mutation. Attracting old-order conservatives and new-day racists, the exploration of hereditary differences also included liberals like Pearson, H. S. Jennings, and Cyril Burt and socialists like J. B. S. Haldane and Hermann J. Muller (Chase 1977; Cravens 1978; Fredrickson 1965, 199–216; Gould 2002, 418–426; M. Haller 1963; Kevles 1985; Ludmerer 1972; Paul 1995; Pastore 1949).

Often associated (although not always ideologically) with social Darwinism and the growing interest in heredity was a concern for race purification and human perfection. Galton had first used the term *eugenics* in 1883, and this term became applied to the movement it inspired. Between 1890 and 1920, the eugenics movement gained the interest of virtually all American scientists working on problems of heredity. At the same time, it captured the curiosity of philanthropists, social scientists, and physicians while also drawing a devoted, if not large, public following, including optimists who saw in eugenics a solution to social problems through better human breeding. During its period of scientific respectability, which ended soon after World War I, the movement attracted people from across the political spectrum, from the Ku Klux Klan and National Socialists to various left-wingers. Although it always maintained a progressive wing, its linkage with reactionary ideology sustained the movement and shapes our perception of it today. After 1920, when some scientists began to disassociate themselves from eugenics, the movement still had enough respectability and financial support to keep itself going, but enthusiasm for it among most academic scientists had waned by the beginning of World War II, only to find a new beginning after the war in its active, if publically subdued, support for sterilization (Gallagher 1999; M. Haller 1963; Hasain 1996; Kevles 1985; Leonard 2005; Paul 1995; Pickens 1968; A. Stern 2005). Even in 1934, Leon Whitney, executive secretary of the American Eugenics Society, boasted: "Eugenics is being taught now in three-quarters of our 500 colleges

and universities, and in many high and preparatory schools," and the public remained aware of eugenics through magazine writings, Sunday morning sermons,
and "better-baby" and "fitter-family" contests sponsored by various eugenicists.
Likewise, social reformers like the Massachusetts physician Clarence Gamble promoted eugenic sterilization well into the 1960s (Dorey 1999; Glenna et al. 2007;
Grinspoon 2013; Rosen 2004; L. Whitney 1934, 288).

The principal goal of the eugenics movement was the translation of scientific
information about heredity into social policies that would lead to the prevention
of human stock prone to degeneracy. Complementing this goal was the belief in
euthenics, a science that promoted the reproduction of superior human stock. Race
purification advocates stressed that through the prevention of inferior stock and
the reproduction of good stock, problems that had always plagued human beings—
poverty, crime and vice, unwanted children, insanity, and feeblemindedness—
could be eliminated. "Purebreeding" would not merely ameliorate these social
problems, not merely sustain their victims while ensuring a new generation of
victims, but would end them. Science, not sentimental goodwill or public paternalism, would lead the way to a truly effective means of social change. Margaret
Sanger and Charles Henderson, Theodore Roosevelt and Woodrow Wilson, Andrew
Carnegie and Mary Harriman, E. A. Ross and Franklin Giddings, G. Stanley Hall and
E. G. Boring, David Starr Jordan and Luther Burbank, Washington Gladden and
Walter Rauschenbusch—all progressives (of one form or another)—were during
part or most of their public lives attracted to and supportive of eugenics (Leonard
2003, 2005; see also Childs 2001; Hasain 1996; Sklansky 2002, 195–203).

The cult of the self-made man grounded in the potentiality of science to lib-
erate human beings from ignorance and outdated beliefs was not the only tradition shaping American consciousness at the turn of the century. Alger and Marden
might point to the payoff of hard work, optimism, and risk-taking, but intense
social stress at the end of the century frustrated the adoption of these values. The
deepest depression in American history (to that time), beginning in 1893; the massive shifting of textile jobs from Northern to Southern states; labor unrest, with
strikes by coal miners in Pennsylvania and Ohio, garment workers in New York, and
railroad workers throughout the Midwest; the alarm created by Coxey's Army; the
rise of Jim Crow in reaction to hard times; the enormous immigration of Eastern
Europeans and the corresponding demands for immigrant restriction; and the generation and concentration of great wealth in the hands of a few "robber barons"—all
proved to many Americans even before the devastation of World War I the frailty
of success and optimism. For many, the period was exciting and challenging; for
others, it was frightening and destructive (Folsom 1991, 148–186).

If the optimists had their Horatio Algers and Herbert Spencers, the pessimists,
too, had both their popular spokespersons and intellectual advocates. Old-guard
conservatives like Henry Adams saw little good in the nouveaux riches Americans
with their high hopes and low brows. Writers, artists, and intellectuals loosely
known as Naturalists, whose attraction to science enlightened their art but left
them melancholy about human nature, saw science as the unraveler of a dark and
unmanageable side of human existence.

Ironically, both pessimists and optimists of the period were drawn to the same social currents: social Darwinism, a preoccupation with heredity, and eugenics. But pessimists reacted differently to them, not in the intensity of their faith in employing these tools for the service of the social order but in how they drew on them to understand what they believed was the rapid degeneration of order, traditional social arrangements, and, indeed, Western civilization. Not unlike the progressives of the period, some pessimists hoped to "improve" the social order by stemming the tide of irrationality and degeneracy. If things could not get better, at least destruction might be postponed. For other pessimists, however, destruction could not be postponed; rather, out of destruction, they believed, must come a new world order based on a superindividuality. Linked with old-order values, images, and traditions, this new order would be based on the will and power of those with special, superior endowments. Thus, late nineteenth-century pessimism, like optimism, had its own irony.

By 1917, the pessimistic outlook seems to have prevailed. It was most evident in how Americans responded to racial and immigration issues. As early as the 1840s, Americans had shown concern for the odd ways and peculiarities of the immigrant. After 1890, the increase of swarthy Eastern Europeans, mostly Catholic or Jewish, only served to heighten the concern. Following immigrant restrictions in the 1880s, Congress created the office of Superintendent of Immigration in 1891, opened Ellis Island the next year, and, in the midst of economic depression in 1897, passed a literacy requirement for immigrants that was, however, vetoed by President Cleveland. In 1891, some citizens in New Orleans lynched eleven immigrants newly arrived from Italy. Three years later, several recent Harvard graduates formed the Immigrant Restriction League. Anti-immigration sentiment was further fueled by international racist perspectives. American and European imperialism reflected the sentiment of "the white man's burden." Kipling's 1899 poem of the same title was read and supported by Americans from Theodore Roosevelt to Jack London, from Samuel Gompers to Booker T. Washington to Andrew Carnegie. When Leon Czolgosz shot and killed President William McKinley in 1901, Americans were enraged but not shocked. After all, most immigrants were known to be, or to have the potential for being, anarchists (Dolmage 2011; Fairchild 2003; Higham 1963; Knox 1914; Ludmerer 1972).

The twentieth century only increased the willingness of Congress to slow the influx of foreigners. By 1900, one out of every seven Americans was foreign-born. In the great cities of the east, this ratio was even narrower. With the support of poorly organized labor and better organized business, Congress enacted the Immigration Restriction Act of 1924. With business having all the cheap labor it could absorb and labor afraid of more competition for jobs, Congress finished off what had started three decades earlier as a campaign among American bluebloods fearing racial and cultural impurity.

To be sure, racism's history in America went back to the Virginia colony. The brand of racism that began to develop after the Civil War, however, had its nadir in the 1890s. Jim Crow might have had its origins in slavery, but economic depression, immigrant influx, and competition between working-class whites and blacks in the 1890s gave this racism its particular form—a form that would persist well into the twentieth century. Thus, the *Plessy v. Ferguson* ruling in 1896 made complete sense in the social context of the period. Racist sentiment, of course, permeated American consciousness, overlapping with native white fears not only of blacks but also of Eastern Europeans, Mexicans and Central Americans, and East Asians. These fears found their sustenance among intellectuals and social welfare advocates of the period.

Even before Thomas Dixon's novel *The Clansman* (1905), the basis of America's first epic film, *Birth of a Nation* (1915), portrayed noble white Southerners defending their superior, albeit broken, way of life against atavistic black rapists and their conniving Yankee "toe holders," the literature of racism had stirred the anxieties of many Americans in popular magazines and novels. From politicians and preachers, Americans became absorbed in Jim Crow. Added to the American literature were the writings of the British-turned-German publicist Houston Chamberlain (1911) and France's Comte Joseph-Arthur de Gobineau (1915), which only increased white American curiosity about and concern for what both writers claimed were the intellectually inferior but physically strong and promiscuous dark races. Later, the writings of Madison Grant (1916, 1930, 1933), Lothrop Stoddard (1920, 1923, 1924), Charles Davenport (1911; Davenport and Steggerda 1929), Samuel J. Holmes (1921), Albert Edward Wiggam (1922, 1925), and others integrated Jim Crow with European racism to create a unique early twentieth-century American racism. No longer limited to blacks, this Americanized European racism linked Dixon's clansman to Chamberlain's myth of Aryan superiority (see also Dixon 1902).

Between 1890 and 1930, the racism encouraged by popular literature became reflected in the lynching of blacks and "foreigners." Both the literature and the lynching became acceptable. William Graham Sumner, a conservative, and E. A. Ross, a liberal, although horrified by the murdering of blacks, both accepted the fate bestowed on "oxlike men . . . descendants to those who always stayed behind" (Degler 1991, 13–19; Gossett 1965, 272–273; Leonard 2003, 2005; E. Ross 1914, 286; Sklansky 2002, 193–202).

In addition to revealing itself in the country's attitudes toward race and immigration, America's multifaceted pessimism also found expression in other movements. Known in America and in Europe as Naturalism, a new, secular perspective saw within urban American society the loss of innocence, spontaneity, and ultimately freedom. In the writings of Theodore Dreiser, Jack London, Frank Norris, and Steven Crane, and of Europeans like Joseph Conrad, Thomas Hardy, and Matthew Arnold; and in the paintings of artists such as Winslow Homer (*The Gulf Stream*) and Thomas Eakins (*Between Rounds*), heroes or heroines were overshadowed by forces bigger than themselves. Reality embodied in grim and grimy city life made heroes of ordinary people, all trying to survive and get ahead, and all at the mercy of forces that could destroy them. In this portrayal of survival of the fittest, understanding the scientific conclusions of social Darwinism did not engender the sort of optimism Spencer had implied. Being free, the essence of the liberal spirit, left Americans at the beginning of the new century confronting forces over which they had only limited control. Linked with racist sentiment of the time, some American Naturalists saw hordes of immigrants, promiscuous blacks, and mindless European radicals challenging the freedoms and traditions cherished by native white Americans. Most Naturalists, principally the Europeans, were not at all optimistic about the ability of individuals to change the course of urban, mindless industrialization. Americans like Norris, Dreiser, and London, while more hopeful, were nonetheless realistic about the ugliness, cruelty, and impersonality of modern life. Unlike Christian fundamentalists of the period, they had no way out. The only transcendence they could muster was either in a hope for a greater awareness from the shock caused by their novels or in a longing for the mythological purity embodied in a primitive Aryanism. From Grimm's fairy tales to Wagner's operas, from Klimt's murals to Mahler's music, from London's novels to Madison Grant's essays, from the wave of anti-urban, outdoor camping to a growing domestic militarism, this desire for transcending modern superficiality and modern ennui for a pure, primitive, "manly" essence became a secular, if incomplete, escape from the world of the mundane, ugly, and flaccid here-and-now. In Europe, of course, this desire emphasized a hyper individualistic philosophy of strongmen, which in its most distorted form provided an intellectual justification for an emerging National Socialism. In America, it manifested itself as an ever-frustrated strongman, like Jay Gatsby, whose sense of superiority ultimately destroyed him.

In this maelstrom of perspectives, some pointing to human weal and some to human woe, views about *mental defectives*, a term that began to be used for feeble minds (eventually replacing it), began to change dramatically. Along with these new views, of course, came calls for new social policies to deal with the newly defined problem. Redefined in the context of new social aspirations and fears, mental defectives in the first decade of the new century began to be seen in more places, in greater numbers, and associated with more and more social problems. Partly of science and partly not, the new social policies advocated by professionals, supported by philanthropists, and legislated by elected officials put mental defectives on the most prominent public agenda they had ever enjoyed. Unlike any other time in American history, the fear of them and the pity for them were at their most extreme. Were mental defectives the greatest source of human vice, misery, and corruption, staining the social fabric with their amoral, promiscuous stupidity? Or were they perpetual children, who only needed happiness and love to adjust to a confusing social order?

CONSTRUCTING THE MENACE OF THE FEEBLEMINDED

With one important exception, the period 1890–1910 was one of solidifying and expanding old policies, not creating new ones. The exception, special education, although becoming a national issue among professionals and philanthropists, remained primarily a local concern. The expansion of old policies and the development of an important new one nevertheless inaugurated a level of urgency more intense than in any other period in the history of intellectual disability in America. Reaching a near hysterical pitch between 1910 and 1920, this urgency moved the field in new, if not always consistent, directions. By World War I, the image of feeble minds created by professionals in the previous decades had shifted to a view of mental defectives that, unlike previous views, began to penetrate American consciousness. More than a shift of labels, the new term suggested new meaning and the necessity for a new social response. The pitiable, but potentially productive, antebellum idiot and the burdensome imbecile of the post-Civil War years gave way to the menacing and increasingly well-known defective of the teens. What made this new image so threatening and ensured acute concerns and shrill warnings was the increasing insistence in the first and second decades of the new century that mental defectives, in their amorality and fecundity, were not only linked with social vices but indeed were the most prominent and persistent cause of those vices. Graduating from being merely associated with social vices to being their fundamental cause, mental defectives became a menace, the control of which was an urgent necessity for existing and future generations.

This apparently dramatic shift, from a burden to a menace, had antecedents in professional and sociopolitical developments in the 1890s and early 1900s. Never idle, superintendents were quick to manipulate the anxieties created by rapidly changing social and economic conditions in America. Never in control of those conditions, however, the superintendents were not always able to shape policies free from unexpected consequences. Their own positions in the institution, too, led them to public pronouncements sometimes incongruent with their personal feelings. The menacing mental defective of whom they spoke with such opprobrium was surely not the same sweet defective they referred to in their private correspondence and autobiographies. These contradictory expressions (between the public rhetoric and the private remembrances) never freed the superintendents from the inconsistencies of the policies they supported between 1890 and 1920. Others not in day-to-day contact with defective minds could make claims about the menacing feeble mind without misgivings or inconsistencies. Although the apparent effects of heredity and the fears of uncontrolled vice suspended their personal feelings for a time, most superintendents still knew the names and faces of specific people under their care. By 1920, their rhetoric had begun to subside even as the mindsets and policies they had so vigorously championed lingered. Indeed, the histrionic rhetoric of the previous decade found expression in the routine of established policies of the 1920s and later decades.

Total Institutionalization

By 1900, virtually all superintendents acknowledged that mental defectives safely in the confines of the institution were not a menace to society. J. M. Murdoch (1909), superintendent of the Western Pennsylvania Institution for the Feeble-Minded, in a report to the National Conference of Charities and Correction with the ominous title "Quarantine Mental Defectives," claimed that efforts to prevent feeblemindedness through institutional segregation would "prevent more misery, pauperism, degeneracy and crime and do more for the upbuilding of our race than any other measure within the power of man." Although sometimes troublesome, particularly if they were high grades of childbearing age, such defectives were controllable in the institution. Some superintendents, like Elwyn Institute's Martin Barr, had hoped for and even written about the total institutionalization of all feeble minds. Before meetings of the American Association for the Study of the Feeble-Minded and before groups in Pennsylvania, Barr (1902*b*) was enthusiastic about the prospect:

> As one by one our institutions become patriarchal, having received successive generations of defectives, we find growing upon the pages of their reports a clearly implied interrogation; "We have trained, for—what?"
>
> Without formal expression emanating from our association as a body there is yet, I believe, a concensus [*sic*] that abandons the hope long cherished of a return of the imbecile to the world.
>
> Now if this conviction arrived at through long experience and much disappointment involves principles affecting the progress of our work and the welfare of children and of society, ought we to be backward in declaring it? And in failing to do so do we not rather underestimate the value of our association to science and to the world at large? If we do not speak authoritatively upon the subject, who shall? And how, then, are legislators and others to be enlightened as to the futility of hopes which the very progress of our work has tended to foster? Indeed, I think we need to write it very large, in characters that he who runs may read, to convince the world that by permanent segregation only is the imbecile to be safe-guarded from certain deterioration and society from depredation, contamination, and increase of a pernicious element....
>
> An ideal spot might be found—either on one of the newly acquired islands, the unoccupied lands of the Atlantic seaboard, or the far West which, under proper regulations, could be made a true haven of irresponsibility, and deriving its population as it would from the trained workers from the institutions throughout the country, might become in time almost if not entirely self-sustaining.

If this goal of total, permanent institutionalization was to succeed, it would have to be, among other things, financially appealing to state lawmakers. Calling for a "third epoch in our history" (the first being Seguin's "experimental" school and the second the custodial institution), Barr (1897; see also 1898) drew on familiar as well as new themes. "Community life," as he labeled this epoch, consisted of communities of feeble minds housed by grade and segregated from society on a reservation or an island or in some other isolated place. Self-sufficient and nearly self-operated, the "feebleminded communities" would have imbeciles trained to care for idio-imbeciles, idiots, and epileptics. Moral imbeciles would be desexed and would join ordinary imbeciles in the care of the institution. By establishing these communities, society could "avert general and widespread calamity" caused by sexually promiscuous, licentious imbeciles. Also, the third epoch would provide a Utopian environment where feeble minds of all grades "in the possession of an assured freedom—always under careful direction and supervision—enjoy happiness and protection in lieu of ignorance, degradation, and ignominy."

A year later, Barr (1898, 487–488) justified the morality of this total incarceration in *International Journal of Ethics*. To an audience of ethicists, he argued that, just as the United States "government is caring for the deaf-mute, the Indian, and the negro; then why should it not care for this race which is once more helpless and more aggressive, which is incapable of self-preservation and fast becoming a standing peril to the nation?" There was open land in the West and undeveloped acreage in the East that could be used for "permanent sequestration under happiest conditions." If the deaf-mute, the Indian, and the Negro could be segregated from ordinary society for their own happiness, then so should the feebleminded receive the same privilege.

And what were the future benefits of this "total community"? Barr claimed that it would take feeble minds who were not productive out of society, where they were "not conducive to the national prosperity." Also, it would remove them from the common schools, which must function to "train people for social living." In the institution rather than in the work force or the school, high-grades would acquire their "productive potential," and low-grades would receive the constant care that neither the productive family nor the school could give. To this future of communities for virtually all mental defectives, the Association of Medical Officers must focus its efforts. Barr (1899) admonished its membership:

> One hundred thousand of the feebleminded in the United States alone, constantly increasing by birth and immigration, and not one-tenth provided for in institutions. The rest crowd our schools, walk our streets and fill alike jails and positions of trust, reproducing their kind and vitiating the moral atmosphere. Science and experience have searched them out and classified them as here presented, but hundreds of their brethren are desolating homes, paralyzing the energies of normal people, or suffer in prison cells, the innocent perpetrators not of crime, but of motiveless acts.

Although he had acknowledged the place of public schools in differentiating feebleminded from normal children and in training some of them before they reached childbearing age, Barr had continued to see the state institution as the principal locus of care and protection. The local school, Barr stressed, should function to differentiate normals from abnormals, not to care and protect the latter. By 1914, Johnson in Indiana; his brother-in-law E. R. Johnstone, the director at Vineland in New Jersey; and others were seeing a more important, if secondary, role for the public schools: "We are beginning with the assumption that a number of feebleminded children, up to the time of puberty, may properly be cared for in their own homes. To this end we are promoting special classes in the public schools" (Johnson 1914). In good homes and with proper training in special classes, preadolescent mental defectives and "backward children" could be socialized to enter the protection of the state facility at puberty. Special classes and special schools would become the "preparatory schools" and the *leitmotiv* of the institution.

Special Education

Special education for children whom educators believed could not comply with the demands of public schools began in the United States in the 1890s. Closely associated with it was a rapid increase in the number of states adding or strengthening compulsory public school attendance laws. Before the Civil War, only Massachusetts had required some form of mandatory school attendance. Between 1865 and 1882, six more states added compulsory attendance laws; between 1883 and 1889, nine states; and between 1890 and 1907, eleven more states. By 1907, the only states without mandatory attendance laws were in the South, but by 1918 they had passed them.

Following the lead of Massachusetts in requiring school attendance, most states' earliest requirements were lax, having exemptions for poor families, families involved in agriculture, and families with sick or disabled children. Given these liberal rules, public school attendance was sporadic, and habitual truancy was common and, until the 1880s, usually overlooked. By the 1880s, state legislatures first in the Northeast and then in the Midwest began to strengthen their requirements for attendance. Leading the way in 1873 was again Massachusetts. Its third compulsory attendance law required local school boards to develop plans to enforce the law.

Although most state laws remained weak until the turn of the century, the tightening of compulsory attendance requirements paralleled the diminution of child labor in American industry. As immigration expanded between 1890 and 1910 and a large pool of adult labor began to supplant child labor, state after state began to find alternative places for working-class children. By 1890, courts began to recognize the rights of states to provide schools for children. Interestingly enough, most decisions of that decade assumed public education was for the protection and safety of the community and not for the benefit of the child or a child's right. School attendance laws in the states in the Midwest and South dependent on farming and the Southern states with growing textile industries, where there was still a demand for child labor, were slower to come and easier to ignore (Good 1962, 375–379; J. Jones 1992, 158–165).

With states adding and enforcing compulsory school attendance laws, it was only a short time before local school boards were extending the length of the school year and the number of grades of required attendance. The earliest public schools provided for twelve-week school years for children between the ages of eight and fourteen. By 1880, many states had added fourteen- and fifteen-year-olds, and some states had extended their requirements to eighteen-year-olds, thus initiating required high school attendance. At the same time, most states began to develop a late September to early June school year (Good 1962, 380; see also Sarason and Doris 1979, 240–279).

Compulsory attendance laws enacted in the last half of the century and enforced in the century's last decade provided the context for the creation of special education. As Lawrence Cremin (1961, 127–128) put it, "Compulsory school attendance marked a new era in the history of American education. The crippled, the blind, the deaf, the sick, the slow-witted, and the needy arrived in growing numbers. Thousands of recalcitrants and incorrigibles who in former times might have dropped out of school now became public charges for a minimum period." He went on, "Compulsory schooling provided both the problem and the opportunity of the progressives; its very existence inexorably conditioned every attempt at educational innovation during the decades preceding World War I." Although Cremin noted that in previous times "the slow-witted" had often dropped out of school, he might have added that often they never attended public schools in the first place.

Most schools exempted the obviously disabled. If parents did not want to send their children to public schools because they were idiotic or slow, school officials had little motivation to demand attendance, especially if the parents' assessment was apparent. The obviously impaired remained at home or were placed in institutions.

Beginning in the 1880s and particularly in the 1890s, public schools began to receive among their enlarging pool of pupils children who were not obviously feeble-minded but "slow and backward," as defined by school officials. Within the context of the newly emerging public schools with their stricter attendance laws, students who previously had not attended school but otherwise appeared to be normal were now part of the school population. Not yet influenced by the writings of John Dewey or the growing emphasis on vocational education, most teachers of the period dealt with the rapid increase in pupils by teaching what they knew—traditional academic subjects. Emphasis remained as it always had more on the subject of instruction than on its method. Even in the primary grades, where instructional methods were of greater concern, the goal was still academic and the methods still emphasized rote memorization and drills. Some teachers might be "natural teachers," but no one particularly knew why. Few up to this time had thought much about how to teach. The impact of large numbers of children would, in the 1890s, change this emphasis.

At first, educators did not emphasize a distinction between students who would not and those who could not learn. Not surprisingly, difficult and apparently delinquent children were often identified as slow and apparently mentally defective children. Reports of teacher frustration, class disruption, and educational inefficiency began to appear. No doubt the impetus for change, the reports were also a rationale for new policies that were matters of convenience.

Whether new problems or large numbers of new pupils were the greatest impetus for creating segregated classes and segregated schools was not entirely clear even to the pioneer special educators of the 1890s. Around 1895, Mary McDowell organized a "vacation school for feebleminded children" at the University of Chicago's settlement house. Supported by the Chicago Women's Club, the school operated in the summer and emphasized its work with "backward" children, most of whom were immigrants having difficulties in the public schools (Powell 1900; Wilson 1928, 25–35). In 1893, Will S. Monroe, a Stanford researcher, sent letters to several hundred public school teachers in California asking them to record information about their pupils. The teachers accumulated data on 10,842 students, noting irregularities of pupils' features, movement, or speech and whether they were maimed or paralyzed, had a history of fits, exhibited low nutrition, or were mentally dull, feebleminded, imbecilic, or idiotic. In his report on the survey (1894), Monroe stated that almost 9 percent of all pupils fell into the category of mentally dull, another 2 percent were feebleminded, but only 6 of the 10,842 students were considered imbeciles or idiots. Anticipating questions raised by mental testers more than a decade later, Monroe asked, "But what of the remaining eight or nine per cent who are yet much below the general average [but are not feeble minded]? Are they to over-crowd our special institutions, by adding to the states' burden? Or are they to remain a hindrance to the 90 or more per cent of normal children of the community?" Answering his own questions, he stated:

In the larger cities and towns, some segregation would be possible, where a specialist might take small classes of the "mentally dull" and "feebly-gifted mentally" and give them such individual instruction as their peculiar defect required. In Norway, I am told, there are such schools for exceptional children, and that in these schools no teacher is permitted to have more than 12 children in her care. Why not have such schools in the United States?

As Monroe and others knew, European schools had already created special instruction for slow learners in reaction to their compulsory attendance laws. By 1900, Prussia, the Scandinavian countries, England, Switzerland, and Austria had created such classes. In 1896, school administrators in Providence, Rhode Island, opened the first public special education class in the United States. Beginning with fifteen higher grade pupils, the class opened in a fire station (Providence School Committee 1896–97). Soon, one city after another followed with classes in Springfield, Massachusetts, in 1897; Chicago, in 1898; Boston, in 1899; New York, in 1900; Philadelphia, in 1901; Los Angeles, in 1902; Detroit, in 1903; and Washington, D.C., Bridgeport, Connecticut, and Rochester in 1906 (Wallin 1914). By 1913, 108 cities had special classes and special schools; ten years later, more than sixty additional cities had added classes and schools. In 1923, 33,971 students were in the nation's various special education programs (Fernald 1924; M. Haller 1963, 95; Osgood 2000, 57–59, 127–146). Growth continued until the Great Depression, resuming after World War II (Crissey 1975).

Interest in the special classes and schools spread as they began to multiply and expand (Figure 5.1, Figure 5.2, Figure 5.3). At the beginning of 1918, the *Survey*

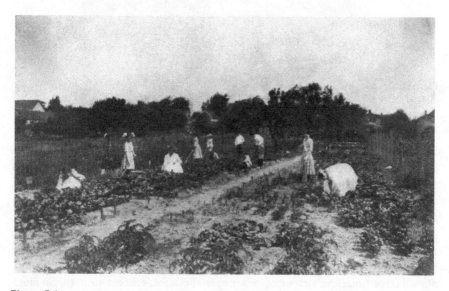

Figure 5.1:
Special classes, Rochester, ca. 1910. (From the *Journal of Psycho-Asthenics*, 1912)

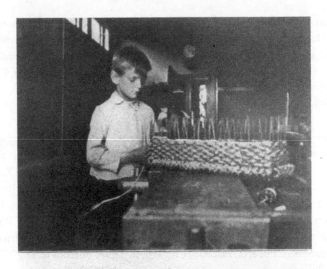

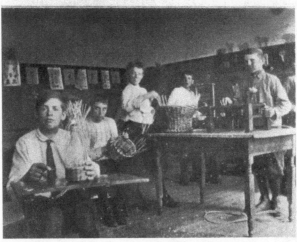

Figure 5.2:
Special classes, Rochester, ca. 1910. (From the *Journal of Psycho-Asthenics*, 1912)

headlined an anonymously written article, "The Passing of the Dunce's Stool." Its author noted: "Special classes have grown so rapidly of late that few states have any carefully worked out program with respect to them" ("The Passing of the Dunce's Stool" 1918). Commenting on a study conducted by the Massachusetts League for Preventive Work, the article's author noted a survey of fifty school systems. Twelve had classes exclusively for feeble minds, thirteen for backward children, and sixteen for both feeble minds and the backward; nine had programs in which pupils were given extra help in regular classes. The author concluded that virtually all large American cities had either special classes, schools, or both. So much attention seemed to be focused on the "special child," a term that teachers and

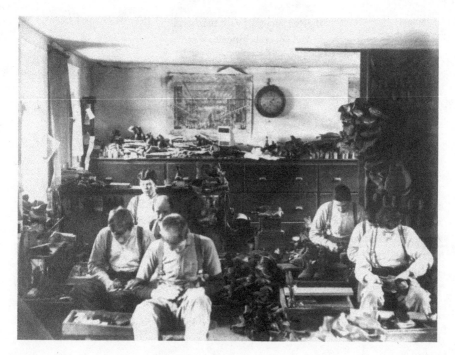

Figures 5.3:
Special classes, Rochester, ca. 1910. (From the *Jurnal of Psycho-Asthenics*, 1912)

school administrators were just beginning to use, that one teacher, May Ayres, was prompted to write a satirical poem, "The Wail of the Well," which appeared in the *American School Board Journal* (cited in Johnstone 1923, 79–80):

> Johnny Jones has lost a leg,
>   Fanny's deaf and dumb,
> Marie has epileptic fits,
>   Tom's eyes are on the bum,
> Sadie stutters when she talks,
>   Mabel has T.B.
> Morris is a splendid case of
>   Imbecility.
> Billy Brown's a truant,
>   And Harold is a thief;
> Teddy's parents give him dope,
>   And so he came to grief.
>
> Gwendolin's a millionaire,
>   Jerald is a fool;
> So everyone of these darned kids
>   Goes to a special school.

They've specially nice teachers,
   And special things to wear,
And special time to play in,
   And special kind of air;
They've special lunches, right in school,
   While I—it makes me wild!
I haven't any specialities—
   I'm just a normal child.

Although the poem reflected the diversity of problems dealt with by special education, most specially educated children were slow learners, and it was to them that
special educators directed most of their attention. By 1900, these slow learners
were divided into two general categories: the mentally deficient and the backward.
Added to these groups were disorderly students, many, if not most, of whom educators believed fell in the backward category (Fernald 1904a). As Lydia G. Chace
reported in 1904, imbecile and idiotic children were for the most part cared for
in the institution, not in the school. At New York's Public School No. 1 on the
Lower East Side, school officials in 1902 began a special class for backward boys
"whose backwardness was directly related to a physical or a mental defect." Chace
(1904) noted:

> The chief aim is to create in the boys a love of work so that when they go out into
> the world, they will not join the ranks of the criminal class. For this reason, ev-
> erything is related to manual training and made subordinate to it. They always
> have some subject as a center; at the present it is the farm. In woodwork, they are
> making a house and barn, fences, furniture, and flower-boxes. They are weaving
> the rugs for the floor. . . . They went to the country for the soil to plant their min-
> iature fields, and sent to Washington for the seeds.

Chace left little doubt that school officials believed that the school system should
control pupils perceived to be incapable of controlling themselves (even to the point
of making "farmers" out of Lower East Siders).

The control of deficient and backward children, most of whom school officials
believed were also misbehavers or prone to bad behavior, became a growing concern of educators in the early years of the new century. Most public school teachers
believed such children learned differently than normal children. Since teachers had
more experience in these matters than any other group, it was assumed they were
right. Consequently, veteran teachers with few exceptions complained about their
inadequacy in teaching slow, backward, and often misbehaving children. Their feelings, in turn, also reinforced a context of inadequacy among new teachers. Most
teachers simply gave up. A Providence school official commented, "Our teachers
in the regular schools found so much relief when disorderly pupils were transferred to the disciplinary schools, that they were not slow to request the removal
of the backward or mentally deficient children, who were receiving comparatively

little benefit in their schools, to the same school for special instruction" (cited in Rochefort 1981).

Almost any classroom in the United States in the first decade of the new century had at least a few students characterized as laggards. According to classroom teachers, they were called various names by their classmates: nincompoop, half-wit, blockhead, dimwit, numskull, cork-brained, dumb Dora, dunce, dolt, cretin, jackass, harebrained, stupid, ignoramus, dunkerhead, mooncalf, thickheaded, dull-ard, hick, lowbrow, ding-a-ling, dingbat, knucklehead, flathead, moonraker, pump-kin head. More often than not, teachers claimed, these children became the butt of classroom teasing, pranks, and cruelty. Added to their feelings of inadequacy in controlling slow children, public school teachers felt sorry for them. In their frus-tration and pity, they began to claim they could do little for slow children other than protect them from cruelty. Not surprisingly, they eagerly supported special classes.[2]

By 1900, public school officials were calling for specially trained teachers to teach in the newly organized special classes. Before Boston opened its first special classes in 1899, school officials had sent several teachers scheduled to teach in them to the Massachusetts School for the Feeble-Minded at Waltham and to the Elwyn Institute in Pennsylvania. For three months, beginning special education teachers received instruction in Seguin's physiological methods, but most of their time was spent as apprentice teachers in the existing institutional classes (Chace 1904).

The first formal training for public school teachers began at the Training School at Vineland, New Jersey, in 1904 (Johnstone 1909; "Summer School for Teachers" 1904). Begun at the initiation of its superintendent E. R. Johnstone and his lead teacher, Mary Morrison Nash, the school operated for six weeks in the summer. Eventually, it attracted teachers from the entire nation and from several foreign countries. After 1910, with Johnstone's growing interest in the development of in-stitutions in the South, several teachers from that region were usually among the summer school's graduates. Other facilities also followed Vineland's lead in offering summer courses for public school teachers. In 1914, Vineland opened a demonstra-tion summer school in conjunction with New York University. Seventy-five pupils from Vineland were enrolled in the summer for the benefit of about eighty student teachers (Byers 1934, 48–52). The following fall, New York University began a two-year certificate program for public school teachers under Meta Anderson, who had been a graduate of the Vineland summer school ("Teachers for the Feebleminded" 1914; see also Sarason and Doris 1979, 317–320).

In another decade, with the integration of psychological testing in teacher edu-cation training, normal schools and university education departments would initi-ate programs for teachers interested in special education, thus replacing the state institution as the central location for such training. Nevertheless, between 1904 and 1930, the institutions remained the most important location for the training of special education teachers and also for the extension of institutional perspec-tives to local educators. In her presidential address to the National Conference of Charities and Correction in 1910, even Jane Addams (1910), not otherwise known for her interest in mental deficiency, recognized the linkage of the institution with the public school:

> For although the public schools in America are quite free from the odor of charity, and were inaugurated and conducted as a matter of public policy, they are greatly indebted to the educational results obtained from the care of defective and delinquent children. Certainly the training of the brain through the coordinating muscles, was first painstakingly worked out by those dealing with children whose minds could not be approached through conventional methods of education.

The first two decades were a heady time for superintendents interested in extending their influence to local school systems. Most schools were interested. Although they cannot now be credited with initiating the special education movement, the superintendents must be given their due in sustaining it. At professional conferences, at state teachers' meetings, before local civic clubs and churches, superintendents advocated for public support of the special classes. Their knowledge about mental deficiency also gave them a monopoly on firsthand information about the problem, which they willingly shared. In their public advocacy and their training of teachers, they influenced the development of a movement—special education—over which they had little direct control. Sometimes their advice moved beyond the local and state level. In 1914, Julia Lathrop, then director of the Children's Bureau in the US Department of Labor, wrote W. H. C. Smith, with whom she had developed a close working relationship from her days at Hull House and on the Illinois Board of State Charities, in a letter headed "CONFIDENTIAL":

> President Wilson is greatly interested in the problems of the feebleminded and has asked the Bureau of Education and the Children's Bureau to join in formulating a plan for an exhaustive study. This letter to you is preliminary to my own effort to prepare a plan for such work as would fall to the share of the Children's Bureau. . . .
> I hope it is not asking too much to beg you to lay your mind to this subject and to make any suggestions that you will. This is a preliminary inquiry on my part, and I shall regard your reply as confidentially as you please, and I warn you that I shall be likely to return again. (Beverly Farm Records, letter from Julia C. Lathrop to W. H. C. Smith, May 4, 1914)[3]

The influence of the superintendents had never been so valued.

Going beyond influence, some, like Martin Barr, integrated local special classes into their schemes of the total institutionalization of all mental defectives. In an 1899 speech to the National Education Association, Barr (1899) acknowledged that, before puberty, many mental defectives could be trained more efficiently in local schools than in large institutions. What was important, he insisted, was that local special education officials coordinate with state and private institutions to prepare mental defectives for what must be their lifelong protection. The local school, even under the best conditions, however, was not the appropriate place for mentally defectives after they reached puberty, when protection became more important than training.

Also in 1899, Walter Fernald (1904*b*) claimed that the overwhelming influence of heredity made attempts to teach traditional reading and writing to mental defectives futile. He acknowledged, however, that learning, although not book learning, was possible for mental defectives in public schools. During this period, he was consulting with Boston and Springfield public schools. In a paper before the American Association for the Study of the Feeble-Minded, he emphasized the protection of the mentally deficient, the same concern expressed by Barr five years earlier (Fernald 1904*b*). Special education could not become a substitute for the institution. His rationale was a familiar one:

> From all the information that I could gather it seems to me that the nearly ten years' experience with the special classes have not proved that a large proportion of feebleminded children can be so educated and trained in the special classes as to be able to support themselves by their own efforts and wages; or that they become wholesome or desirable members of a modern community.
>
> I believe that careful observation and study of the life history of large numbers of these specially trained pupils will show the need of life-long protection and assistance.

Three years later he wrote:

> Perhaps the chief function of these classes in America has been to demonstrate that the community is not the place for an adult imbecile. A defective boy or a defective girl may be tolerated, but an adult human being, with the mind of a child and the body and passions of an adult, is a foreign body in any community. These classes have demonstrated perhaps more graphically than ever before the fact that while they will improve under training and education perhaps to the point of usefulness and self-respect not obtained hitherto, yet when adult life is reached some provision must be made to protect not only these people themselves, but the community from the consequences of their incapacity. (Fernald 1907)

De-emphasizing the distinction between mental defect and backwardness, Fernald insisted that the institution would always be necessary for both. No matter how well trained, defective children in local special education classes would become defective adults.

If the state institution must be the eventual outcome of local special education, as Barr, Fernald, and most other superintendents began to claim, then training in the public schools must be adapted to that outcome. A committed champion of permanent, total institutionalization, Barr (1904*b*) advised teachers and school administrators to focus exclusively on what he called manual training. The standard academic curriculum was useless to feeble minds. With his emphasis on institutional "community life," Barr (1897) envisioned "communities of skilled artisans working in various trades and applied arts. Here imbeciles, separated from the world and forbidden to marry, shall become self-supporting, self-respecting citizens." Special education could assist in this community life model by beginning manual training early in the students' school experience.

Echoing Barr's position, Mary C. Dunphy (1908), superintendent of the Children's Institution on Randall's Island, insisted that, after training and at graduation from the special school, the mentally defective teenager "should be transferred to a home or colony wherein he can prove his social efficiency by being of use to others and himself." Otherwise, mental deficients would drift inevitably into crime and vice. She added:

> Moral instincts are almost always lacking in the mentally deficients, so even in the ordinary intercourse of home and social life they are a menace to the welfare of the community.
>
> This unfortunate tendency, coupled with the undesirable surroundings in many of their homes and the dangers of the unrestrained play of the streets, tends to nullify any ethical lessons or impressions gained by a few hours in school. Therefore, in the interest of the public weal as well as for their own sakes, it is of paramount importance that atypical children be prevented from coming in contact with those of normal minds, in order that their abnormal personality may not react unfavorably upon the latter.

Emphasizing the interrelationship of public schools and institutions, Fernald, Barr, and A. C. Rogers, among others, became leading advocates of medical diagnosis to identify and segregate deficient and slow children from normal ones. Rogers (1907) noted that too often feeblemindedness, backwardness, and normality were confused, and only slightly less often were other medical conditions inappropriately associated with mental deficiencies. Barr (1904b) insisted that physicians should provide the primary, medical identification and classification for mentally defective children; only then would teachers be allowed to educate these children. Following in the tradition of his predecessor, Isaac Kerlin, Barr believed that only the physician could accurately classify feeblemindedness through observation (Elks 2004). After years of working closely with school systems throughout the Northeast, Fernald (1920, 1922) opened an outpatient diagnostic clinic at his Waltham facility where children were brought for evaluation. In addition, a team of medical experts from the institution traveled throughout Massachusetts to inspect for feeblemindedness and other disabilities among the state's children. Between 1900 and 1920, most superintendents stressed the necessity for medical expertise in the identification of mental deficiency among public school pupils. The prominence of psychometrics and psychologists after 1908 only added to the medical superintendents' insistence on medical diagnosis.

Their emphasis on medical expertise in the burgeoning public schools was, of course, self-serving. In a time when medical standards and training were becoming an issue to the profession, medical superintendents were sensitive about their place in the new world of community-based medicine (McGovern 1985, 162–171; Rosenberg 1987). They knew they had something to offer. Unlike most physicians, they were experts on feeblemindedness. With their years of experience and observation along with their knowledge of the "stigmata of degeneracy," they saw a role for themselves not only in the institution, but also in the growing field of community medicine and, in their case, community psychiatry. Like their alienist colleagues in the insane asylums, now just as likely called state hospitals, the superintendents of state schools—their own new name for their institutions—were trying to free themselves from the professional stigma of institutionalization. The public schools, then, became an opportunity for sharing their institutional expertise in local settings and for bringing local interest to the institutions.

As noted earlier, one avenue for establishing this linkage was the training program for public school teachers. Another was research. Leading the way in research was the Elwyn Institute in Pennsylvania. Two of Isaac Kerlin's protégés, Martin Barr and A. W. Wilmarth, carried out significant pathological research at Elwyn. Barr also did important work on cerebral meningitis. Finally, Elwyn became the site for the much-heralded, if soon discredited, experiments in craniectomy and craniotomy. By the end of the century, others, too, were adding research facilities as they could find funds and equipment to do so. Not surprisingly, most of this research reflected the pathological and etiological interests of the medical superintendents (Barr 1892; Keen 1892; Kerlin 1888, 1892c; Norbury 1892, 1894; Wilmarth 1892, 1894).

The Social Construction of Testing and Eugenics

In 1899, A. C. Rogers became the first superintendent to conduct psychological research. A. R. T. Wylie, a pharmacist at Rogers's Minnesota facility, had completed a psychology doctorate at the College of Wooster. In addition to his pharmaceutical duties, Wylie carried out research on "mental pathology." Emphasizing sense and reaction-time measurements typical of the "brass instrument psychology" of the period, Wylie reported his research to the American Association for the Study of the Feeble-Minded and published in its journal (Wylie 1900a, 1900b, 1902, 1903). After Wylie later pursued medical training, eventually becoming the superintendent of the North Dakota Institution for the Feeble-Minded, Rogers hired Frederick Kuhlmann, a recent graduate of the Clark University psychology program, to continue similar studies (Popplestone and McPherson 1984).

If Rogers led the way for psychology's entrance into institutional research, E. R. Johnstone in New Jersey launched it in directions that would not only revolutionize the field but would also change it from an "armchair" appendage of philosophy to an independent discipline. Not a researcher himself, Johnstone, like Isaac Kerlin of an earlier generation, was an organizer, an administrator, and a good salesman. With seemingly boundless energy, Johnstone, who had never graduated from college, manipulated and cajoled professionals, politicians, and the public into taking an interest in mental deficiency. Although he received less credit than others, he was directly responsible for most changes taking place in the field.

In 1894, Edward Ransome Johnstone had been teaching literature in a Cincinnati high school when his wife's brother, Alexander Johnson, superintendent of the Indiana School for the Feeble-Minded, hired him to be head teacher of the institution's school. The two men worked well together, Johnstone initiating several changes at the Indiana facility. In 1898, with Johnson's blessing, he accepted the vice principal's position at the New Jersey Training School for Feeble-Minded Children at Vineland (later known as the Training School at Vineland). In 1900, at the death of the school's founder, Olin Garrison, Johnstone at the age of thirty became principal and head of the institution, a position he held until his death in 1946. When Johnson resigned as superintendent of the Indiana school in 1903, Johnstone was then the only superintendent of a major facility who was not a physician, and he remained throughout most of his career one of the few superintendents without medical training (Byers 1934; Eadline 1963).

In 1901, the new principal attended a child-study meeting in Newark. Founded by G. Stanley Hall, the child-study movement reflected the influence of the Clark University faculty on public education of the period. Indeed, until around 1910, when John Dewey's and Edward Thorndike's work became better known, Hall's child-study groups were the center of educational thought in the United States (Danforth 2008; D. Ross 1972, 364–365). Johnstone had become involved in the movement. With him at the meeting were Earl Barnes, a well-known Philadelphia educator, and Henry H. Goddard, a member of the psychology department at the Pennsylvania State Normal School at Westchester. On the train back to Philadelphia, the three talked about mutual interests and exchanged gossip. Out of their camaraderie, they decided to join together as "consulting paidologists," a group of like-minded educators who would share ideas about mental deficiency and "carry on investigations into [the] mental condition and capacity of . . . [feebleminded] children" ("Training School at Vineland" 1963).

By 1904, the group had become the Feebleminded Club. Meeting twice annually, at first in Philadelphia but eventually at Vineland, the club grew to include prominent educators and philanthropists from New Jersey and Pennsylvania. In 1903, the idea of training public school teachers had led to the creation of the first classes the next summer. In 1904, the group was influential in starting the *Training School Bulletin*. As J. E. Wallace Wallin (1953) recalled at its fiftieth anniversary celebration, the Feebleminded Club had provided a place where members could "swap ideas, tell the latest yarns, discuss informally the questions of the day and the fray, and peer at one another in the dining room through a pall of tobacco smoke." In 1905, the club began to discuss expanding the summer school for teachers into a learning laboratory in order to conduct research useful to the public schools. In 1906, the research department of the Training School at Vineland was born (Byers 1934, 40; Leiby 1967, 106).

Johnstone, with the blessing of its principal backer and fellow Feebleminded Club member, Samuel S. Fels, the Philadelphia soap manufacturer, hired Goddard to head the new research laboratory at Vineland. Tired of the drudgery of large and numerous classes at Westchester and due a sabbatical leave during the next academic year, Goddard was eager to have the opportunity to begin research at a facility he already knew. Since 1901, he had regularly consulted at Vineland and, as a charter member of the club, had visited it frequently. Fels, a backer of several philanthropic enterprises and also a loyal supporter of progressive and usually Democratic politicians and causes, stipulated that Goddard and Johnstone meet quarterly with him about the activities of the research department. He insisted, too, that his contributions would be made only on a quarterly basis. Future funding, he reminded Goddard and Johnstone, depended on results. As Stanley Porteus (1969, 64), Goddard's successor at Vineland, remembered: "As far as the Training School was concerned, [Fels] made it clear that his sole interest was research. His concern with the feebleminded was not with their training and welfare, but as he frankly put it—'in getting them off the earth.'"

Goddard's work began in September 1906. Still under the influence of Hall's genetic psychology and of the "brass instrument" methodology also prevalent during the time, his research was not producing the results insisted on by Fels. In his notebook of the period, kept for Johnstone's review, Goddard expressed frustration at accomplishing so little. Like the work of other researchers at the time, his attempts to find an association between "basic human differences" (i.e., sense reactions, temperament and memory, and height and weight) and intellectual differences were going nowhere (American Association for the Study of the Feeble-Minded 1910, 148; Goddard 1907a, 1907b, 1909a; Leiby 1967, 107; Popplestone and McPherson 1984; Zenderland 1998, 71–98).

In the spring of 1908, while traveling in Europe, Goddard met Ovide Decroly, the well-known Belgian educator. Decroly was using a test of intelligence he had first read about in 1905 in articles by Alfred Binet and Theodore Simon in L'année psychologique (1905a, 1905b, 1905c).[4] Decroly gave Goddard copies of one or more of the Binet-Simon articles and his own recently published article for L'année (Decroly and Degand 1906). Binet, a physician whose interest in developmental psychology was in part the result of his reading of G. Stanley Hall, had been hired by the French Ministry of Education to devise a method for screening slow learners in the French public school system. He designed a "higher order" test that measured students' cognitive abilities. Unlike so-called lower order screening popular at the time, Binet and Simon's test appeared to correlate with teachers' opinions of the intellectual levels of their pupils. From 1905 until his death in 1911, Binet stressed that the test he and his colleague had devised gave an accurate measurement of intelligence. Nevertheless, intelligence, he insisted, was a pliant structure that could be developed through good health and educational instruction and in a good environment (J. Brown 1992; Goddard 1943; Wolf 1973, 80, 160–162, 283–284; Zenderland 1998, 92–98).

In 1943, Goddard recalled that at first he had not taken the articles seriously. Nevertheless, shortly after the start of the new school year, he began to use his own translation of the test on inmates at Vineland (Goddard 1943). After several months, Goddard began to appreciate the potential for getting the kind of results expected by Johnstone and Fels. In the July 1908 issue of the Training School Bulletin, he casually mentioned Binet's work, giving it no special prominence (Goddard 1908c). By the end of the year, however, he had published an article in the bulletin solely devoted to the Binet and Simon intelligence tests (Goddard 1908a).

From 1908 to 1910, Goddard presented his findings to the American Association for the Study of the Feeble-Minded, showing his growing confidence in the test (Goddard 1908c, 1909b, 1910c). Almost immediately, other psychologists became interested in the test. Most prominent were other graduates of the Clark program—Edmund Huey, Lewis M. Terman, Arnold Gesell, and also J. E. Wallace Wallin, who had done postgraduate work at Clark (Minton 1988, 21–29; D. Ross 1972, 352). Soon, these psychologists and others were replicating the test and making their own adjustments and refinements to it, as the important tool they all saw it to be. Many new intelligence tests were soon born, some of which, like Terman's Stanford-Binet, received greater prominence. As early as 1921, the publishers Henry Holt, J. B. Lippincott, World Book, and Houghton Mifflin had displays at the Second International Exhibition of Eugenics in New York. Each had published its own intelligence tests and was competing for a growing market (J. Brown 1992; Laughlin 1923).

For their own part, Goddard and Johnstone more than any other figures in the early history of the Binet-Simon test broadcasted its potential. Thousands of people became fascinated by the test, but most employed it while ignoring Binet's insistence on the pliancy of intelligence. Beginning in the Vineland summer school of 1909, Goddard introduced school teachers to his own version (Goddard 1910a, 1910e). For the next twenty-seven years, nearly one thousand teachers learned about this and other versions of the test, and, at least before 1930, they were expected to know how to administer and interpret them. Coming from every state in the union and from several foreign countries, these teachers spread the Vineland enthusiasm for the test to school systems nationwide and abroad. It became, Joseph Byers remembered, a "missionary enterprise" (Byers 1934, 48–52). By 1913, 72 percent of examinations for special education classes in the United States were Binet tests, and more than 50 percent of the examiners were special educators, most of whom were Vineland graduates. "Most of the teachers became trail blazers in their home communities. Many rose to positions of leadership," Wallin (1953) remembered. In 1913, Charles Bernstein began a summer school for public school teachers, which included instructors from Vineland, at the Rome State School. By 1935, he had sent another one thousand testers among the uninitiated (*Herald*, August 1, 1921, August 1, 1926; Riggs 1936, 32, 52, 97).

Surpassing the hopes of the medical superintendents, Goddard and his psychological associates linked the school and the institution through the training of school teachers in the technology of intelligence testing. In so doing, they gave the institution greater prominence. Local teachers and public officials looked to Vineland as a mecca of research for special education (Brown and Genheimer 1969; Hill 1945). Professionals caught up in the frenetic praise for and curiosity about the new test were also quick to elevate Goddard to prominence. In 1914, the American Association for the Study of the Feeble-Minded made him its president, the first member who was not a superintendent to be so honored. His numerous writings, including his magnum opus, *Feeble-Mindedness: Its Causes and Consequences* (1914), were lauded in professional and popular journals and newspapers during the teens. Back at Vineland, Fels was pleased, at least for a time. Goddard's quarterly reports were showing promise. By 1911, the Vineland Research Laboratory had grown to a staff of seventeen. In 1913, when a new and larger building replaced the institution's aging and inadequate hospital, Goddard's one-room lab moved to more spacious quarters in the old three-storied hospital (Byers 1934, 71).

The Binet-Simon test, as crucial as it was to Goddard's career and Vineland's prestige, contributed to only part of the public's growing recognition of the psychologist and the training school. At the 1910 meeting of the Association for the Study of the Feeble-Minded, in addition to reporting on his continued work on the Binet test, Goddard also discussed his continued work on backward children (Goddard 1908b, 1909c). Until this time, such children for the most part had been considered amenable to treatment. F. M. Powell (1900) of the Iowa State School represented the view of most superintendents and school officials: "This class does not include children with such marked deficiencies that they cannot be brought up to the ordinary standard of intelligence; they are normal, but impeded or embarrassed in mental growth, owing to psychical or physical impairment or neglect." They belonged not in an institution but in public schools, where they should receive special and extra attention. They should be examined by a physician, Powell added, and not be put in classes with normally progressing children, although they should be allowed to have opportunities to commingle with them. A. C. Rogers (1907) was even more optimistic about the improvability of backward children. But other superintendents, like Fernald, Barr, and Rogers, had been concerned not about the improvability of backward children but about the ability of backward teenagers and adults to avoid vice, crime, and childbearing.

Beginning in 1909, Goddard began to modify the superintendents' views on the improvability of backward pupils. A class of children existed, he claimed, probably 2 percent of all school-aged children, who looked in most respects like ordinary children but who were mentally deficient. Often labeled backward, dull, or slow, they were certainly brighter than children traditionally recognized as feebleminded, but they were still abnormal. "Will the backward child outgrow its backwardness?" Goddard asked in an article with the same title (Goddard 1909c; see also Goddard 1908b, 1910b, 1911b, 1911c). His testing and recent pedigree studies revealed that their abnormality was a permanent one. Because of their prevalence and the distinctiveness and permanence of their condition, these children required a new label. In Great Britain, Goddard noted, authorities called these children *feebleminded*. In the United States, however, this term was already used generically to refer to all grades of mental deficiency. *Backward*, too, would not do since it implied a temporary impairment. Thus, Goddard proposed the term *moron*.

Between 1910 and World War I, the moron served several functions. First, it transformed Kerlin's moral imbecile into an expanded and fully recognized member of the family of mental defectives. Second, it provided a linkage between mental defect and new understandings about heredity. Third, it provided a new insight into the nature and consequences of social problems traditionally associated with mental deficiency. Finally, it reinvigorated old policies and shaped new ones to deal with these problems. Ironically, these policies would endure even after the new assumptions about heredity and about the causes of social problems were questioned and ultimately found wanting.

The new testing tool discovered by Goddard in 1908 led to a new classification of mental deficiency and also to a new understanding of the relationship between moral behavior and intellect. Intertwined with both the new category and the new relationship was Goddard's interest in heredity, which was most prominently revealed in his 1912 book *The Kallikak Family* (Goddard 1912c). The Binet-Simon test, the moron, and the Kallikaks were the result of Goddard's and Vineland's frenzy of activity between 1908 and 1912. The medical superintendents recognized the value of the changes occurring and, despite some professional uneasiness about the new *psychological* tools, were not reluctant to champion them for their own purposes.

In 1908, Fernald (1909) expressed a view typical of his colleagues in other facilities:

> Cases of imbecility with criminal propensities—"criminals who have committed no crime"—will be recognized at an early age before they have acquired facility in crime, and permanently taken out of the community and given life-long care and supervision in special institutions.... Every imbecile, especially the higher-grade imbecile, is a potential criminal, needing only the proper environment and opportunity for the development and expression of his criminal tendencies. The unrecognized imbecile is a most dangerous element in the community. From a biological standpoint the imbecile is an inferior human being.

This harsh view held by Fernald and others was the prelude to a new, liberal, rationalized, and scientifically objective means of dealing with groups of citizens unable to adapt to the newly emerging contours of American life in the early part of the century. Although observations of pathological degeneracy and case studies of moral imbecility had proved useful to the expansion of the hospital-modeled institution of the 1880s and 1890s, in the face of rapid twentieth-century change these constructions were becoming less useful and less scientifically sound. A threat had to exist in order to expand and sustain the institution, but this threat also had to remain within the parameters of scientific respectability. Goddard, again, was the innovator.

Goddard's primary contributions to the social construction of mental disability in the 1910s were his redefinition of mental deficiency to include the moron, his studies of mental deficiency's association with Mendelian heredity, and his novel claims for the linkage of mental deficiency and crime. In 1909, the year after he introduced the Binet test to an American audience, Goddard addressed the American Association for the Study of the Feeble-Minded on the issue of the classification of mental deficiency. For Goddard, medical classification schemes like those championed by the medical superintendents were imprecise and too eclectic. The only characteristic shared by all mentally deficient people was a deficient intellect. An etiology relying on medical categories was inadequate because the catagories failed to account physiologically for this deficiency. Other schemes based on lower order motor control also, although perhaps showing future promise, were for the moment inadequate. Mental tests of higher order faculties, however, provided a precise, generalizable, and reliable means of classifying all forms of mental deficiency (Goddard 1909*b*; see also Noll, Smith, and Wehmeyer 2013; Zenderland 1998, 2004).

The American Association for the Study of the Feeble-Minded, taken by the potential of Goddard's claims, appointed a committee "for the purpose of considering classification of the mentally deficient and to make recommendations for the adoption of some uniform classification and report at the next meeting" (American Association for the Study of the Feeble-Minded 1910, 146). Among the five members appointed to the committee were Goddard and Fernald. At the association's meeting in 1910 at the Lincoln school, Goddard presented the committee's new scheme ("Report of Committee on Classification" 1910; see also figure 4.1). In it, Goddard suggested using the term *feeblemindedness* to designate all forms of mental deficiency. *Idiots* referred to individuals with a mental age of two years and less; *imbeciles*, three to seven years; and *morons*, eight to twelve years. The effects of this classification scheme were to replace Kerlin's now outdated system, to introduce a new category of feebleminded people—the moron—and, by doing so, to enlarge the projection of mental deficiency in the general population to at least 2 percent from less than 1 percent. For Goddard, Kerlin's moral imbecile had captured neither the extent nor the character of high-grade mental deficiency. Morons were a common occurrence, not an unusual one. Morons were also an example not of polymorphous degenerative heredity but of Mendelian heredity, the focus of many younger scientists of the period.

Cultivated generally by the times and specifically by his mentor, G. Stanley Hall, Goddard's interest in intelligence was never isolated from his interest in heredity. In 1910, the same year he published the results of his work on the Binet test and created the category of moron, Goddard (1910*d*) published an important paper in the *American Breeders' Magazine*. Charles Davenport, director of the genetics laboratory at Cold Spring Harbor, was impressed by the article's content and had it republished in the first bulletin of the Eugenics Record Office. This article was to begin Goddard's close association with a community of scholars, politicians, and industrialists interested in the issue of "better breeding," or eugenics.

In some respects, Goddard's views on the hereditary basis of feeblemindedness resembled those held by degenerative theorists like Kerlin and Barr. For example, like the degenerativists, he linked feeblemindedness with social vices: poverty, backwardness, crime, prostitution, delinquency, and drunkardness. He departed from the earlier theorists in his view of cause and effect. For the degenerativists, social vices were clearly associated with feeblemindedness, but their manifestation and rate of occurrence were hardly predictable or regular. Given his enthusiasm over results from testing and from new pedigree studies, Goddard was more convinced than the earlier theorists about the causal relationship between social vice and mental deficiency. The linkage, he came to see, was simple. At least two-thirds of all feeblemindedness was the result of hereditary factors, what he called the "cancerous growth of bad protoplasm." Added to this was the apparent fact that a high proportion of social vices was linked with feeblemindedness. His preliminary studies suggested that crime did not cause the feebleminded to inherit feeblemindedness; logic would indicate, therefore, that feeblemindedness affected rates of crime. Thus, the association between social vice and mental deficiency held by the degenerativists shifted under Goddard's guidance to a causal relationship (see also Gelb 1995; Goddard 1910b; Goddard and Hill 1911; Willrich 1998).

This new causal relationship, of course, easily ushered in a new conceptualization of mental deficiency. Mentally deficient people, especially those who were morons, were no longer merely a social *burden*, they were now a social *menace*. The menace rhetoric already being touted by the superintendents fit Goddard's newly emerging views. Along with the change from burden to menace came the claim that mentally deficient people were breeding at an even greater rate than the degenerativists had earlier believed. According to Goddard, the rate among morons was at least twice the rate of the general population.

For a solution to this problem, Goddard turned to his eugenical compatriots. In 1911, he proposed two directions for the social control of the feebleminded (Goddard 1911a). One involved testing the feebleminded with the Binet scale, placing them in either segregated institutions or in segregated classes depending on their criminal tendencies, and prohibiting them by law from marrying. The other, more Draconian solution would ensure the prevention of new feeble minds: institutionalize all defectives of reproductive age to prevent their breeding and, if necessary, sterilize them. Although the data presented in his earliest articles were still inconclusive, by 1912, Goddard was beginning to get results that he believed strengthened his assumptions about the menace and multiplication of the feebleminded. The culmination of these findings was his study of the Kallikaks.

In 1912, Goddard published *The Kallikak Family: A Study in the Heredity of Feeble-Mindedness*. In it, he traced the lineage of an eight-year-old girl who had entered the Training School at Vineland in 1910. He gave the girl the fictitious name "Deborah Kallikak," the surname being a combination of the Greek words *kallos*, "good," and *kakos*, "bad." To develop his research, Goddard relied on the "pedigree" findings of his assistant, Elizabeth Kite. Kite, a social worker at the school, had used the memories of elderly family members to construct Deborah's family tree. Although these memories were often vague and frequently based on the stories passed down from even older generations of Kallikaks, Kite and Goddard soon believed that they had discovered a dramatic example of generational inferiority.

According to Goddard (who published under his own name and not with Kite[5]), Deborah's degeneracy had its origins during the American Revolution. Her great-great-great grandfather, "Martin Kallikak," had been a soldier in the colonial forces. On leave from "one of the taverns frequented by the militia he met a feebleminded girl by whom he became the father of a feebleminded son" (Goddard 1912c, 18). The son took his father's first and last names, but as an adult he was known as "Old Horror." This *kakos* ancestor, Goddard tells us, produced 143 feebleminded progeny, along with dozens of epileptics, alcoholics, prostitutes, and common criminals. Illegitimate births from this line were routine; poverty was the norm. For Goddard, the names of Old Horror's descendants reflected their low station: "Old Sal" and "Old Moll." Deborah, then, was only the most recent example of a long line of degenerates.

Had Goddard's story ended there it would have differed little from other pedigree studies that had preceded it. Through family memories and records, however, he discovered that Martin, the revolutionary soldier, had returned from the war and married an upstanding Quaker. Together, Goddard tells his readers, they produced a line of respectable, law-abiding, and successful citizens. The *kakos* line of the family, then, had a corresponding *kallos* line.

Before Goddard's discovery of the Kallikak family, the causal link between vice and intellectual disability was still problematic. After all, the relationship between the two factors could just as easily be related to the environment, a claim acknowledged earlier by Dugdale in his study of the Jukes. If it could be demonstrated, however, that inferior stock remained inferior throughout a family's lineage and that such stock consistently engaged in a variety of social vices, one would have, Goddard believed, a case for the immutable effects of simple Mendelian heredity. Feeblemindedness, then, became a transmissible genetic flaw. In the story of the Kallikaks, Goddard found his demonstration, and with it he began to shape a new view of the mentally deficient offender.

According to Goddard, urban filth, poverty, and disease were not the causes of the blight of Deborah Kallikak. Rather, her great-great-great grandfather's one-time peccadillo had ruined her and many other generations of Kallikaks: "No matter where we traced them, whether in the prosperous rural district, in the city slums to which some had drifted, or in the more remote mountain regions ... an appalling amount of defectiveness was everywhere found." Goddard concluded that "if all of the slum districts of our cities were removed tomorrow and model tenements built in their places, we would still have slums in a week's time, because we have these mentally defective people who can never be taught to live otherwise than as they have been living" (Goddard 1912c, 70–71). Added to the effects of heredity was the fecundity of the feebleminded. Goddard noted: "There are Kallikak families all about us. They are multiplying at twice the rate of the general population, and not until we recognize this fact, and work on this basis, will we begin to solve [our] social problems" (Goddard 1912c, 70–71).

To solve the social problem of the Kallikaks, Goddard turned to familiar solutions: marriage restriction, segregation, and sterilization. As an institutionally based psychologist, it is not surprising that he was most favorably disposed to segregation (Goddard 1912d). Marriage restriction alone had only a small effect. "By segregation or sterilization," he told the 1913 Illinois Conference of Charities and Correction, "... we could, in a generation or two, reduce the number of our dependent classes enormously and save from a fourth to a half of the expense of our criminals, our paupers, to say nothing of the moral degradation and disease engendered by our prostitutes" (Goddard 1913b, 11). All in all, Goddard believed, less procreation meant less feeblemindedness and thereby less social instability.

Although the creation of the moron in 1910 provided a potential justification for the expansion of special school and institutional populations, and also for the growth of psychologists' presence in the field of mental deficiency, the very claims for both the morons' vast numbers and their potential for increase in the general population led the field away from Barr's policy of total institutionalization. The menace of the feebleminded was principally the threat of millions of morons, most of whom were not in the institution. These members of the higher grade of feeble-minded individuals made up a sizable part of the lower class population. At the same time, they were increasing because of their sexual fecundity and because of immigration. Accordingly, morons were becoming more and more of a drain on society because of their propensity toward social vice. They were out there among us, and they were doing bad things. Although the superintendents used the threat of the moron to enlarge existing institutions and build new ones, they also abandoned their dream of institutionalizing all feeble minds. Ironically, the threat they constructed to sustain their policy of total institutionalization would in its apparent magnitude eliminate the policy. By 1913, as just over half the states had enacted marriage restriction acts, the superintendents had come to see that the menace of the feebleminded had to be fought on several fronts (Davenport 1913).

Goddard's moron would live on in popular literature and in the public's conscience for at least four decades after the 1920s. In the 1930s, "little moron" jokes would (along with Polack jokes, both of which had their origins in Goddard's testings) become all the rage. Their popularity would continue even into the late 1970s, when "sped" (a contraction of "special education") jokes, a new version of an older "sick joke" genre, would supplant them (Barrick 1980; Baughman 1943).

By 1928, in the face of vocal opposition, Goddard would "recant" his earlier claims about the moron (Goddard 1928). Evidence suggests that his change of heart was more a matter of form than substance (see J. Smith 1985, 66–80; J. Smith and Wehmeyer 2012). Nevertheless, by 1928, like most of his colleagues, Goddard seemed convinced that the cognitive and social dimensions of the moronic classification were firmly enough in place to make the frenetic rhetoric of the preceding decade unnecessary. Now, in both the institution and in the community, liberal social policies supported not only by medical experts but also by psychologists could be *routinely* carried out. Morons no longer had to be exclusively seen as a menace; they could now be a joke, too (P. Ryan 1997).

SPREADING THE THREAT OF MENTAL DEFICIENCY

Routinization, however, did not come overnight. Between 1908 and 1920, the rhetoric of the "menace of the feebleminded" became increasingly shrill in annual meetings of the American Association for the Study of the Feeble-Minded and the National Conference of Charities and Correction. In edition after edition of the *Survey* and in popular magazines and daily newspapers, speakers and writers warned of a national calamity if states did not take immediate steps to curtail the multiplication, the liberties, and the immigration of morons. Ironically, this alarm was occurring after the dramatic growth of the institutions in the previous decade. In 1890, there were twenty public and four private institutions in the United States. In 1903, there were twenty-eight public and fourteen private facilities. In 1890, the population in institutions for feeble minds was 5,254 inmates. By 1903, it had increased to 14,347. Discharges because of death or transfers accounted for only

8.5 percent of the total population change in 1904. Thus, new admissions, along with the trend toward lifelong institutionalization, not turnover, accounted for the major part of this dramatic increase in institutional populations (Koren 1906).

Despite this increase, superintendents remained convinced that large numbers of mental defectives were still in the population. They noted that most of the insane and paupers were receiving institutional care at state expense (e.g., Johnson 1914; also Koren 1906). The feebleminded, however, were still lagging behind. The 1904 census enumerations indicated that 16,551 almshouse inmates were feebleminded. Even discounting some probable confusion between senility and feeblemindedness by almshouse officials, this number indicated to superintendents and their social welfare supporters that more feeble minds were being served in poorhouses than in institutions. Although the 1904 census had only counted feeble minds in institutions, there was every reason to believe that, as previous censuses had indicated, many defectives in American communities were receiving no training, care, or control. Indeed, even before Goddard's introduction of the moron, most experts in the field estimated that 150,000 people in the United States were feebleminded and needed institutional care (Koren 1906). When Goddard introduced the idea of the moron and began to suggest that this group of previously unidentified feeble minds was the most dangerous and prevalent type of mental defective, he placed before the superintendents a grave and threatening picture. With only one-tenth of the national population of idiots and imbeciles receiving services, Goddard insisted that morons, a category larger by far than either of the other two types of feeble minds, must be added to the pool of uncontrolled clientele. By 1910, the numbers of feeble minds seemed enormous.

Added to these specific and immediate concerns was the linkage of feeblemindedness with immigration. During 1907, the year after Goddard began his work at Vineland, the United States admitted the highest number of immigrants in its history. When several major banks failed that same year, causing a deep, albeit brief, financial panic, the superfluous place of the immigrant in American business seemed more apparent than ever. Calls for immigration restrictions continued to increase from blueblood nativists, American labor, and eugenicists. More than in previous decades, the 1904 census report on institutionalized citizens drew feeble minds into the picture of immigration restriction in a more urgent and pressing way. Data from that census indicated that of the 12,155 white inmates in institutions for mental defectives, 33 percent were from families in which either one or both parents were foreign-born. The parentage of 22 percent was unknown, leaving only 45 percent of inmates with known native parentage (Koren 1906, table 3).

In the context of growing concern about the influx of immigrants, census data about the propensity of feeblemindedness among immigrants seemed to confirm what superintendents, philanthropists, and some politicians had been claiming for several decades: immigration was responsible for much of the increase in feeblemindedness. Typical of her colleagues, Alice Mott (1894) had claimed: "Our foreign-born inhabitants and those of foreign parentage are thirty-four percent of the whole population; but they furnish over fifty percent of our defectives." From her perspective in the public schools, the linkage of immigration and feeblemindedness looked even more alarming than it did for the superintendents. E. J. Emerick (1917) in his presidential address to the American Association for the Study of the Feeble-Minded warned against the free admission of immigrants, an alarming number of whom were mentally deficient. In 1882, Congress had barred the admission of lunatics and idiots and, in 1903, of epileptics (Kamin 1974, 15–28). Obviously, critics a decade later contended, some of these sorts were, despite the restrictions, getting in, and many more were being born to newly admitted immigrants. In February 1912, the Chamber of Commerce of New York State sent the Commissioner of Immigration a resolution urging the exclusion of feebleminded immigrants, reflecting the public insistence for more fail-proof restrictions ("Chamber of Commerce" 1912; see also Knox 1914). In 1917, when Congress considered legislation to bar "persons of constitutional psychopathic inferiority," superintendents were nearly unanimous in their support.

Data provided by Goddard beginning in 1912, the same year that *The Kallikak Family* appeared, not only lent support to this growing fear of defective strangers but also provided a tool for their efficient detection. With funding from the philanthropists Bayard Cutting and Bleeker VanWagenen and using trained field workers like Elizabeth Kite, Goddard began giving Binet tests to immigrants on Ellis Island. Soon he reported to Samuel Fels and to the American Association for the Study of the Feeble-Minded that the Binet scale could detect mental defectives more quickly and more accurately than methods being used by physicians (Goddard 1912a, 1912b, 1913a; see also Dolmage 2011; Knox 1914). Not all physicians agreed with Goddard's conclusion (e.g., Sprague 1913), but word of his work and findings began to filter through the social welfare community.

In 1917, Goddard presented what he characterized as shocking data: as many as 40 to 50 percent of immigrants were feebleminded. The data might seem outrageous, he acknowledged, but the tests were conclusive (Goddard 1917a, 1917b). When the *Survey* reported the findings, many in the social welfare community were astounded, but most were prepared to believe the author of *The Kallikak Family*. "If you had gone to Ellis Island shortly before the war began and placed your hand at random on one of the aliens waiting to be examined by government inspectors," the *Survey* writer stressed, "you would very likely have found that your choice was feebleminded" ("Two Immigrants Out of Five Feebleminded" 1917; see also Knox 1914; Richardson 2011). But Goddard had his critics. The New York Council of Jewish Women, for example, recognized that Goddard's definition of "normal intelligence" was meaningless, given his claim for massive feeblemindedness among immigrants (Winkler and Sachs 1917).[6] Yet the effects of his reports, despite the criticism, would remain. Even after Goddard had departed Vineland for Ohio, the purveyors of immigrant restriction—Harry Laughlin, Davenport, and Grant, Wiggam, and Stoddard—used Goddard's findings to argue their case (e.g., Stoddard 1923, 96–97). Both Warren G. Harding and Calvin Coolidge made the restriction of immigrants (many of whom, they reminded audiences, were defective) a campaign theme in their successful run for the White House (Coolidge 1921; Degler 1991, 42–43; Fairchild 2003; Gossett 1965, 404–405; McDonagh 2001).

In 1924, the Johnson-Lodge Immigration Act did what previous laws had not done. It restricted by quotas, not by conditions, setting nationality quotas at 2 percent of the 1890 level. Once again, the superintendents, although only a small part of the anti-immigration chorus, raised their voices in support. Even as late as 1945, E. Arthur Whitney (1945), successor to Kerlin and Barr at Elwyn Institute and one of the most influential superintendents of the period, claimed that certain nationalities produced more defective stock than others. "A thorough screening by the immigration authorities," he claimed, "would eliminate not only the mental defectives but those of mental defective or psychopathic stock who will be clamoring for admission now that World War II is at an end." Not until 1965 did Congress reverse its earlier prohibitive legislation against the immigration of feebleminded persons or families with feebleminded members (Boggs 1975, 444–445; Fairchild 2003).

By 1910, broadcasting the "menace of the feebleminded," a term that seemed to capture the convergence of various concerns about the multiplication of and social threat posed by feeble minds, had become even more urgent. The American Association for the Study of the Feeble-Minded had proved to be a forum for the superintendents' ideas and concerns. The National Conference of Charities and Correction had provided a means for expanding the superintendents' position within the burgeoning social welfare community. And the *Survey*, published by the Russell Sage Foundation, began after 1910 to be a source for the transmission of the message of the menace of the feebleminded to educated laypersons interested in social welfare. However, even though the associations and the journal had provided a disciplinary matrix for the field, they had had little influence on either the general public or legislators. With the growing interest in immigration restriction, eugenics, and the "white man's burden," coupled with the dilemmas presented by widespread public schooling, superintendents found themselves after 1910 in positions of newfound influence. Before citizens' groups and to elected officials, they presented the message of the menace of the feebleminded. Several of them were especially influential—Walter Fernald in New England; Charles Bernstein and Charles Little in New York; A. C. Rogers, E. J. Emerick, and A. W. Wilmarth in the Midwest; Martin Barr and J. M. Murdoch in Pennsylvania; F. O. Butler on the West Coast. None of these men was as important in spreading the threat of mental defect as the Committee on Provision for the Feeble-Minded.

Founded in December 1914, the committee had its antecedents in the previous decade and, like several other new developments of the period, was the brainchild of E. R. Johnstone. As early as 1906, Johnstone had seen the potential for such an organization. He told an audience of the National Conference of Charities and Correction:

> Greater efforts must be made to have the great public know of the defectives, so that we shall not be accused of having axes to grind when we ask for more provision for them. Institution men must encourage visits, give out information and indeed, conduct a campaign of education, so that in the first place the unwillingness of parents to send their children shall be changed to eagerness, and then will follow the demands of public opinion and concessions of legislatures. (Johnstone 1906)

Two years later, before the same group, he anticipated another important direction. With its annual conference in Richmond, Virginia, Johnstone (1908) took the opportunity to address the need for institutions for feeble minds in the South. Focusing specifically on Virginia, Johnstone emphasized the need for services in public schools, the medical inspection of school-aged children, and the development "along progressive lines" of a state facility. He warned his audience of juvenile reform schools and brothels filled with feeble minds. He reminded them of the Jukes, now seen to be victims of hereditary degeneracy. He told them of more recent pedigree studies, for example, the Ross family of Indiana, the family of Lucy X in Pennsylvania, and the Jackson whites and the Jackson blacks in New Jersey, all tainted by hereditary flaws and all perpetrators of various troublesome and seemingly intractable social problems. The problems were multiple, and their recurrence was inevitable. The feebleminded of Virginia, he pleaded, would continue to be sources of problems until the state made provisions to segregate them in public schools before puberty, in state institutions at puberty. Virginia could be a leader in the South, he insisted. At the same meeting, Alexander Johnson (1908), then executive director of the conference, echoed his brother-in-law's call. Concerned Virginians must advocate for a state institution to prevent the ongoing reproduction of degenerate, crime-prone feeble minds.

It was, of course, around the same period that Goddard began his use of intelligence testing, created the moron, began work on *The Kallikak Family* (1912c), and came to the attention of Charles Davenport. In 1904, Davenport had received funding from Andrew Carnegie to found the Laboratory for Experimental Evolution at Cold Spring Harbor, New York. One of the first biologists to appreciate the revolutionary implications of Mendel's work, Davenport introduced translations of works by the European botanists and geneticists Karl Correns and Hugo de Vries to American scientists (Rosenberg 1961). Shifting his evolutionary interests from the study of plants and animals to human beings, Davenport became aware of Goddard's research, probably around the time he joined the American Association for the Study of the Feeble-Minded in 1909. At the 1909 meeting of the American Breeders' Association, Davenport was influential in establishing the Committee on Eugenics, which selected David Starr Jordan, the chancellor of Stanford University, as its first chair and appointed Davenport its secretary.[7]

The same year the Committee on Eugenics voted to establish a subcommittee on the heredity of the feebleminded. A. C. Rogers chaired the subcommittee and Goddard was its secretary. Its four additional members included J. C. Carson, H. H. Donaldson, Walter Fernald, and J. M. Murdoch. All members, except for Goddard, were prominent superintendents (M. Haller 1963, 62–65).

In December 1909, Goddard, as secretary of the subcommittee, sent letters to superintendents of private and public institutions throughout the nation asking them to supply data about the hereditary status of their inmates. In the midst of his work on the Kallikaks, Goddard's request to the superintendents reflected not only his own interests but also the superintendents' own assumptions about the hereditary degeneracy of their clientele (Beverly Farm Records, letter from Henry H. Goddard to W. H. C. Smith, December 4, 1909).

Impressed with Goddard's work, Davenport had been influential in placing him in the secretary's position on a subcommittee otherwise dominated by medical superintendents. More important in shaping both their careers, Davenport published as the first bulletin of the newly established Eugenics Record Office Goddard and Johnstone's paper "Inheritance of Feeble-Mindedness," which had been delivered at the first meeting of the eugenics section of the 1910 meeting of the American Breeders' Association (Davenport 1910; Goddard 1910d). A committee of the American Association for the Study of the Feeble-Minded consisting of Goddard; Johnstone; Rogers; William Healy (then of Chicago); William T. Shanahan of the Epileptic Colony at Sonyea, New York; and David F. Weeks of the facility for epileptics at Skillman, New Jersey standardized a plan for charting pedigrees. At the association's 1910 meeting at the Illinois Asylum (where Goddard introduced the moron), the members enthusiastically adopted the plan. With few changes, Davenport published the plan as the second bulletin of the Eugenics Record Office, thus providing dissemination for this new tool in the codification of hereditary feeblemindedness (Davenport et al. 1911).

Goddard's relationship with Davenport was a symbiotic one. Goddard's interest in heredity went back at least to his work with G. Stanley Hall; Davenport's to the Harvard biology department. Their mutual, overlapping interest was important to their desire to understand human aberrations and do something to stop their occurrence. By 1909, it seemed clear to both that feeblemindedness was a unitary genetic flaw. Feebleminded people, they became convinced, were products of traits passed on in predictable regularity over generations. Given the simple nature of the flaw, they insisted, it would be possible to eliminate feeblemindedness by eliminating reproduction among the feebleminded. W. M. Hays (1910, 223), in the first edition of the *American Breeders' Magazine*, summed up the enthusiasm generated by Goddard's findings: "The article of Doctor Goddard, of New Jersey, on page 165, reporting investigations into the heredity of feeblemindedness, may be epoch-making in drawing attention of Mendelian students to the importance of investigation of unit characters in man."

It was in this context that Davenport first approached Mary Averell Harriman in 1910. The previous year, Harriman had inherited the fortune of her railroad magnate husband, E. H. Harriman. Added to her own, this fortune made her one of America's wealthiest and most influential citizens (Campbell 1971; "Harriman, Mary Williamson Averell" 1933). Probably influenced by her daughter, Mary (later Mrs. C. C. Rumsey), who had studied under Davenport at Cold Spring Harbor, Harriman in February agreed to fund the study of human evolution at Davenport's laboratory (see Allen 1986; Largent 2008, 50–68; Pauly 2000, 214–227). Soon thereafter, the Eugenics Record Office was born. Over the next decade, the office published several reports concentrating on the study of the pedigrees of degenerate, criminal, poor, and always feebleminded families. Often done under the auspices of superintendents of institutions for feeble minds, these reports were championed by the American Association for the Study of the Feeble-Minded at their annual meetings, in their journal, and in their communications with legislators, community leaders, and among themselves. Likewise, Davenport and his colleagues became frequent contributors to the association's journal. Although extending beyond Goddard and Johnstone's focus, the work of Davenport and the Eugenics Record Office became fully integrated with the interests of the superintendents after 1910.

Harriman's support of eugenical research took a less prominent (but from the perspective of social policy an ultimately more important) turn in December 1914, when she agreed to fund the Committee on Provision for the Feeble-Minded. As the major backer of the Eugenics Record Office, Harriman had received timely information of the committee's workings over the preceding four years. In 1913, she became a member of the board of managers of Letchworth Village, a position she held until her death in 1932 (New York State, Department of Mental Hygiene 1948, 104). One of her several country homes even adjoined Letchworth Village. Both her financial backing of the Eugenics Record Office and her membership on the Letchworth Village board ensured her place in the disciplinary (albeit lay-disciplinary) network of intellectual disability services. As such, she was also well aware of Goddard's research at Vineland, where she was soon to be involved in a new project. The seeds of this project had been planted almost two years earlier.

In February 1913, Johnstone hired his brother-in-law, Alexander Johnson, to be executive director of Vineland's extension division. In 1903, after several years of political controversy, Johnson, who earlier had launched Johnstone's career in the field of mental deficiency, had resigned as superintendent of the Indiana School for the Feeble-Minded. After a stint teaching at the New York School of Philanthropy, Johnson became general secretary of the National Conference of Charities and Correction. There, among other things, he championed the cause of mental defectives. As part of his activities with the conference, Johnson began lecturing to state conferences and other state and local groups on the theme of the menace of the feebleminded. During 1911 and 1912, he concentrated his speaking engagements in the Southern states. In 1912, he addressed the Southern Sociological Congress and, over the next decade, continued to present papers to that association. Even before being hired to take over the Vineland's extension division, then, Johnson had shown interest in and developed relationships with philanthropic and academic personages in the South (Byers 1934, 75–84; Johnson 1923, 399–407).

Johnson filled a position held by Johnstone and Goddard since 1910. Having grown beyond their capacity to tend to it, the extension division had become an important source of social policy change in New Jersey. Under Johnstone and Goddard, the department of extension surveyed conditions in the state, using field workers to seek out and assess the conditions of the feebleminded. In 1911, under prodding from Vineland staff and supporters, the New Jersey legislature, with the enthusiastic support of Governor Woodrow Wilson, authorized statewide special education classes and mandated eugenic sterilization for certain categories of adult feeble minds. In 1914, at the urging of the extension division, the legislature, with the support of Governor James F. Fielder, Wilson's successor, appointed a commission on the care of mental defectives. The commission recommended the permanent segregation of the state's mental defectives and authorized the establishment of widespread farm colonies to handle the anticipated influx of institutionalized clientele. Johnson, already familiar with issues associated with feeblemindedness, assumed his new position not only to relieve Johnstone of the increasing responsibilities of the extension division but also to enlarge its work beyond New Jersey (Johnstone 1914; Leiby 1967, 109; McPhee 1968, 47–54).

To accomplish this end, Johnstone and Johnson knew the extension department needed additional funding. In the fall of 1914, Davenport, already intimately involved in the Vineland activities, made arrangements for a meeting with Mrs. Harriman. Not so much to convince her of the efficacy of the undertaking—she was already convinced—but to launch the enterprise on a truly national footing, Davenport along with Johnstone called prominent leaders in the field of mental deficiency to meet with Vineland staff and backers at Harriman's home on December 18, 1914.[8] By the spring of 1915, the committee had issued a statement of purpose: "To disseminate knowledge concerning the extension and menace of feeblemindedness, and initiate methods for its control and ultimate eradication from the American people" ("A Committee to Eradicate Feeblemindedness" 1915). Elected to the committee's board of directors were the New York psychiatrist Milton J. Greenman, chair; Johnstone, secretary; and the philanthropist Bayard Cutting, treasurer.[9] Leaving his post as New Jersey Commissioner of Charities, Byers became the committee's executive secretary, and Johnson assumed the position of field secretary (Byers 1934, 75–84; Johnson 1923, 393–400).

At first hoping to use the newspapers to launch their campaign, Byers and Johnson found most dailies too preoccupied with World War I to devote the kind of attention to mental deficiency that they wanted. Given this fact, they turned most of their attention to the lecture circuit. For the next three and a half years, Byers attended to committee business and Johnson toured the nation promoting the message of the menace of the feebleminded to any group ready to listen. Soon, as Byers (1934, 82) remarked, "The whole country seemed to [be] becoming feebleminded-conscious." By 1918, the committee had operations in thirty-three states, some of which had active state and local chapters usually made up of prominent citizens. In New York, for example, the state committee included socialites Mrs. Charles Dana Gibson (the original "Gibson Girl"), Mrs. William K. Vanderbilt, and Eleanor Johnson. Under their influence, the city of New York increased funding for the Randall's Island institution by more than $500,000; had the institution's longtime director, Mary C. Dunphy, replaced with one to its own liking; and instituted easier requirements for the permanent segregation of the city's mental defectives ("A Half-Million Dollars for Randall's Island" 1915). In 1923, members of the New York committee would join with other state social welfare advocates to support a $50 million state bond issue for New York institutions. Among their six-point platform was point three: "To protect the community from dangerous mental defectives" (*Herald*, November 1, 1923, 1).

In other states, too, Johnson's efforts were paying off. By 1918, nine states, mostly in the South, had opened facilities; five states with what the committee perceived to be inadequate facilities opened additional ones; and four states expanded existing institutions. In addition to the creation and expansion of institutional services, the committee was responsible for the development of special classes in virtually all thirty-three states where it worked ("The Folly of Freedom for Fools," 1918; Johnson 1923, 413–417; Ramsay [ca. 1920]; Whitten 1967, 17–19).

Crucial to Johnson's goal was moving the message of the menace of the feeble-minded beyond the confines of the social welfare community where, by 1914, the issue was well understood, to the general public, where, he believed, it was not. In 1923, he recalled:

> In the minds of the general public there was a vague idea that there does exist a "problem of the feebleminded," that there are many of them and that something should be done. But they were usually or frequently confused with the Insane. There was no general knowledge of the relations between feeblemindedness and poverty and crime; there was plentiful ignorance of what proper care means; of the possibilities of training; of the colony plan and how much of benefit it might bring; of the degree to which thousands of imbeciles and morons, otherwise helpless or dependent, or hurtful to social order, might be made safe, useful and happy; of the methods of sterilization and segregation. There was evident need of a wide presentation of the facts, the results of experiment, in a popular, positive, objective way; not merely as it had been done to social workers at national and state conferences; but to the general public. The task was to force upon the attention of the whole people the facts we knew; to convince them of the validity of our methods and of the duty of every state to its feebleminded; and to induce each to discharge that duty fully. (Johnson 1923, 393)

Before like-minded colleagues and supporters, Johnstone (1914) talked of the propaganda value of Johnson's work. Articles in the popular press about feeblemindedness and crime; feeblemindedness and "the assassination of prominent people"; feeblemindedness and inebriety, insanity, syphilitics, prostitutes, and other sex offenders; feeblemindedness and "tramps, paupers, homeless men and women, the drunkards and drug fiends, and the inefficients" were all relevant to the propaganda activities of the extension division and later the Committee on Provision. This information, he insisted, should be collected and widely disseminated.

By the beginning of 1916, Johnson felt confident his goal was being accomplished. During his first three years of work, he had visited every city and town in New Jersey, speaking to nearly 20,000 people in 111 lectures, most of which included stereoscopic illustrations. Working with the state committee on provision for the feebleminded, Johnson had persuaded the New Jersey legislature to enact a medical inspection law to detect feeblemindedness in public schools, a sterilization statute, and a law prohibiting marriage of the insane or feebleminded persons; appropriate funds for special school classes; give the courts the authority to compel admission to state institutions for feeble minds; and authorize the parole of sterilized inmates from state facilities (Johnstone 1914). Johnson did not confine himself to New Jersey. He gave 250 lectures, traveling as far north as Montreal and Newfoundland, as far south as New Orleans and Texas, and west to Illinois.

After the formation of the national committee, he lectured in 350 cities and towns, in several more than once. He estimated giving 1,100 lectures between 1915 and 1918 to 250,000 people in all parts of the nation. These audiences included:

> general public meetings; legislative assemblies and committees; state universities; colleges, medical schools, theological seminaries, state normal schools, summer schools for teachers, high schools, teachers' institutes, parent-teachers' associations; church congregations at Sunday services and prayer meetings, ministers' meetings, Sunday-schools, and Bible classes; schools of social work in seven different cities; chambers of commerce, business men's associations: Rotary, Kiwanis, Lions and other lunch clubs; women's clubs, local, state, and national, and national councils of women; national and state conferences of charities; conferences of health officers and of county officials, and conferences on mental hygiene; social workers' clubs, immigrants' national associations; juvenile protection associations; civic leagues; settlements; state meetings of Kings' daughters; eugenics education meetings; audiences in motion picture shows, and others. (Johnson 1923, 396–397)

Johnson was especially proud of his speeches at American universities and colleges. Between 1913 and 1918, he gave ninety-five lectures to groups of students in seventy-two different cities in twenty-eight states. He estimated a total student audience of 20,000 (Johnson 1923, 399).

Of the various sections of the nation in which he worked, Johnson seemed most proud of his efforts in the South. Although English by birth, Johnson seemed to get along especially well with Southerners. In Arkansas, South Carolina, Mississippi, and Virginia, Johnson devoted much time and energy, but other states of the region also felt his presence. Gaining entree through women's groups and churches, he organized lectures before all sorts of voluntary associations and legislative committees. Preaching the menace of the feebleminded message, he soon found attentive audiences. Aware that the war had driven the prices of cotton and tobacco to record highs, he knew Southern legislators were in atypically generous moods. Fear and high prices had their effect, as one Southern state after another appropriated funds for state institutions, and Southern communities began special education classes (Johnson 1923, 415; Ramsay [ca. 1920]; Whitten 1967, 17–19; Noll 1995, 2005).

Between 1914 and 1923, nine Southern states founded institutions for feeble minds. None housed African American inmates. Not until 1939, when Virginia opened the all-black Petersburg State Colony, did black people enter such public facilities in the South. As Steven Noll (1991, 133, 143) noted: "The apocalyptic expressions of physicians and superintendents concerning the 'menace of the feebleminded' rarely, if ever, mentioned race. . . . With control enforced by legalized segregation, there appeared little need for institutions for the feebleminded to further control black deviants." Ironically, as Noll observed, prohibited from institutions, blacks (for a time) escaped "the indignities of compulsory eugenic sterilization."

In other states where services for mental defectives had existed for several decades, the committee mobilized support for the expansion of services. Using

warnings associated with the "menace of the feebleminded," these state committees often hired field workers to do state pedigree studies to demonstrate the results of inadequate prevention (e.g., Butler 1907, 1923; see also Bix 1997; Hahn
1980). In 1908, Johnstone (1908) reported on the Ross family, the family of Lucy
X, and the Jackson whites and Jackson blacks. Albert E. Winship (1900) linked
the Jukes of an earlier era with his "Edwards clan." Elizabeth Kite (1912*a*, 1912*b*,
1913), Goddard's colleague on the Kallikak study, published a series of articles on
"The Pineys" in the *Survey* (see also McPhee 1968, 47–54). The Boston physician
Charles P. Putnam wrote about the Corwin family (Committee on Protection of the
Feeble-Minded 1913). Arthur H. Estabrook and Charles Davenport (Davenport 1912;
Estabrook and Davenport 1912) published *The Nam Family* and Estabrook (1916)
followed with his reanalysis of the Juke family. In 1912, Davenport and Florence
H. Danielson (1912) published *The Hill Folk*. Mary S. Kostir (1916) followed with her
study of the "Family of Sam Sixty," and, the same year, the Eugenics Record Office
published Anna W. Finlayson's "The Dack Family" (Finlayson 1916). Shortly after
A. C. Rogers' death, Maud Merrill published their *Dwellers in the Vale of Siddem* (A.
Rogers and Merrill 1919). Mina A. Sessions (1918) also came out with her study of
the Hickory family (Harkins 2004).

Even into the 1920s, these studies were regularly and frequently conducted.
Wilhelmine E. Key (1920, 1923) of the Race Betterment Foundation of Battle Creek,
Michigan, studied six generations of Pennsylvania degenerates known as the Rufer
family. At the Second International Congress of Eugenics in 1921, Estabrook (1923;
see also N. Deutsch 2009) reported his study of the tribe of Ishmael, the "American
gypsies" whom Oscar McCulloch had first identified nearly forty years earlier. At the
same congress, held at the American Museum of Natural History in September and
October 1921, Estabrook exhibited a booth of "cacogenic families," where pedigree
charts and photographs of twelve notoriously degenerate families were displayed.
Nearly ten thousand visitors viewed this and other exhibits in conjunction with
the congress's activities. The exhibits were funded by a grant of $2,500 from Mary
Averell Harriman (Laughlin 1923). Two years later, E. R. Johnstone (1923, 101–116)
reported on "Kate and Her Family" and the family of "Old Iz and Hanner Anne." In
1926, Estabrook and Ivan E. McDougle (1926) published *Mongrel Virginians: The Win
Tribe*. In Vermont, the zoologist Henry F. Perkins published his study of the "degenerate" Pirate family (Gallagher 1999, 81–83). In 1931, Eleanor Rowland Wembridge
(1931) published *Life among the Lowbrows*, in which she took the scientific pedigree
study to its most popular limit. Recounting the lives of several mental defectives,
she pictured her studies as sometimes lovable, sometimes threatening, but always
hopelessly stupid. Published by Houghton Mifflin, the book sold well in the popular
book-buying market. Even as late as 1936, Jack Manne wrote about the "A Hollow
Family" and the "B Hollow Family" (Manne 1936). What Dugdale and McCulloch
began in the previous century burgeoned into a national pastime after Goddard's
1912 study. In state after state and community after community, in rural areas and
in urban ones, feeble minds were now viewed as a frequent, permanent, and growing
menace.[10]

Emphasizing a theme first made prominent by Goddard, these pedigree studies also reinforced a belief in the linkage of rapidly multiplying mental defectives and a host of social problems: crime, prostitution, abuse of charity, juvenile delinquency, venereal diseases, illegitimate births, and drunkenness. Lay committees in state after state and community after community, echoing the earlier warnings of the superintendents, called for immediate and permanent controls for defective minds, especially moronic defective minds. A 1915 study including pedigree investigations by the Cincinnati Juvenile Protective Association (Figure 5.4) was typical of most. The association warned:

> The moron group is the most serious menace to society. The idiot and the imbecile, because of their low degree of intelligence are easily recognized. They usually do not look normal and are often physically repellant. The moron, however, can pass as normal among laymen. Like a twelve-year-old child, he can understand instructions and perform fairly intricate tasks. He can read and write, feed and clothe himself, can take an interest and discuss the events which transpire about him, but no matter what his physical age and size, he is always a child in his power of discrimination, of self-control, of planning and of initiative. *To leave him on his own resources out in the community, forced to compete with his normal fellows in*

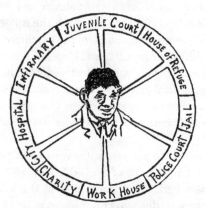

THE FEEBLE-MINDED

OR THE

HUB TO OUR WHEEL OF VICE, CRIME AND PAUPERISM

Cincinnati's Problem

Figure 5.4:
"Cincinnati's Problem," 1915. Cover of *The Feeble-Minded*, a pamphlet distributed by the Juvenile Protective Association of Cincinnati. (Courtesy of the Ohio History Connection)

industry, to live up to the standard of morals evolved from the complexities of modern
civilization, when he has not the inherent qualities necessary to enable him to do so,
results in the ne'er-do-well, the unemployable, the vicious, the immoral or the criminal.
(Juvenile Protective Association of Cincinnati 1915, 7; emphasis in the original)

By 1918, the last year of its existence, the Committee on Provision for the Feeble-Minded had accomplished a remarkable feat. In less than four years, it had influenced the expansion of state institutionalization and local special classes to an extent never before seen. Although some scientific discomfort with its claims about the "menace of the feebleminded" was already surfacing, its message still evoked praise in lay and academic circles (see, e.g. English 1922).

In 1917, for example, after the army refused to fund a proposed intelligence testing program for new recruits, the committee began subsidizing the work of Goddard, Robert M. Yerkes, Lewis Terman, and other psychologists on what eventually became known as the army "Alpha" and "Beta" tests. Housed at the Training School at Vineland, these psychometricians saw an opportunity to expand their newly developed tool. By the end of the war, they had tested 1.75 million men and concluded that 40 percent of the white male population was feebleminded. Although critics like Walter Lippmann later raised questions about the meaning of "average intelligence" given such a high percentage of feeblemindedness, the army tests would both launch the field of applied psychology and affirm Americans' growing confidence in psychology's ability to measure general intelligence (Brigham 1923; Brown 1992, 109–125; Burnham 1968; DuBois 1970, 61–66; Gould 1981, 192–199; Lippmann 1922a, 1922b, 1923; Minton 1988, 64–74; J. Trent 1982, 135–139; see also Darrow 1926).

By 1918, the mental hygiene movement, which had begun in 1908 with the publication of Clifford Beers's influential book *The Mind That Found Itself* (Beers 1908), had through the machinations of Greenman, Salmon, and Fernald taken the wind out of the committee's sails. Uncomfortable with the influence of psychologists like Goddard and social workers like Johnson, the psychiatrists on the committee persuaded backers to shift their loyalties and largess. Their opposition was not so much directed at the psychologists' most effective tools, the intelligence tests, as it was at their growing national prominence. In December 1914, Fernald had been in Mrs. Harriman's parlor at the creation of the Committee on Provision for the Feeble-Minded. By the following July, however, he was warning W. H. C. Smith:

> I suspect that they will try to put over at the meeting in San Francisco [of the American Association for the Study of the Feeble-Minded] a vote of approval of the Vineland Extension work. I shall not be present at the Association meeting this year. The Committee on this project is made up of Dr. [A. C] Rogers and you with myself as Chairman.
>
> Personally, I do not believe we ought to endorse this or any other movement whose future is uncertain, and not yet worked out. Of course, I should be glad if your opinion agreed with mine. If it does will you not write to Dr. Rogers to that effect? . . . I think we want to be cautious what we endorse.

Two weeks later, after a reply from Smith, Fernald wrote again:

I thank you for your very kind letter of the 20th and am delighted if you think you feel as I do.

I am sure we all feel that extending the work of the feebleminded cannot be turned over to any one institution or one group of people but that all agencies that have the right point of view, should receive our interest and our approval. (Beverly Farm Records, letters from Walter E. Fernald to W. H. C. Smith, July 17, 1915; July 31, 1915)

Seeing in the mental hygiene movement a way to enlarge their influence, especially outside the parameters of the state institution, these medical superintendents began to distance themselves from what they began (quite quickly) to see as the excessive hyperbole of the psychologically and eugenically based Vineland message. After the war, when some began to hint that Goddard's research was "just too good," the psychiatrists, through the mental hygiene movement, pulled the plug on the Vineland spotlight. In 1918, Ohio State University offered Goddard a position in its psychology department. By that time, Milton J. Greenman, a psychiatrist on the board of the Committee on Provision, as much because of professional jealousy as of scientific uneasiness with Goddard's pedigree findings and conclusions, convinced Samuel Fels that Goddard's work was scientifically weak. Soon thereafter Fels wished Goddard well in his new efforts in Ohio (Porteus 1969, 68; see also Gelb 1999). Johnson also moved on to his next "adventure," this time with the American Red Cross. Thus, in 1918, the two principal purveyors of the menace of the feebleminded left Vineland and their sources of funding. The momentum begun by their efforts would take another decade to subside. The postwar Red scare, anti-immigration agitation, and the results of the army Alpha testing would, among other things, sustain the menace rhetoric despite the absence of the Committee on Provision for the Feeble-Minded (Bagley 1924). And, of course, superintendents trying to maintain their newly won appropriations would take up the efforts in their individual states. But the frenetic energy was soon to dissipate, and, with the emergence of the mental hygiene movement, the menace of the feebleminded would be transformed into a new message—one emphasizing adjustment and adaptation, one eventually transforming the menacing feeble mind into a maladjusted perpetual defective.

CONCLUSION

The rhetoric of "the menace of the feebleminded," which emerged in the first decade of the twentieth century and continued into the third, was relatively short-lived among the medical superintendents. By 1920, most medical men (and occasionally medical women) had begun to distance themselves from the menace message and its link to eugenics. In part, this distancing was the result of the very claims made by the eugenicists for the enormity of feeblemindedness. Since there were so many of them, how could all feeble minds be segregated in institutions? In part, however, the distancing was the result of the medical superintendents' discomfort with the success of their nonmedical colleagues in spreading the message of the menace of the feebleminded throughout the nation, in opening new institutions, and in acquiring funds from influential and rich Americans. By distancing themselves from what they had so recently helped to create, they were separating themselves from a challenge to their own authority and influence.

In the place of eugenics, these medical superintendents turned to the new psychiatry with its emphasis on mental hygiene, the language of adjustment and adaptation, and community-based services. To be sure, the shift was quite sudden. As late as 1908, Walter Fernald (1909, 17, 33), for example, had warned in no uncertain terms: "The unrecognized imbecile is a most dangerous element in the community. . . . From a biological standpoint the imbecile is an inferior human being." Facing the threat of the nonmedically dominated Committee on Provision for the Feeble-Minded, however, he quickly changed his position, finding that feeble minds could, after all, adjust to community placement (1919, 1924). His "change of heart" about menacing feeble minds in communities and eugenics was also a change of head. Fernald and his colleagues at other public facilities for feeble minds had supported the Committee on Provision as it gained legitimacy. They joined in its successful campaign to use the threat of the menace of the feebleminded to get new and bigger legislative appropriations. As the committee's influence grew, however, medical superintendents like Fernald turned against it, instead linking their futures to the emerging mental hygiene movement and its vision of community services.

As dramatic and successful as the Committee on Provision had been, then, in its very success it hid the greater success of the old guard in keeping the vision of feeblemindedness within its own professional purview. As such, feeblemindedness would remain with the superintendents—at least for a time.

The superintendents' motives in first supporting and then opposing the menace of the feebleminded point to the complexity of institutional social control. On the one hand, there were few incidents in the history of deviance in America in which plans for control were more deliberate. For a time, superintendents, social welfare luminaries, and old-money and new-moneyed philanthropists joined to develop a theme that they carried to both lecture halls and legislative assemblies. Given the linkage between the class fears among American bluebloods and a variety of emerging professional classes interested in "cashing in" on those fears, the forces behind control were clear: a social threat had to be removed from society and prevented from re-emerging.[11]

There can be little doubt that this linkage played an important part in shaping the intensity of the menace rhetoric and its results. On the other hand, the linkage cannot explain the short life of the movement. Faced with challenges to their prominence in controlling their own facilities and the wider "disciplinary matrix" of feeblemindedness, along with their eagerness to join fellow psychiatrists in expanding their professional influence outside the asylum to the community, medical superintendents began to distance themselves from the rhetoric of control associated with eugenics and its program for the various "threats to America." The very abruptness of this shift in perspective after 1920 demonstrated that even the most apparently conspiratorial control had within it internal institutional and professional dynamics and contradictions.

For the medical superintendents, it turned out to be the best of all possible courses. From 1900 to 1920, when they were active in the menace of the feeble-minded movement, superintendents gained more prominence and institutional power than they had ever before known. Presidents, governors, university professors, and philanthropists were seeking them out. With their new and larger legislative appropriations and their growing respect among fellow psychiatrists, medical superintendents could, in the 1920s, turn their backs on eugenics and formulate a new vision of an adaptable and adjustable feeble mind. They could do so because the rhetoric of the new vision easily turned to routine. As such, they were in a better position to maintain their own authority in even more rationalized, routinized facilities. Put another way, superintendents of the period knew as well as Max Weber that *charismatic* control of the sort embodied in "the menace of the feebleminded" could initiate new patterns and degrees of authority but could not sustain authority in the language of mental hygiene's adaptation and adjustment; thus, superintendents *routinized* their newfound institutional authority and public prominence and also looked to the community to expand both. One of America's most prominent examples of woe in the first two decades of the new century, feebleminded Americans would find themselves reconstructed as examples of the human weal in the 1920s. The change, of course, had nothing to do with them.

NOTES

1. Nora Groce (1992) wrote about the reaction of Job's Harbor, a small Massachusetts coastal town, to Millard Fillmore Hathaway, who lived from 1858 to 1921. From the recollections of the townspeople, Groce reconstructed the attributes of Hathaway that led him to become the "town fool" of Job's Harbor. Groce noted that most of the citizens of the town had great affection for Hathaway and maintained a self-imposed limit on the amount and intensity of teasing they forced him to endure, and Hathaway, as Groce pointed out, was quite skilled at getting along. Despite the townsfolk's affection, he froze to death one winter. Groce's study (albeit involving only one case and done retrospectively) suggests that, in some small towns and rural areas, citizens may not have absorbed the success-failure norm that was developing in urban America.

2. This construction of intellectual disability among school teachers in the first part of the twentieth century can be appreciated in a circular sent in 1912 by the North Carolina Teachers Association to "every grade teacher in North Carolina." It was in this period that the state began to discover mental defectives in the public schools. The circular read:

Fellow Teacher:

Rid your room of mental deficients. You owe it to the enormous majority of normal pupils. You owe it to the deficients who are entitled to special education. You owe it to the tax payers on whom these deficients, when adults, unless specially educated, will be a burden. Finally, you owe it to yourself. You can no more do your grade work properly with a deficient child in your room than you could do it were a blind or a deaf and dumb child put into it.

For the protection of your own professional character, take the action which we urge. We need not add that there is even a distinct personal award in the removal of a wholly unwarranted wear and tear upon your nerves. (North Carolina State Archives, Department of Public Instruction, correspondence, January–March 1912, A–F)

3. Woodrow Wilson was not the only president interested in feeblemindedness in the contexts of immigration restriction and eugenics. Theodore Roosevelt (1904) had written favorably about eugenics. Warren G. Harding advocated immigrant restriction in his 1920 campaign, and Calvin Coolidge (1921) warned Americans about racial degeneracy because of racial inbreeding (see Gossett 1965, 404–405).

4. More than three decades later, Goddard (1943) recalled only one 1905 article by Binet and Simon. Actually three articles by them appeared in the 1905 edition of *L'année psychologique*.

5. The place of women, like Kite, as eugenics field workers is detailed in Bix (1997).

6. Sixty-four years later, Stephen Jay Gould (1981, 165) also recognized what he called Goddard's "unconscious statements of prejudice."

7. Other members included Alexander Graham Bell, Luther Burbank, W. E. Castle, Charles R. Henderson, J. Arthur Thomson, W. L. Tower, H. J. Webber, C. E. Woodruff, and Frederick A. Woods, all successful representatives of business, science, and academia.

8. In attendance were secretaries of four state boards of charity: R. W. Kelso of Massachusetts, Joseph T. Martin of Virginia, Amos W. Butler of Indiana, and Joseph Byers of New Jersey. Also attending were several superintendents: Walter Fernald of the Massachusetts Training School, Charles Little of Letchworth Village in New York (on whose board Harriman served), J. Moorehead Murdoch of the Pennsylvania State Training School at Polk, A. C. Rogers of Minnesota, and E. R. Johnstone of the Vineland facility, all of whom were also in town to hold a public hearing on plans for the new state facility known as Letchworth Village (New York State, State Senate 1915). Other Vineland representatives included four of its board members: the philanthropists Bleeker VanWagenen, Samuel S. Fels, and R. Bayard Cutting and the psychiatrist Milton J. Greenman, along with Alexander Johnson. Joining these interested parties were Charles B. Davenport; Harry V. Osborne, judge of the recently established juvenile court of Newark, New Jersey; Franklin B. Kirkbride, a trustee of Letchworth Village; and Jerome D. Greene and Mina M. Bruere, both of Manhattan. The next month, two of those in attendance, Cutting and Fels, joined with the philanthropist Maurice Ayars to commit additional funds to the project.

9. Other board members included Harry Osborne, Mrs. C. C. Rumsey (née Mary Harriman, daughter of Mrs. E. H. Harriman), the psychiatrist Thomas Salmon, and socialites Bleeker VanWagenen and Caroline Wittpenn.

10. Nicole H. Rafter (1988) brought together a collection of eleven of these eugenic family studies. She holds that the eugenicists were "professionals involved in the

new business of social control," adding that "the family studies did more than extend professional horizons. They also validated that extension, giving it rationale, scientific authority, an aura of expertise and objectivity, the family-tree technology, and [a] claim to community service" (Rafter 1988, 14–15, 16).

11. On the linkage of class fears and the emerging professional classes, see Bledstein (1976).

CHAPTER 6

Sterilization, Parole, and Routinization

During the Great War, American farmers had never had it so good. Mild weather and increased demand ensured high prices. Feeding the home front, the "boys over there," and much of Western Europe made American farmers prosperous. In 1920, things began to change, however, and change quickly. Total farm net income dropped from more than $10 billion in 1919 to $9 billion in 1920 and then to $4 billion in 1921. By 1925, most farm commodities were selling at prewar or even lower prices. Farmers who had borrowed money during the war to expand their output began to lag behind in their loan payments and face default because of bumper crops and low prices. Veterans returning home found farms no longer prosperous and were drawn to the cities by growing industries. After all, one in every five American families owned an automobile, and the ratio of haves to have-nots appeared to be narrowing. If the soldier farm-boy could see Paris, why not Detroit or Pittsburgh or Cincinnati? The Great Depression, generally acknowledged as beginning with the crash of 1929, actually hit rural America nearly a decade earlier (Daniels 1966, 146; Garraty 1987, 52–84; C. Meyer 2007, 111–172).

Increasing numbers of farmers began to abandon their farms, especially in the Northeast and upper Midwest, selling or renting their land holdings at deflated prices. Their descendants, now often in the city, were even more eager to dispose of their not-so-profitable real estate. For superintendents of state schools for mental defectives or the mentally deficient (two of the choice terms of the period), this cheap land was a blessing. In upstate New York, in western Massachusetts, in central Ohio, and in the newly opened Southern facilities, superintendents like Charles Bernstein, George L. Wallace, F. L. Keiser, and others were buying and renting land as fast as they could acquire the funds to do so. In 1915, for example, the Illinois Asylum for Feeble-Minded Children in the farm-rich center of the state had 520 acres of purchased or leased land; by 1920, it controlled nearly 900 acres; and, by 1930, 1,140 acres (Bateman, Selby, and Currey 1920; Illinois Department of Public Welfare 1930, 126).

What the superintendents had for decades called for and what the Committee on Provision for the Feeble-Minded had so effectively aroused was the public support for more new institutions and bigger existing ones. By 1923, the figures were even more astonishing than the superintendents had dared hope for a decade earlier. In 1923, the American Association for the Study of the Feeble-Minded compiled an "incomplete list of State and private institutions" and published the listing in its 1924 proceedings. According to the association's findings, there were fifty-eight public facilities. Forty-two of the forty-eight states had at least one public institution for mentally deficient people. Several states had two facilities, and a few (Massachusetts, New Jersey, and Pennsylvania) had three. New York boasted six (American Association for the Study of the Feeble-Minded 1924, 365–373). Even more astonishing than the growth and size of public facilities was the multiplication of private institutions. In 1900, there had been about ten private facilities; by 1923, there were eighty.

Few doubted that American institutions were segregated by socioeconomic class (Table 6.1). Even as early as the 1870s, public institutions were becoming facilities for the children and siblings of America's working class, poor, and immigrants. By 1910, all public institutions for feebleminded people were primarily housing lower class Americans.[1] When the state of New York, for example, planned for what it saw as its premiere school for feeble minds, Letchworth Village, it took for granted that "the majority of feebleminded persons belong[ed] to families in adverse circumstances" (New York State, State Senate 1915, 8). From the opening of the school at Barre in western Massachusetts and Seguin's school in Manhattan, the well-off could send their children to private schools where education would be stressed while (especially by the end of the century) lifetime care could be assured.

Private schools went by many names: home, farm, private school, institution, school of adjustment, academy, hospital, psychopathic institute, psychological school, and training school. They identified their clientele in several ways— backward youth, retarded children, the backward, defectives, backward and inefficient children, subnormal children, the feebleminded, and those needing

---

Table 6.1. COMPARISON OF THE SOCIOECONOMIC CLASS OF APPLICANTS AND ADMISSIONS TO THE LINCOLN STATE SCHOOL, 1888–1906

	Parents' Ability to Pay Expenses[a]					
	Able Not		Able		No Report	
Dates[b]	Applied (%)	Admitted (%)	Applied (%)	Admitted (%)	Applied (%)	Admitted (%)
1888–89	52 (52)	28 (47)	40 (40)	24 (41)	8 (8)	7 (12)
1901	42 (42)	25 (37)	55 (55)	42 (62)	3 (3)	1 (1)
1905–66	82 (41)	74 (41)	111 (55)	98 (55)	7 (4)	7 (4)

Source: These data come from admission application books of the Lincoln State School and Colony, Illinois State Archives, Record No. 254.4. Each admission book contains 100 applications.
[a]The form asks, "Are the parents able to furnish the child with clothing and pay expenses of transportation?"
[b]Dates represent record numbers 2101–2200 (1888–89), 3000–3099 (1901), and 5305–5505 (1905–06).

adjustment. Although some remained day schools and philosophies differed among them, most private schools were unlike their public counterparts in only two ways— their size and their resources. Most private schools had fewer than five hundred inmates. Several were much smaller. Only a few, like the Elwyn Institute and the Training School at Vineland, were larger. All private schools, of course, charged tuition. Sometimes tuitions varied by the ability of a family to pay. Before the admission of an inmate, the operator (usually a physician or an educator) determined a fee and from time to time renegotiated charges. High prices during World War I, for example, caused most private operators to demand higher tuitions (e.g., Beverly Farm Record, unsorted letters from families to W. H. C. Smith 1917–19). Public institutions charged fees, but only to a small proportion of their clientele. Only after World War II did public institutions begin a more aggressive attempt to collect fees from families who could pay. Private institutions, of course, could also be more selective in admitting clientele.

W. H. C. Smith's admission ledger, for example, contained a record of each request for admission to Beverly Farm from its opening in 1897 until 1911. Most entries listed the disposition of the request and the reason for admitting or denying admission. Smith refused to admit clientele to his private "farm" who, as he defined them, had "gross habits" and were uncontrollable misbehavers. He also declined the admission of African Americans and people whose relatives' financial situation appeared unstable (Beverly Farm Records, Application Book #1 1897–1911).

Despite these differences, private facilities, like their public counterparts, shared a common understanding of mental deficiency and the necessity of providing custody for many defectives. Not surprisingly, relatives who could afford them looked to private facilities to provide private custody. The menace of the feebleminded rhetoric left few postwar Americans proud of having a defective family member. This imposed humiliation, embarrassment, and grief could best be assuaged by the absence of the defective family member. If one could afford it, private care made the transition less problematic and, of course, more private. Public facilities had to take all sorts; private ones did not. In 1851, the Rowells family, well-to-do neighbors of John Greenleaf Whittier, had no reluctance acknowledging in their local newspaper their good feelings about their son's education at Samuel G. Howe's publicly funded school (see Chapter 1). By 1920, few prosperous Americans felt comfortable advertising their personal calamity. Although the message of the superintendents in the 1920s was becoming less harsh than it had been just a few years earlier, their warnings by now had filtered into the American consciousness. The popular media, still flamed by the popular eugenicists, kept the warnings current (e.g., Haring 1930; Sloss 1912; Wembridge 1926a, 1926b, 1927). At worst, mental defectives were poor, law-breaking, sexually promiscuous, hereditarily tainted lowlifers; at best, they were (or would become in the 1930s) silly "little morons," the stylized jokes of college students, office workers, and, by the 1940s, of most American elementary school students (on the "little moron" joke cycle, see Baughman 1943; Botkin 1944; Davidson 1943; see also Barrick 1980). To have a defective in the family was to be associated with vice, immorality, failure, bad blood, and stupidity. To place that defective in a public facility was to be associated with the lower classes.

In 1930, an article titled "Deficient" appeared in the popular literary magazine *Atlantic Monthly*. The author, Helen Garnsey Haring, whom the magazine's editor described as the "daughter of a mural painter and wife of a professor of history," wrote of her experiences with her son, a mentally deficient twelve-year-old boy. Her "coming out" was unusual for parents during this period. It was probably not accidental that the editor of the magazine made a special point of noting Haring's pedigree (both blood and marital). As the daughter of an artist and wife of an academic, Haring could hardly be associated with hereditary taint. Although acknowledging her son's previous admission to a public institution, Haring was quick to tell her readers that he was now in a private school where special attention was improving, although hardly overcoming, his weak mind. Reflecting a theme that was becoming prominent among professionals in the 1920s, Haring emphasized the emotional impact of having a defective child in the family. "The parents who find themselves, as we did nine years ago," she concluded her article, "suddenly face to face with tragedy, inescapable, can only try to alleviate it with such courage as they can muster and such knowledge as they may gain. But one hopes that public sympathy and cooperation will aid them more in the future than in the past to adjust, to a life they cannot avoid living, these pathetic little outsiders."

After 1920, the focus of mental defect would increasingly be on the middle-class family, on its burden, on its tragedy, and on its ability or inability to cope. Popular attitudes about mental deficiency, cultivated by superintendents and their supporters, convinced prosperous parents not only that having a defective mind in the family was stressful but also that to deal with the stress, families had best give up their defective family member and be silent about it. The attitudes and the silence would linger for several more decades. After all, who wanted to have a source of stress in the family? Who wanted to risk the stability and good name of the family?

Along with the growth in the number of facilities for mental defectives was a dramatic increase in the number of people admitted to institutions. The national picture reflected not only the growth of older public facilities, but also the emergence of new institutions in the South and West. The institutional population of mental defectives in 1904 was 14,347; in 1910, with the spread of the menace of the feebleminded rhetoric, the inmate population had increased to 20,731. In 1915, 5,940 new inmates (including epileptics) were added to the nation's public institutions for mental defectives, and 3,172 were discharged or died, bringing the total to 32,727 (US Department of Commerce 1919). By 1923, seven years after the demise of the Committee on Provision for the Feeble-Minded, the population had reached nearly 43,000 (A. Deutsch 1949, 369).

Data from specific institutions revealed the same pattern of growth. The Rome State Custodial Asylum for Unteachable Idiots opened in New York in 1894. In 1916, its official capacity had reached 1,200, but it housed 1,554 inmates, ranging from a three-month-old infant to an eighty-five-year-old. In 1915, 344 new inmates had been admitted, 65 died, and 146 were discharged. This increase of 133 inmates to the already crowded conditions stressed the capacity of the facility's 200 attendants. The total operating expenditures for the fiscal year ending June 30, 1915 were $228,893, or $12.81 per inmate per month. The Rome asylum had

1,200 acres, or roughly 0.7 acre per inmate (a much smaller holding than that of Letchworth Village, for example, situated on 2,084 acres in Thiells, New York; US Department of Commerce 1919).

The situation at other state facilities was similar. At the Lincoln State School and Colony (the new name for the Illinois State School), 1,888 inmates were crowded into an institution with a capacity of 1,700. In 1915, the school admitted 246 more inmates than were discharged or died. Per inmate monthly costs were $13.24, and the institution had only 520 acres, or less than 0.3 acre per inmate. The population of the Ohio Institution for Feeble-Minded in 1915 was 1,912 with a capacity to expand to 2,200. Like the others, it admitted more inmates than it lost, gaining 180 inmates in 1915. Per inmate costs were $11.80, and its per-inmate acreage was a bit over 0.7 acre. At the Massachusetts School for the Feeble-Minded, the population of 1,610 inmates was nearly 100 over its capacity. During 1915, the facility added 31 inmates to its rolls. It had a monthly expenditure of $16.19 per inmate and claimed one of the most generous acreage ratios, 1.5 acres per inmate (US Department of Commerce 1919).

In addition to the population increases, the public facilities were experiencing an increase in a particular type of clientele—the defective delinquent—which placed even further demands on institutional capacity. Prone to criminal and immoral behavior, morons as they were now called, like their earlier counterparts moral imbeciles, were believed to need institutionalization for their own benefit and the protection of society (Fink 1938, 234–239; New York State, Rome Custodial Asylum 1915, 14; New York State, State Senate 1915, 8).

Pressure on the private schools, although easier to deal with, was no less great. In 1922, Superintendent W. H. C. Smith of Beverly Farm in Illinois reported that since his facility opened in 1897 he had received 3,800 applications but had admitted only 420 children and adults (Beverly Farm Collection, handwritten speech by W. H. C. Smith ca. 1922). Correspondence among private school operators suggested that few had trouble filling their schools (e.g., Beverly Farm Records, letters from C. T. Wilbur to W. H. C. Smith, November 20, 1904 and March 25, 1909). Demand far exceeded supply. Through word of mouth, advertising in educational periodicals, and referrals from superintendents of already overpopulated institutions, newly opened private schools were quickly filled.[2] In both private and public institutions, then, growth was more rapid and persistent than it had ever been.

Prior to this period of explosive growth, superintendents had generally enjoyed long tenures in their public facilities. Doren in Ohio, Wilmarth in Wisconsin, Rogers in Minnesota, Fernald in Massachusetts, Wylie in North Dakota, Mogridge in Iowa, Bernstein and Little in New York, and Murdoch in Pennsylvania (and later in Wisconsin) all had long occupancies at their respective facilities. The institutions they operated thereby became *their* institutions. Although all had problems from time to time with state legislatures, difficult governors, or prying boards of directors, by the standards of their successors, most were given freedom to run their facilities and their personal lives as they saw fit. As such, many of them became involved in local "booster" projects and business deals, linking activities at the institution with both the projects and the deals. Doren, for example, acquired extensive land holdings in and around Columbus. Almost always "land rich and cash poor," he was constantly hounded by creditors and tax collectors. Apparently, he had a penchant for show horses and dogs and had a fine collection of both, some of which he kept at the institution (Doren 1854–1905). A. C. Rogers, too, was involved in several extrainstitutional businesses: in 1908, he became vice president of the Wisconsin Lumber and Cattle Company. He was also a co-owner of the DeSoto Fruit, Agricultural and Manufacturing Company in Americus, Georgia, which required the occasional pilgrimage to look after his holdings there, usually in winter. Unlike most citizens of Minnesota, the inmates of the Minnesota School for the Feeble-minded and Colony for Epileptics rarely suffered for peaches while Rogers had interest in the company (Beverly Farm Records, unsorted letters from A. C. Rogers to W. H. C. Smith, November 29 and 30, 1904; December 6 and 13, 1904; Michels-Peterson 1978).

Neither superintendent saw these activities as unusual, and neither seemed restrained by institutional commitments. If personal business seemed congruent with their institutional business, so, too, were their personal lives and personal eccentricities integrated into the life of the institution. When Kerlin's wife died in 1892, it was widely known around Elwyn that he had had a séance in her bedroom on the night after her death. To Kerlin's disappointment, Mrs. Kerlin kept her silence (Barr 1934). Kerlin's command of Elwyn was so singular that employees feared his infrequent but never predictable 4:00 A.M. inspections "with his large black notebook under his arm" (Barr 1934). At Beverly Farm, W. H. C. and Nellie B. Smith became tour guides for groups going to the newly constructed Panama Canal and to the Grand Canyon. They made other trips to Hawaii and Europe (Beverly Farm Records, unsorted letters, mainly after 1910). Charles Bernstein was an active Rotarian, traveling around the country for meetings and, on one occasion, to Europe for an international conference of the civic club (Riggs 1936, 28, 101). Several other superintendents traveled extensively. None seemed to feel a need to stay close to the institution. What all these otherwise diverse activities had in common was a reflection of the congruity between the superintendents' personal and business lives with the life of the institution. Once they had shaped the institution to reflect their personalities, what they did "personally" became itself an extension of the institution.

What they had created, however, would soon become the undoing of several superintendents. Part of the undoing resulted from the pressure of numbers and the growing complexity of dealing with the care of people with many and varied problems. Part of the undoing resulted from the incongruity between old words and new words, between old commitments and new constructions. Winds of change began to rise as early as 1916: in that year, C. B. Caldwell, the only physician to come out of the 1908 scandal at the Lincoln school blameless, wrote his friend W. H. C. Smith:

> My transfer, which was effective today came as considerable of a surprise in that
> the notice was so short, though I had suspected for some time that a change might
> be made. . . . The recent law for commitment of feebleminded permitted the admission of a conglomeration of persons—defectives of criminal, alcoholic and insane

types—and the resultant disorder from lack of proper facilities to handle them made a decided difference in the work now and as you knew it at Lincoln. (Beverly Farm Records, letter from C. B. Caldwell to W. H. C. Smith, May 1, 1916)

Two years later, Thomas H. Leonard, superintendent at Lincoln, resigned in frustration. He wrote Smith prior to his resignation that the school was "so crowded at the present time that some sections [were] sleeping two in a bed." He went on to complain: "Cook County sent us about fifty-five cases in June; many of them bed patients. . . . Just why they persist in filling up our institution with this class is more than I can explain" (Beverly Farm Records, letter from Thomas H. Leonard to W. H. C. Smith, July 12, 1918). George S. Bliss, superintendent of the Indiana School for Feeble-Minded Youth (formerly the Indiana School for the Feeble-Minded), also resigned that year. The pressure for increasing admissions without additional legislative appropriations along with what he saw as an uncooperative board convinced Bliss that it was time to leave (Beverly Farm Records, letter from George S. Bliss to W. H. C. Smith, January 1, 1920).

In North Carolina, C. Banks McNairy, whose institution had opened only a decade earlier, reported extreme overcrowding and a flood of applications. He wrote Kate Burr Johnson, the commissioner of public welfare:

We have received the boy from Asheville and the one from Pamlico County, and I have also received one from Beaufort. The Asheville boy is a low grade idiot, wild as an animal, the one from Beaufort is an imbecile and an epileptic and the Pamlico County boy is an idiot. Nothing under God's heaven can be done for any of them as I can see. It is just a matter of segregation, food and clothing—the lowest types of animals.

He added, "While I sympathize with all these people and the communities, in the name of high heaven where are we going?" (North Carolina State Archives, State Board of Public Welfare, box 178, Letter from C. Banks McNairy to Kate Burr Johnson, May 23, 1924). In 1925, the Board of Public Welfare decided that McNairy's complaints about conditions at Caswell Training School reflected his too close "personal interest in the work. . . . He wants a part of it all," the board reported (North Carolina State Archives, State Board of Public Welfare, box 178, "Notes on Caswell Training School for Governor McLean," June 15, 1925 [unsigned]). In June, the board fired him.

Finally, in 1919, A. W. Wilmarth resigned from the Wisconsin Home for the Feeble-Minded. One of the nation's most senior superintendents, Wilmarth had received his early training at Elwyn Institute under Kerlin. He had worked as a junior physician there with both Martin Barr and Smith. Like Kerlin and Barr, he was an enthusiastic champion and practitioner of sterilization. After twenty-three years at the Wisconsin facility, Wilmarth, the home's first and only superintendent, found himself growing tired of controversies. He had advocated for a larger institution all his professional life. By 1919, he had seen the fruition of his efforts, but the results were not as he had imagined them to be. Legislative authorization to enlarge his facility had not matched legislative appropriations. His board, too, was becoming increasingly meddlesome and uncooperative. In 1913, the Wisconsin legislature had authorized sterilization to stop the breeding of future generations of mental defectives and to make room for new inmates through the parole of sterilized ones. Yet, protests from the "Catholic element," Wilmarth felt, had undermined his efforts. No longer, he complained, could he control the character and pace of change (Beverly Farm Records, letter from A. W. Wilmarth to W. H. C. Smith, February 25, 1916; December 13, 1919).[3]

FIRST STERILIZATIONS

The growing pressure to take more and more of the state's problems motivated superintendents to turn to sterilization as a means of dealing with institutional overpopulation. Ironically, the eugenics movement along with the IQ test had convinced most superintendents even before the war's end that total institutionalization of all mental defectives was an unrealistic goal. There were just too many morons, most of whom, superintendents came to believe, were breeding at a rate faster than the general population. Before 1918, total institutionalization advocated by most superintendents and sterilization advocated by some had as their purpose the social control of feeble minds. Safe in the institution and sterilized, feeble minds were harmless. The reports of enormous numbers of mental defectives among American recruits in 1917 and 1918, however, made superintendents less sanguine about the prospects of total institutionalization. The already mounting numbers of inmates in their overcrowded facilities also forced most of them to rethink their previous policies. Opposition from some churches, courts, and politicians, along with their own mixed feelings, had also caused superintendents to waver in their support for sterilization. Although much support for the procedure continued, between 1918 and 1927, most superintendents had become cautious about sterilization.

Originally, superintendents had supported sterilization for two other purposes: institutional order and eugenic control. These rationales were related, reflecting institutional needs and social trends. In 1892, as part of his presidential address to the Association of Medical Officers of American Institutions for Idiotic and Feeble-Minded Persons, Isaac Kerlin championed "asexualization" to control "epileptic tendency" and for "the removal of inordinate desires which [are] . . . an offense to the community" (Kerlin 1892c). Kerlin acknowledged that he had allowed the sterilization of one inmate at the Pennsylvania Training School. That case involved the removal of the "procreative organs" of a young woman. Kerlin (1892c) remarked, "When I see the tranquil well ordered life she is leading, her industry and usefulness in the circle in which she moves, and know that surgery has been her salvation from vice and degradation, I am deeply thankful to the benevolent lady whose loyalty to science and comprehensive charity made this operation possible."

In March 1894, F. Hoyt Pilcher, the superintendent of the Kansas State Asylum for Idiotic and Imbecile Youth, began castrating older boys and men who masturbated. By 1895, he had castrated eleven inmates. One of these men, Charles

Billings, died shortly after the operation, leaving some to suspect that the operation caused his death (J. Holman 1966; "Reviving an Old Scandal" 1895). Several medical journals of the period supported or were at least curious about the practice. The local *Winfield Courier* and the larger *Kansas City Times*, however, attacked it. As much to embarrass the Populist governor of Kansas who had appointed Pilcher as to protest Pilcher's actions, these Republican papers headlined "Horrible Story Regarding the Kansas Asylum for Imbecile Youth." The Kansas City paper quoted Charles T. Wilbur: "The individuals practicing it [castration] should be placed in the penitentiary just as quick as possible for such atrocious practices. It was never practiced in institutions in this or other countries" ("Reviving an Old Scandal" 1895). Using the scandal at the Kansas asylum as a campaign issue, Republicans in 1895 elected one of their own as governor, and Pilcher was removed. In 1897, the political tide turned again, and he was appointed to his former position. Taking up where he left off, in the next two years Pilcher performed forty-seven additional castrations on fourteen females and thirty-three males (Cave 1911; Gish 1972, 108–114; J. Holman 1966).[4]

Contrary to Wilbur's claim to the *Kansas City Times*, by 1895, superintendents were becoming interested—albeit cautiously interested - in sterilization. At the 1895 meeting of the Association of Medical Officers of American Institutions for Idiotic and Feeble-Minded Persons, A. C. Rogers discussed a successful case:

> One was a girl who was periodically maniacal, during the intervals she was like ordinary girls. Mentally she was very stupid. She learned next to nothing. From earliest childhood she was noted for outbreaks of passion. She was very sexual and vulgar, was constantly masturbating, would frequently expose herself. . . . We discussed removing her ovaries. . . . The operation was performed; no bad results followed and for six months the girl was better in every way. (Association of Medical Officers 1897, 50)

He added parenthetically, "Gradually she returned to her former habit . . . [and] was sent to the hospital for the insane, as a measure of protection." In his 1897 presidential address to the same association, Martin Barr (1897) devoted the greatest part of his message to the benefits of desexualization. He noted with approval the work of Pilcher in Kansas and the model legislation proposed by DeForest Willard. At this meeting, it was clear that superintendents were aware of the political troubles Pilcher faced in Kansas. Most wanted to avoid similar troubles in their own states. Barr called for the association to help superintendents secure legislation to protect them from liability. A. C. Rogers concurred: "The profession should not shirk its plain responsibility in assisting to shape legislation which, while permitting desexualization, shall hedge the operation by suitable safeguards from abuses" (A. Rogers 1897).

In Pennsylvania, Barr had already begun to advocate for state legislation to permit sterilization. By 1901, the board of the Pennsylvania Training School along with several Philadelphia physicians and surgeons had persuaded the state legislature to pass such a bill. As word about the bill became known in the state, opposition developed, although it was neither widespread nor particularly vocal. When the governor vetoed the bill, Barr and his followers were disappointed. Never that concerned with his own liability, however, Barr continued to sterilize Elwyn clientele, usually by castration, although (in the case of men) after 1900 by vasectomy, a procedure devised in 1899 by Harry C. Sharp, a physician at the Indiana State Reformatory (Barr 1902a, 1904a, 189–197, 1904b; Gugliotta 1998; Reilly 1991, 31–40).

Shortly before and after the turn of the century, the first group of sterilizers were interested in controlling sexual behavior they believed was inappropriate or destructive to the well-being of their inmates. By surgically eliminating the sexual instincts, they could also control behaviors that offended social sensibilities and thereby maintain proper order in the institution. Not surprisingly, most sterilizations were castrations, and the majority were done on idiots and low-grade imbeciles whose "obscene habits" were most bothersome to superintendents and their staff. Legislators, eleemosynary agents, and Sunday-school classes were frequent visitors to the state school; masturbating "low-grade" inmates were hardly images of the state school institutional authorities wanted their visitors to remember. Although most superintendents had interest in heredity, before 1900, they had shown little concern for linking sterilization with eugenic birth control among high-grade morons.[5]

By the end of the first decade of the new century, their interest began to shift. No doubt some of the reason for the shift was opposition from critics who saw sterilization to control behavior as an act of punishment and in violation of the Constitution's prohibition of cruel and unjust punishment. Indeed, controversy about the procedures had persuaded A. C. Rogers along with A. W. Wilmarth of the Wisconsin Home for Feeble-Minded to join Alexander Johnson of the Indiana School for Feeble-Minded Youth and Mattie Gundry of the Gundry Home for Feeble-Minded and Epileptics in Virginia in opposing sterilization as part of their duties on the National Conference of Charities and Correction's Committee on Colonies for and Segregation of Defectives. In their 1903 report, they stated: "We may call on the surgeon for any act upon an individual which is to benefit him. We may not treat him as we do with our cattle, for the benefit of ourselves or of the state" (Johnson 1903).

Ironically, both Rogers and Wilmarth, despite their protests, had previously performed castrations at their institutions. Like that of other superintendents of the period, their personal support for sterilization was tempered by opposition, which occurred so vocally in Kansas and by the 1901 gubernatorial veto in Pennsylvania. E. R. Johnstone (1904) reflected the ambivalence in his 1904 presidential address to the Association of Medical Officers of American Institutions for Idiotic and Feeble-Minded Persons: "Unsexing has been suggested and many strong arguments brought in its favor, but as yet the public knows too little of advantages of the operation and of the social dangers from this class, and so will not agree to the idea."

At the 1902 meeting of the National Conference of Charities and Correction, a year before the Committee on Colonies' report, Barr (1902a) had reaffirmed his support for sterilization as "the most beneficent instrument of law, the surgeon's knife preventing increase." No doubt bristling from the defeat of his model sterilization law in Pennsylvania the year before, Barr had begun to shift his rationale for sterilization. Following the general interest growing among social welfare luminaries, Barr and other superintendents of institutions for feeble minds in the first decade of the new century found a new and more potent rationale for sterilization—"preventing increase." Eugenics promised a better world through better breeding. Technologies developed first by Sharp, who by 1907 had sterilized 465 "guests of the state," also provided a less draconian means for this new end (Gugliotta 1998; Kevles 1985, 93; L. Whitney 1934, 126). No longer would superintendents have to be vulnerable to the accusation that they were punishing inmates merely for offensive behavior.

Although superintendents were never as unanimous in their support for sterilization as they had been for segregation, by 1910, most were at least willing to condone and perform sterilizations under particular circumstances. Fernald, Smith, Bernstein, Johnstone, and Rogers for the most part had opposed the procedure for *eugenic* purposes, although in the midst of the menace of the feebleminded campaigns, some had warmed to eugenic sterilization, especially vasectomies and tubal ligations (e.g., Bernstein 1913; Johnstone 1911). Interestingly enough, Rogers, who in the 1890s had supported castration for behavior control, was less enthusiastic nearly twenty years later about vasectomies and tubal ligations for eugenic social control (A. Rogers 1913).[6]

Others like Wilmarth, Johnstone, and B. W. Baker, superintendent of the New Hampshire School for the Feeble-Minded, who had all previously waffled on the issue, in the midst of the menace of the feebleminded rhetoric joined Barr in advocating sterilization for eugenic control (American Association for the Study of the Feeble-Minded 1918, 28; Johnstone 1911, 6–7; Wilmarth 1918). That Wilmarth in 1916 would openly write his friend Smith about sterilization demonstrated that the public opposition of superintendents like Smith may have been motivated more by fear of repercussions than by personal commitments. Wilmarth wrote:

> Your letter came this morning. We have been doing some "sterilizing." It was hard to get the bill through. It had the quiet, but powerful, opposition of the Catholic element against it, and that is a telling force in this state. Then I waited until the smoke had cleared away before beginning. We have cut the "vas" on 16 boys, to date, and tied both ends so as to destroy continuity. We have noticed no change in their mental characteristics, nor do I expect any. My sole aim was to prevent these boys begetting more of their kind should they leave us through elopement, discharge, or other method of removal.
>
> Now I am preparing a list of young women for operation. We have not fully decided whether to simply cut and tie the tubes, and thus isolate the ovaries, or remove the ovaries, and see if that will diminish sexual excitement. I rather think we will do the last named operation, or perhaps try each method on a part of the girls and compare results (if a change in administration does not remove us from the field of view). Our Dr. Frost, who has charge of our women's side, believes the removal of the ovaries, may in time diminish, or delay, sexual appetites. (Beverly Farm Records, letter from A. W. Wilmarth to W. H. C. Smith, February 25, 1916)

Wilmarth's letter left little doubt that, along with eugenic social control, the control of behavior remained an important aspect of the superintendents' interest in sterilization. It is not insignificant, too, that Wilmarth was more concerned with controlling "sexual excitement" in women than in men.

In 1907, under the prodding of Sharp at the Indiana State Reformatory and Amos Butler at the State Board of Charities, Indiana passed the first sterilization law in the nation. Focusing on habitual criminals and rapists, the law also allowed for the involuntary sterilization of the insane, epileptics, and idiots. In the name of eugenics, eleven more states had by 1917 authorized sterilization procedures. After World War I, fifteen additional states passed legislation authorizing sterilization under some circumstances. In many states, interest in the procedures, of course, was fanned by the superintendents. Wilmarth, for example, joined with a sociologist, E. A. Ross, and a biologist, Michael F. Guyer, both faculty members of the University of Wisconsin and both considered progressives, to lobby for the successful passage of that state's sterilization statute in 1913 (Leonard 2005; Osgood 2001; Vecoli 1960).

Yet the ambivalence of many superintendents paralleled the fate of many state sterilization laws. By 1921, of the fifteen statutes passed, only ten were still law. New York's statute was declared unconstitutional in 1918. After that, laws in New Jersey, Nevada, Michigan, and Indiana were also thrown out by their respective courts. In other states, governors refused to carry out the legislation. In 1911, the governor of Indiana, where the first law had been signed by his predecessor in 1907, declined to release state funds to any institution that performed sterilizations. In Oregon, Vermont, Nebraska, and Idaho, governors vetoed legislation (Laughlin 1923, 1926). By 1918, too, interest in promoting sterilization had waned among the superintendents. Except for Barr, Wilmarth, and Baker, most superintendents began to question, if not the efficacy of sterilization, at least the strident claims made for its eugenic potential.

Some of their emergent concern also resulted from their observations of a growing popular linkage of eugenics and euthanasia. As Martin Pernick (1996) has shown, principally in the decades of the 1910s and 1920s, writings and films popularized euthanizing "defective babies." Thus, extrainstitutional advocates like Charles Davenport and Harry Laughlin, popular eugenicists like Albert Edward Wiggam, and racists like Madison Grant and Lothrop Stoddard were moving, in their advocacy and in their "science," increasingly outside the bounds of respectable biology, medicine, and social science. As they reached the height of their national prominence in the 1920s, these eugenicists with their various "threats to America," along with their occasional support for euthanasia, were losing much of their appeal to superintendents. In place of eugenics, most superintendents were becoming increasingly conscious of their place in the postwar "new psychiatry" with its roots in mainline, *scientific* medicine. Although eugenicists continued for another decade to present papers to the American Association for the Study of the Feeble-Minded and superintendents did not entirely lose their interest in eugenics, most of them after the war looked for a new rationale to rekindle their practice of sterilization. But, as we shall see in Chapter 8, there were exceptions even into the 1970s.

STERILIZATION FOR INSTITUTIONAL
POPULATION CONTROL

In 1924, the foster parents of Carrie Buck, a seventeen-year-old girl, petitioned officials in Charlottesville, Virginia, to commit the teenager to the Virginia Colony for Epileptics and the Feebleminded, where the same court three years earlier had committed her mother, Emma Buck. Carrie was pregnant and unmarried. After arriving at the institution, she gave birth to a daughter, Doris. Three generations of female "imbeciles" (as even the newly born child was labeled) convinced state officials that they should sterilize Carrie.

In 1924, Virginia had enacted legislation allowing the sterilization of certain inmates in state facilities, but the law had remained untested. A court petition to sterilize Carrie Buck, officials believed, would make an especially compelling case. After working its way through lower courts, *Buck v. Bell* was argued before the United States Supreme Court in April 1927 (Lombardo 2003, 2008; Smith and Nelson 1989, 17–88). The next month, Justice Oliver Wendell Holmes rendered the opinion of the court.[7] His next-to-final paragraph of the opinion became familiar to interested parties at the time and has been often quoted since:

> We have seen more than once that the public welfare may call upon the best citizens for their lives. It would be strange if it could not call upon those who already sap the strength of the state for these lesser sacrifices, often not felt to be such by those concerned, in order to prevent our being swamped with incompetence. It is better for all the world, if instead of waiting to execute degenerate offspring for crime, or to let them starve for their imbecility, society can prevent those who are manifestly unfit from continuing their kind. The principle that sustains compulsory vaccination is broad enough to cover cutting the Fallopian tubes. . . . Three generations of imbeciles are enough.

Almost never quoted, however, is an important section of the opinion's final paragraph:

> But, it is said, however it might be if this reasoning were applied generally, it fails when it is confined to the small number who are in the institutions named and is not applied to the multitude . . . . Of course so far as the operations enable those who otherwise must be kept confined to be returned to the world, and thus open the asylum to others, the equality [between institutionalized and noninstitutionalized defectives] aimed at will be more nearly reached. (United States Supreme Court 1927, 207–208)

In 1927, Justice Holmes's decision —one joined by Chief Justice William Howard Taft, and Justices Louis Brandeis and Harlan Fiske Stone —reflected a new and growing interest in sterilization not only for controlling behavior and "controlling defective stock," but also for institutional population control. Before the war, the Committee on Provision for the Feeble-Minded, along with extrainstitutional purveyors of eugenics, had convinced legislatures to build new institutions and expand old ones. Also, child welfare advocates had insisted that mental defectives should no longer be permitted in homes for the poor, as the almshouses were now being called. Although mental defectives had been kept in poorhouses for a century, in the 1920s, several states enacted legislation to prohibit these admissions. Persuaded by both trends, states were now more than ever turning to institutions for mental defectives to solve social problems once dealt with by the almshouses. Many states, too, were following the trend set by Illinois of allowing judges the authority to commit children and adults to such schools. After all, state officials reasoned, the public had spent money to build and expand these facilities, just as superintendents and social welfare authorities had called on it to do, so why should they not be fully utilized?

In the decade between World War I and the Great Depression, the populations of the public institutions continued their prewar expansion. In 1923, their combined population was just under 43,000. By 1926, it was just over 50,000, and, by 1936, institutional population stood at nearly 81,000 (US Department of Commerce 1938, 3). In the midst of this growth, sterilization—now out of favor as a means of eugenic control—took on a new life. Sterilization could be linked with another growing interest of the superintendents: inmate parole and discharge to communities. In the midst of demands to take more and more inmates, superintendents discovered that feeble minds could make it "on the outside" especially if they could not procreate.

Even by 1920, superintendents like Bernstein, Fernald, and Wallace began to see that the demands for institutional admission could only be met by releasing some inmates from the institution. Pioneered by Bernstein, institutional parole became a way of institutional population control. To make parole possible, most superintendents came to believe, sterilizations were necessary. In the community, paroled inmates could not afford to be parents, nor could they be allowed to produce new generations of defectives. Also, most superintendents had doubts about the ability of mental defectives to be good parents, especially away from the supervision of the institution.

Already ruminating over paroles and still intrigued by, if not publicly supportive of, eugenic sterilization, superintendents were freer after the 1927 Supreme Court decision to pursue sterilization for institutional population control. The new interest was soon evident. In his 1927 presidential address to the American Association for the Study of the Feeble-Minded, B. W. Baker (1927), superintendent of the New Hampshire School for the Feeble-Minded, noted with favor the *Buck v. Bell* ruling of the same year. He reminded his colleagues that the Supreme Court had declared sterilization legal for eugenic purposes. He proposed that the association institute a study of sterilization practices and effects. Two years later, George E. McPherson (1929; see also Grinspoon 2013), superintendent of the Belchertown State School in Massachusetts, echoed Baker's enthusiasm. He noted that sterilization was particularly important for "girls" before parole and discharge. In 1920, H. H. Ramsay ([ca. 1920], 13), superintendent of the newly opened Mississippi School and Colony for the Feeble-Minded in rural and remote Jones County, had cautioned that

"sterilization would not be a safe and effective substitute for permanent segregation and control." By 1931, as he was about to leave Mississippi to become the superintendent of the Utah State School, his views on sterilization, like those of his
counterparts in other institutions, had changed. "Selective sterilization," he echoed
in his presidential address to the association, should become "an ally to the parole
system of the institution" (Ramsay 1931, 295).

In 1930, Harvey M. Watkins (1930) of the Polk State School in Pennsylvania
summarized the growing consensus in his paper "Selective Sterilization." After
noting the approximately 10,000 "successful" procedures carried out, Watkins reminded his audience that sterilization had saved thousands of taxpayer dollars by
allowing for parole. Parole meant better care for inmates who truly needed institutional care, and sterilization had allowed those who could make it "on the outside"
to be free from the constraints of parenthood. Such freedom, he believed, proved
to be a blessing to mental defectives in the community and to the community now
freed from worry about future defectives. To those like his now-deceased colleague,
Walter Fernald, who had claimed that vasectomies and tubal ligations merely led
to sexual promiscuity, Watkins produced data that he believed made such concerns
unwarranted. Finally, confirming the growing support for sterilization, Watkins
presented the results of a questionnaire on sterilization he had sent to 317 members of the association. Of the 227 replies, 80 percent favored the use of sterilization. Only sixteen responses indicated disapproval of the procedure. Obviously,
the once wavering membership had, by 1930, become favorably disposed to sterilization. Watkins concluded: "The time has arrived when this Association should
give consideration to this further step in dealing with the mental defective. Its
membership approves. The public demands. Justice to the individual defective requests, and thirty years of experimentation warrants its adoption as part of a broad
and conservative program." In his presidential address to the association in 1932,
Watkins (1930) made the linkage between sterilization and parole even more explicit: "Sterilization should be looked upon not as a panacea or as a cure-all but as
having a limited selected field and application to a limited group who, after suitable
training and education, are eligible for parole." The following year, at the annual
meeting of the American Association on Mental Deficiency, the new name for the
American Association for the Study of the Feeble-Minded, B. O. Whitten, superintendent of the South Carolina State Training School, criticized the Committee on
Program for failing to include a session on sterilization (American Association on
Mental Deficiency 1933, 391). After 1933, there would be few such omissions.

In 1934, officials of the Third Reich began what would eventually be the sterilization of 400,000 Germans, or 1 in every 100 citizens. Two decades earlier, a German
translation of *The Kallikak Family* had appeared, and American pedigree studies
were well known to Germans, indeed, precipitating *asoziale familien* studies both in
pre-Nazi Germany and after 1932. Proto-Nazis and Nazis alike praised American
sterilization laws. In 1936, the University of Heidelberg awarded Harry Laughlin
an honorary doctorate in medicine. Until his death in 1942, Laughlin would advocate against the lifting of the 1924 immigration quotas, thus becoming part of a
movement in America to refuse entry to Jews trying to escape the Holocaust (Allen

1986; Bruinius 2007, 255–264, 280–295; Chase 1977, 353; Hassencahl 1969; Kuhl 1994, 40–42, 86–88; Proctor 1988, 99–100). Medical superintendents (along with most respectable American scientists) may have rejected the excesses of the eugenics movement, but its effects had devastating, if unintended, consequences.

The same year that the German mass sterilizations began, Leon F. Whitney (1934) published *The Case for Sterilization*. Whitney was at the time the executive secretary of the American Eugenics Society. Assuming an apparently more moderate tone than American eugenicists of previous decades, Whitney rejected as naive the old notion that feeblemindedness was a simple Mendelian trait. Feeblemindedness was more complex, linked to a number of hereditary factors.[8] Echoing the superintendents' new views on sterilization, Whitney claimed that the procedures ensured the mentally deficient their place in the community. Institutions, he insisted, should train mentally defective children and keep low grades. High-grade trained adults could do just as well in the community, provided they were sterile. Especially given the effects of the economic depression, sterilized adults outside of the institution could save resources needed for other indigent citizens. Adding a final twist, Whitney suggested a method of "voluntary" sterilization, one that would avoid the negative connotations now being associated in some American minds with the German legislation: "Give them the necessary information and instruction and let them decide for themselves whether to have a few children or many. . . . Here is a nice shiny automobile; and here is a baby. . . . Which will the morons choose?" (Whitney 1934, 275).

The "choice" of Mr. and Mrs. Moron, of course, had nothing to do with the matter. Viewed in professional circles and in the popular media as incompetent, child-like potential parents, morons and high-grade imbeciles were sterilized to make them ready for community placement or parole, a new policy to relieve the crowded conditions of public institutions, now stressed as never before by the Great Depression. Most institutional authorities told mental defectives nothing before they sterilized them or, as with Carrie Buck, lied to them about the procedure (see Block 2000; Gould 1984, 335–336; Lombardo 2008; Smith and Nelson 1989).

LAYING THE FOUNDATIONS FOR PAROLE

As the Great Depression lingered through the 1930s, the need for parole assumed an even greater urgency. Hard times only increased demands on institutions. But hard times also made the parole of inmates, even sterilized inmates, harder to accomplish. State officials might believe they could save costs by paroling and discharging sterilized inmates, as Whitney and most superintendents predicted; but what were inmates to do once they were paroled? Like the vision of productivity held by Howe and Hervey Wilbur in the 1840s and 1850s that had been disrupted by the Panic of 1857 and the Civil War, the vision of parole in the 1920s would be quickly frustrated by an economic system in crisis in the 1930s. This time, the crisis would be a truly deep one, and it would be followed by the social disruption of another world war. After the 1930s, parole would wane; sterilization would not.

The seeds of opposition to the eugenics movement, not only among superintendents, most of whom were identifying themselves with the emerging "new psychiatry" of the postwar years, but also among other disciplines and professions, were sown even as eugenics reached the height of its notoriety. As Charles Davenport was setting up his offices at Cold Spring Harbor around 1908, Thomas Hunt Morgan began breeding fruit flies in his lab at Columbia. Like many biologists of the time, Morgan was initially attracted to and involved in the eugenics movement, only breaking with Davenport in 1915. Yet when opposition arose in the prewar period, it tended, like that of Morgan's, to be private and cautious (Cravens 1978, 159–188; Kevles 1985, 122).[9]

By the first half of the 1920s, psychiatry, too, began to shift from a unit-character explanation of insanity to a multicausal one. Prior to World War I, eugenics had thoroughly fascinated most American psychiatrists. Unlike the institutional alienists of an earlier generation, however, this group of psychiatrists had held both to August Weismann's theory of "germ plasm" immutability and to Mendelian theories of inheritance. Human characteristics, they had believed, were not affected by exogenous factors, and the transmission of those immutable characteristics followed simple and predictable rules (Sicherman 1967, 347–359).

Aaron Rosanoff, a psychiatrist at King's Park State Hospital in New York, had been a leading proponent of this position. In 1911, Rosanoff and his research associates published two articles, one in the *Journal of Nervous and Mental Diseases* and the other in the *American Journal of Insanity*. Charles Davenport reprinted the articles the same year as bulletins three and five of the Eugenics Record Office (Rosanoff and Cannon 1911; Rosanoff and Orr 1911). In both articles, Rosanoff traced the pedigree of patients at King's Park and concluded that insanity was a unitary, degenerative characteristic following simple Mendelian laws of heredity. These pedigree studies had lent empirical verification to psychiatry's fascination with eugenics.

Although not as involved with eugenic research as Rosanoff, other American psychiatrists had been just as enthusiastic about the possible impact of eugenics on mental disease and deficiency. Throughout the 1910s, psychiatrists in the two leading psychiatric organizations of the time—the American Medico-Psychological Association (predecessor of the American Psychiatric Association) and the Mental Hygiene Association—had devoted annual meeting time and journal space to the issue. At the American Medico-Psychological Association's annual meetings of 1914, 1915, and 1917, presidential addresses focused on the relationship between mental defect and eugenics. In his 1914 address, for example, Carlos MacDonald (1914) had insisted that "there was a need for arrest[ing], in a decade or two, the reproduction of mental defective persons, as surely as we could stamp out smallpox if every person in the world could be successfully vaccinated." Like their Medico-Psychological counterparts, Adolf Meyer, Walter Fernald, and other leaders in the mental hygiene movement affirmed the salubrious potential of eugenics.

By 1915, however, Rosanoff began to doubt some of the claims made by the Cold Spring Harbor group, particularly as they applied eugenics to immigration. In that year, Rosanoff (1915) suggested that the proclivity to insanity among immigrants was more the result of emigration than heredity. Others, too, like William Healy, began to question the eugenic association between various social problems and mental disability. In 1913, Edith Spaulding and Healy (1913) had published findings of a study of 668 delinquents. They concluded that there was "no proof of the existence of hereditary criminalistic traits, as such." In 1915, Healy (1915) published *The Individual Delinquent*, in which he claimed that delinquency was associated with mental disability principally as a result of environmental factors. If any hereditary linkage between mental disability and crime existed, Healy claimed, it was at most slight (J. Trent 1987).

Also that year, Walter Fernald (1919) began a study of patients at the Massachusetts School for the Feeble-Minded who had left the institution and had been living in communities. Quite to his surprise, Fernald claimed, he found that most of these discharged patients were functioning well. In 1917, Adolf Meyer (1917), certainly one of the most popular and respected champions of mental hygiene, began to distance himself from the eugenics movement. Finally, in January 1917, Abraham Myerson (1917a, 1917b, see also Hexter and Myerson 1924), a Boston psychiatrist, published the first of two lengthy articles entitled "Psychiatric Family Studies," launching his career-long attack on the political agenda of the eugenicists (J. Trent 2001). The title of Healy's (1918) address to the 1918 meeting of the American Association for the Study of the Feeble-Minded summed up the emerging new vision among psychiatrists: "Normalities of the Feeble-Minded."

Together these studies, doubts, and new professional visions began to dismantle two important claims made by eugenicists of the period: the causative relationship between social vice and mental disability and the inevitable fecundity of the feebleminded outside of the segregated institution. Once the cognitive doubts set in among professional circles, the eugenics movement lost much of its influence as a respectable scientific enterprise. By the end of the 1920s, meetings and journals of the American Medico-Psychological Association and the Mental Hygiene Association began to have fewer eugenic topics. Heredity in these circles was increasingly discussed more as an issue of genetics than eugenics. After 1909, too, American psychiatry began to feel Freud's impact and directed its gaze away from heredity. By the 1920s, the psychology of *adjustment*, embodied in the scientific calm of the mental hygiene movement and the "new psychiatry," had begun to supplant the earlier decade's short-lived fascination with eugenics and with the alarmist rhetoric that accompanied it (White 1917).

The cognitive doubts, then, were accompanied by factors linked to the growing disciplinary matrix of the new psychiatry. As noted in Chapter 5, Fernald, Rogers, and Smith were all interested in limiting the influence of the Committee on Provision for the Feeble-Minded, which had been closely linked with the Cold Spring Harbor group. Eugenics, they began to believe, had become a science taken up by not-so-good biologists, psychologists, and social workers. Especially when those nonmedical sorts made claims about mental disease and defect and received widespread public attention and philanthropic cash, medical superintendents felt their turf threatened. Eugenicists had advocated for policies and procedures emphasizing the confinement of and restrictions on mental defectives, and, at first, institutional superintendents had seen in the movement a way to attract public attention and support for their financially starved facilities. Even before 1920, however, *institutional* superintendents saw in mental hygiene and the new psychiatry ways of enlarging their spheres of influence to *extrainstitutional* settings.

Almost from the beginning, then, there had been professional uneasiness about the purpose, potential, and power of eugenics. The whisperings had begun even before the war and became obvious after it. As early as 1912, Jessie D. Hodder, superintendent of the Massachusetts Prison Reformatory for Women and a pioneer in psychiatric social work, wrote Julia Lathrop at Hull House about summer school classes at Harvard University given by William Healy, then director of Chicago's Juvenile Psychopathic Institute. "A good many people in the class, Vineland fed," she wrote, "wanted more of just the same thing, and I think in the beginning were upset as people who believe that there is some absolute method in the world always will be" (quoted in Dummer 1948). Hodder had been specifically incensed by Goddard's linkage of mental defect with crime and delinquency (Eggers 1986).

By 1916, Fernald had begun lobbying behind the scenes against the Committee on Provision for the Feeble-Minded even before his 1917 studies "officially" marked his opposition to total institutionalization and the eugenics movement. Bernstein often talked about the eugenics movement as "not made up of medical men." After Martin Barr went in 1919 to consult at the recently opened Caswell Training School in North Carolina, he gloated to W. H. C. Smith about taking over a role once held by the social worker Alexander Johnson. Johnson, Barr reported, was still "working over the feeble wound" of the demise of the Committee on Provision (Beverly Farm Records, letter from M. W. Barr to W. H. C. Smith, January 28, 1919; see also North Carolina State Archives, State Board of Public Welfare, letter from C. Banks McNary to Mrs. Clarence Johnson, June 19, 1920). Although they might turn to cognitive rationales to denounce the excessive rhetoric of the eugenicists, many of the superintendents were motivated *first* by social and professional interests to distance themselves from the methods and message of their once favored colleagues.

What the institutional superintendents began to sense around the time of World War I was the potential of moving their influence outside of the confines of the state facility to the community. Before this time, psychiatrists had been alienists, men and women who had lived their lives and found their professional mission within the borders of their own institutions and within the circle of their fellow superintendents. The "new psychiatry," grounded in mental hygiene's emphasis on prevention, child-guidance clinics, and psychiatrists working in juvenile courts, schools, general hospitals, and private practice, had as its focus communities (Grob 1983, 108–178; K. Jones 1999, 62–119; Nehring 2004). In communities, ordinary people had problems coping with and adapting to day-to-day conditions. Although differences arose among them about the most efficient ways of solving these problems, psychiatrists in the 1920s saw the eugenicists' message of restriction and confinement as increasingly antithetical to their new vision of community psychiatry and to their place in it. Their turning away from eugenics, then, fit their new message and their new professional interests and self-image.

COLONIES AND PAROLE, DEPRESSION AND WAR

The interest of superintendents in paroling inmates paralleled their newfound interest in sterilization. Their rationale for justifying this new shift in policy and perspective emerged from their rejection of eugenics and their growing attraction to the mental hygiene movement with its emphasis on *social adjustment* and *social adaptation*. Not since the earliest efforts of Hervey Wilbur, Samuel Gridley Howe, and Henry Knight had superintendents supported the discharge of educated inmates from the institution to *adjust* to local communities, working in local industries or on family farms. After the late 1850s, Wilbur, Howe, Knight, and each of their successors had abandoned the policy of community reintegration. From time to time, superintendents discharged inmates to their families but not to fend for themselves in the world. Between the 1850s and World War I, inmates had received education to live in the shelter of the institution, protected from the world and the world from them. If the mental hygiene movement provided a new cognitive rationale for a new vision of adaptation and adjustment, sterilization provided a new means to that end.

The only "intermediate" facility created by superintendents before 1900 had been the farm colony. Begun at the Syracuse asylum in 1882 for the growing number of men who were unable to leave the still-designated "educational" school, the earliest farm colonies were signs of the emerging post-Civil War custodial policy overtaking public charitable facilities. In 1893, the Indiana School for Feeble-Minded Youth opened a similar colony (Davies 1923, 109–110). Not until 1899, with the beginning of the farm colony at the Massachusetts School for Feeble-Minded and Fernald's articles about the colony, did farm colonies attract national attention, spurring other institutions to develop them. Without exception, all remained appendages of the institution, often supplying it produce, dairy products, and meat. Superintendents sent "boys" from the institution to these colonies, where, living under the supervision of a farm couple, they grew crops; tended cattle, pigs, and chickens; and kept out of trouble. Almost all superintendents agreed: farm colonies had proved to be a good place for delinquents who otherwise caused problems in the institution.

The farm colony, of course, was never truly *intermediary*. It had not been created as a stepping stone to the community. If an inmate left the colony, it was usually to return to the institution. In the midst of the superintendents' turn-of-the-century commitment to total institutionalization, no serious thought was given to returning inmates to the community.[10]

As other superintendents were doing, Charles Bernstein, the superintendent of the Rome State Custodial Asylum for Unteachable Idiots, opened his first farm colony in 1906, three years after assuming his position at the asylum. Near the institutional grounds, the Brush colony resembled in size, practice, and purpose Fernald's Templeton colony opened in 1899. Yet, from the beginning of his work at Rome, Bernstein held views that made him out of line with other superintendents and social welfare advocates.[11] These views would affect his outlook on farm colonies.

As its title suggested, the Rome asylum was opened in 1894 as New York's institution for custodial defectives. Partly because inmates of all grades were being admitted to the Rome facility and partly because of his own discomfort with the label, Bernstein soon requested his board drop "unreachable idiots" from the institution's title. Although his predecessor had kept all wards of the institution locked, Bernstein had them unlocked except for those housing delinquents. By 1904, he began "industrial training" while insisting that traditional academic work was useless (American Association for the Study of the Feeble-Minded 1905; "Bernstein Dies" 1942).

When Bernstein opened the Brush colony in 1906, then, there was every indication that his reformist bent would also shape his plans for the new colony. Soon, the Brush colony was working well, and Bernstein was acquiring new farms. In 1914, he opened the first domestic colony for "girls" and in 1917 opened a colony for female inmates who worked in factories. By 1928, he had opened fifteen colonies for women; in the 1920s, he added several colonies for children, so-called junior colonies. At the time of his death in 1942, he had founded sixty-two colonies in rural and small-town settings for men, women, and children (Figure 6.1).

If he had done nothing else with his colonies, Bernstein would have been remembered for their number and diversity but not more. In 1912, however, he persuaded the state legislature to give him the authority to discharge inmates (R. Wilbur 1969, 17–18). Shortly afterward, Bernstein began a policy of paroling inmates, after a time of useful work and good behavior in the colony, to work on privately owned farms. At first, most farmers who took inmates were well-known to the institution and had worked with the inmates on a trial basis, when "boys were farmed out" during

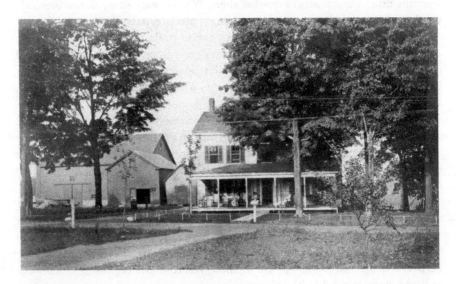

Figure 6.1:
Brush farm colony at the Rome State School in New York, 1936. (From James C. Riggs's *Hello Doctor: A Brief Biography of Charles Bernstein*, 1936)

harvest time (Davies 1923, 116–117). Bernstein was careful not to parole inmates whom he believed were habitual offenders of institutional and colony rules. Before the Depression, he maintained a "trial" period between parole and final discharge.

In 1922, the sociologist Stanley P. Davies (1923, 114–115), described colonies from which parolees were discharged: "They are distinguished by their unusually trim and tidy appearance. Run-down farms have rapidly taken on a new aspect when they have been converted to this (as yet) rather novel use. . . . The earlier farm colonies had been, after the first year, entirely self sustaining, covering from the value of their products both the rental or interest on the investment, etc., and the maintenance."

Between 1906 and 1914, Bernstein started four more colonies for men. Already, paroling men to local farms was raising eyebrows among his fellow superintendents (e.g., American Association for the Study of the Feeble-Minded 1917). In 1914, two years after the publication of Goddard's *The Kallikak Family* and in the midst of calls for controlling the menacing feebleminded, he opened an urban colony for women. Most were aghast (Riggs 1936, 115, 119). Set up in Rome about two miles from the institution, the colony had mentally defective women "available for domestic working, sewing, etc. by day, week, or month" (Rome Custodial Announcement, October 7, 1914, quoted in Davies 1923, 134; see Figure 6.2). Living with the women was a "house mother" and providing institutional supervision was a social worker, Inez F. Stebbins, Bernstein's sister-in-law. In 1916, Bernstein opened a second female colony. After the war began in Europe, he started a colony near the Utica Knitting Mills, where twenty-four women began to work. Women from the colony or those discharged to the community after parole continued working there after the war (Davies 1923, 138).

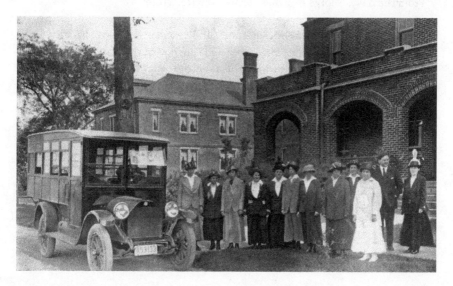

Figure 6.2:
Domestic workers with Charles Bernstein at the Rome State School in New York, ca. 1925. (From James C. Riggs's *Hello Doctor: A Brief Biography of Charles Bernstein*, 1936)

By 1917, just three years after opening his first colony for women, Bernstein had paroled seventy-seven female inmates, sixty-three of whom were eventually discharged. By 1922, he had begun eighteen more female colonies. One-third of all adult females assigned to the Rome institution were by that year in colonies (Davies 1923, 138–145).

Both before the war, when he was the only superintendent with a policy of parole and discharge, and after it, when other superintendents began to develop an interest, Bernstein missed few opportunities to spread his faith in paroles to state and national groups. As part of this outreach, he sent his institution's monthly newspaper, *The Herald,* throughout New York. In virtually every issue before 1933, he included letters from paroled and discharged inmates. He especially valued letters from discharged women. Showing that they could adjust to independence, maintain work, and even get married and raise normal children, Bernstein printed letter after letter of success stories from inmates adapting "on the outside." In November 1914, Evelyn Ulrich wrote from the recently opened first colony for women:

> I have been working in two places since I have been here. Tell Frances Cooper I will write to her just as soon as I can and give her my love. Miss Bayne will you please come down and see our little cottage? I am getting to be some cook and also are all the rest of the girls. Sunday I went out to work for the first time to stay with some children.
>
> I am giving them music, I mean the girls every evening to make everybody happy here, if it isn't the Piano it is the music box. I am trying my very best to stay outside. I will always remember what you have told me. (*Herald,* November 1914, 3)

From the navy, George Brown, a former inmate, wrote:

> Just a few lines to let you know that I am still alive and in the best of health. I am now in the U.S. Navy. I enlisted July 9th and I am now at the Training Station at Newport, R.I. and expect to leave here on a ship next week for France.
>
> This is a fine place down here. There are about 10,000 boys down here. There isn't a chance to get lonesome. There are a lot of boys in your institution who I think if they were in the navy it would make a man of them.
>
> I was considered feeble-minded once, but I was given the chance to prove that I was not. I am now in a place where you have to have a strong mind and be quick witted. I am proud to say that I am just as good as any of them. The reason for me getting out of the hole that I once got in is that I made a fool out of the ones that tried to make a fool out of me. You must remember me, the kind of a boy that I was, so if there are any others like me, give them a chance, they will make good. (*Herald,* September 1917, 6)

Another former inmate now in the army wrote:

> Camp life seems to suit me, for up to the present I am in good health and spirits and always ready at meal times. We are well taken care of here and nobody

seems to have any complaints to make. I am trying to get a few days furlough at Christmas and if I have time shall try to visit my friends at the institution. (*Herald,* January 1918, 4)

Several colony inmates wrote about the pleasure they had felt in the colonies and for their work. "We all enjoyed ourselves at the New Year's Dance very much indeed," wrote Lulu Hefferman, "and would like to thank Dr. Bernstein for letting us go up. We were all glad to get back to our home. . . . We are anxious to get back into the mill as we heard they missed us for the day and a half we were away. That shows us we are wanted in the mill. We will make up for lost time" (*Herald,* February 1920, "supplement"). James A. Albrecht wrote: "Just a line from an old-timer. I am a nurse down here taking care of T.B.'s for the Sante Fe Railroad. I am getting along O.K." (*Herald,* December 1921, 4). Other inmates reintegrated themselves in local schools, some taking subjects not usually associated with mental deficiency. Muriel Draisley, for example, wrote:

I have just received my report card Friday, so I thought I'd let you know my marks. Algebra, three; Civics, three; English, two; Latin, four; Gym, three and Citizenship, two. On the back of the card it told what the marks stood for and I will copy it for you. Group one includes those whose work is of highest excellency, a distinction reached by few in a class, group two those whose work while not perfect is still so excellent that it is decidely [sic] above the average of good work. (*Herald,* December 1921, 4)

Several discharged inmates wrote about their home lives "on the outside." Most were women; many had married and had had children. Lottie Stellman H. (as the *Herald* identified her) penned, "I am writing you to let you know that I am getting along pretty well now. Just before Christmas my husband was sick with the pneumonia but he got along all right and now he is working again. My two children had pneumonia and Thomas died just before Easter. I have a good husband and he helps me with the work at home" (*Herald,* June 1924, 47). Another discharged inmate, Doris Caley, wrote:

My husband has been out working on a wreck on the railroad all night and he has not come home for his breakfast yet. Dr. Bernstein, I only wish that every girl or woman that gets married nowadays could have as good a man as I have, then they would not have any fault to find with him and their [sic] would be no trouble if they do what is right. I am working a bed-spread for my bed and have learned to make shirts for my husband and have learned to do other things in the line of sewing that I did not know before.

Shortly before the depression, John F. Sieroloski, an inmate at the Hilman colony, wrote of life there:

Today we was out plowing and we plowed up some of the biggest stones you ever did see, and it took 10 of us boys to get one of them out of the ground.

Altogether we dug a number of stones weighing around 200 to 400 lbs. each, but there is One Big Stone we will have to use a team of horses to move it from its place first thing in the morning.

I was doing cooking here for awhile in the house only I got so I did not like it so they gave me a better position outside as a teamster and general farm hand.

I and John Bogan are two very good wood choppers and are today claiming the championship class; as real up-to-date woodsmen; and challenge any young man with physical experience and a good ax to try us out.

We have a victrola here, and a few good pieces and go for long hikes every Sunday afternoon and for a nice long ride over at Taberg, N.Y. or Rome, N.Y. wherever the people of the colony wish to travel in their car. (*Herald*, June 1929, 2)

Beginning in 1919, Bernstein initiated a "colony week." Each summer, usually in June, colony inmates came to the institution for a week of demonstrations, games, and socializing. Discharged and paroled inmates were also invited, and usually dozens joined in the reunion. During the same period, at least one edition each year of the *Herald* was devoted exclusively to colonies and parole (e.g., *Herald*, March 1919). Each issue of the newspaper also published many letters from colony inmates and discharges, serving as an incentive for inmates in the institution.

Through his colony parole and discharge program, Bernstein could demonstrate to state legislators and social welfare officials his commitment to saving the state money and finding a way to admit more clientele to the institution. The issue of overhead was as old as the institutions. All superintendents had justified new policies on the basis of savings to taxpayers. Bernstein, like Johnson and Fernald before him, was eager to point out that most colonies paid their own way. Some even provided surplus produce, dairy products, and meat for the institution. After 1928, too, Bernstein found a kindred spirit in Governor Franklin D. Roosevelt. Although Bernstein could play to members of various New York political parties, he worked well with Roosevelt, who, along with Eleanor Roosevelt, made annual visits to the institution. Roosevelt, a gentleman farmer himself, had advocated for "back to the farm" policies, especially after the Depression worsened. Bernstein's reclamation of abandoned farms fit closely with Roosevelt's interest in resettling depression-ridden city folk on New York farms (Garraty 1987, 82, 123, 131, 199).

Bernstein also justified his colonies by linking them to parole and discharge from the institution. Colonies provided a transition, a half-way setting, between the institution and the local community. Many inmates, he believed, entered the institution merely because of maladjustment in their homes and local communities. Following the growing theme of the postwar mental hygiene movement in whose association he was an active member, Bernstein stressed the issues of *adjustment* and *adaptation*. Most inmates were not a product of bad genes. Bad genes required bad environments to make bad people. Free mental defectives from the slums, poor health, and social stress, and they could become good citizens. This was true, he believed, of women as well as of men. To assume, as most did before 1917 (and as many did after), that female mental defectives were prone to licentious behavior and were particularly vulnerable to the sexual advances of wily men was to fail to recognize that moral behavior and good citizenship were natural to no one. All people, including mental defectives, had to *learn* cautious and upright behavior if they were to live prudent and productive lives (Kline 2001; Odem 1995; Ordover 2003; Rembis 2011; J. Trent 1986; Vogt 2012).

As the tide of opinion began to turn after 1917, Bernstein's opinion became even bolder. Of eugenics he wrote:

> During these twenty years I have observed the trend of scientific opinion fluctuating between the two extremes of assigning as the causative factor of mental deficiency at one epoch faulty environment and at another defective parentage. Today the modern eugenics movement which is principally led by sociologists and psychologists, many of whom have little or no insight into the pathological conditions underlying many of these defects, teaches that all, or nearly all mental defect is to be attributed to heredity or to faulty parentage, this teaching being based principally on the fact that so many of these defectives are found in localized communities or afflicted families and groups.
>
> On reflection the thought occurs, does one any more inherit mental and nervous peculiarities and state of mind or physical attitudes than they do their various physical malformations and religious or political beliefs?

In reaction to the concern of eugenicists and superintendents about marriage among mental defectives, he shocked both groups:

> We are the more thoroughly convinced . . . that, with our limited knowledge of and the many more or less misleading theories pertaining to the eugenics aspect of the work with the so-called mental defectives and borderline cases of feeble-minded, eugenics considerations should not constitute the principal or controlling factor or consideration when we come to pass on paroles and discharges, and even though marriage and reproduction ensue, still we are not deterred in continuing this hopeful practice . . . for in many instances we have seen such matings bring forth children the equal of so-called non-tainted stock, and too, the percentage of such normal children not below the average of normal offspring from what are commonly accepted as normal human beings. (Bernstein 1921)

There is little doubt that Bernstein's civil libertarianism and emphasis on the social origins of personal and social problems were sincere. For at least fifteen years among his fellow superintendents, his voice of caution in the face of the eugenics alarm was singular. But it would be wrong, too, to ignore Bernstein's repeated acknowledgment that colonization, parole, and community discharge were policies that represented responses to the large number of requests for admission to the institution, exaggerated first by a world war and later by a serious economic depression. Put another way, Bernstein's persistent faith in the influence of a good environment to shape human nature for the better fit well with a necessary policy change, given social and economic conditions after 1917.

As noted earlier in the chapter, after 1917, superintendents began to shift from an emphasis on the "menace of the feebleminded" to themes of adapting and adjusting mental defectives for institutional and extrainstitutional environments. Bernstein's fellow superintendents, who had always (albeit cautiously) respected him, began after 1917 to take him seriously. Fernald, Wallace, even fellow New Yorker, Charles Little, and many of the younger superintendents began to visit Rome, later sending their staffs. Some of the Southern institutions that had originally sent their personnel to Vineland for training began in the 1920s to look to Rome. The Rome summer school for teachers, with its emphasis on colonies, began to attract pupils from all over the United States and from abroad, and state and national commissions visited Rome to observe its colonies and parole system. After 1925, not only did E. R. Johnstone begin to make visits and to send his Vineland staff to Rome, but even Charles Davenport traveled there.

As the dream of total institutionalization faded in the 1920s, even the most committed old-guard eugenicists became interested in what began to be known as the "Rome Plan." In 1923, when the National Committee on Mental Hygiene published Stanley P. Davies's (1923) sociological dissertation, *Social Control of the Feeble-Minded*, done at Columbia under Franklin Giddings, Bernstein's efforts were given an even wider audience. Devoting two chapters to Rome, Davies described the positive results of colonies and parole. In so doing, he challenged the eugenicists' fears of the fecundity and immorality of feeble minds. Even more important, he provided an intellectual rationale for the new and growing emphasis on mental defect as an issue of social adaptation and adjustment. Mental defectives, he insisted, were a social problem not because of a natural propensity to degeneracy, immorality, or fecundity but rather because of their failure to adapt and adjust to their given environment, institutional or not.

By 1925, most institutions were trying colonies and parole, especially public facilities pressured to take new inmates. Paroling law-abiding, well-adjusted, trained morons and even high-grade imbeciles opened public institutions for mental defectives of all grades whose applications for admission filled every superintendent's filing cabinets. With their populations increasing annually, superintendents began to see Bernstein's policy of parole—a policy they had only ten years earlier looked on as foolish—as a way to make room for the new demand.

Although early in his career Bernstein acknowledged that in a few circumstances the use of sterilization was proper, he was uneasy with the recurring interest in the procedures that was developing after 1927. His discomfort was not unaffected by what he regarded as a medical procedure being promoted by people who were not physicians—that is, the eugenicists—and were, he believed, interlopers in matters best left to medicine. Although Bernstein did not support sterilization in most cases, most superintendents followed his lead in paroling and discharging inmates only with the reassurance provided by sterilization.

After 1933, the year of the German sterilization laws and in the depth of the depression, no superintendent insisted on sterilizing every inmate, although most had come to see sterilization as necessary for inmates ready for discharge. If they worried about the likelihood of sexual impropriety outside of marriage, especially among female discharges, or if they suspected that inmates of either sex would transmit hereditary degeneracy, superintendents usually recommended it. Lloyd N. Yepsen (1934; see also P. Ryan 2007), then with the New Jersey Department of Institutions and Agencies, reflected the consensus emerging among superintendents at the 1934 meeting of the American Association on Mental Deficiency:

> Throughout the country we are witnessing a demand for reduction in taxes.... Nearly every institution in the country is living on sustenance appropriations....
>
> Will the new social order be easier for the feebleminded? Will it be easier for him to adjust in the future than it is for him to adjust now? Will he find the planned future will take him into consideration? ... Recent surveys have shown that individuals who have been effective up until recently are certain to be casualties in the future. There is no place for individuals who were effectively placed some years ago. The number of unplaceable youths every year amounts to three-quarters of a million.

In light of these prospects, Yepsen asked, "What can we do for them?" Three of his suggestions revealed the impact of the Depression on shifts in the meaning now being given to sterilization and to parole and discharge:

> Marriage should be discouraged but when consummated should be made as near childless as possible.
>
> Permissive and selective sterilization should be encouraged if the continuance of neuropathic families is to be discouraged....
>
> The institutionally trained should be, when possible, returned to their homes under planned supervision. This "graduation" will make available the specialized training to additional children in need of such training.

For Yepsen and others, sterilization was becoming a requirement for most placements outside the institution, and "placement outside the institution" was, when it occurred at all, becoming more and more a matter of returning inmates to their families, not to productive work.

At the same meeting of the American Association on Mental Deficiency, L. Potter Harshman (1934), a psychiatrist at the Fort Wayne State School (formerly the Indiana School for Feeble-Minded Youth), reported on sterilizations in Indiana. The state, he noted, had passed its second sterilization statute in 1927, twenty years after the passage of its first. Although community placement was the most important factor in sterilizing inmates at the Fort Wayne State School, institutional officials performed most sterilizations on males and females under the age of sixteen years. Harshman provided an explanation:

> Many of our cases are observed over several months before a decision is reached. It may be quite desirable to wait until the patients have been fully trained, reached their I.Q. prediction and are ready to go out on parole. But a review of the releases and discharges as well as the escapees from the ordinary school for feebleminded

makes us believe that many cases can have the operation done as a routine on admission and then when unexpected releases take place or furloughs are granted it is not necessary to abide the time of operation. This makes for a more flexible movement of population.

In the discussion that followed Harshman's paper, several superintendents joined the theme of the *routine of* sterilization. Although the levels of participation varied, especially among those states that had statutes and those that did not have them, superintendents had, by the Depression, routinely linked parole and discharge with sterilization. J. M. Murdoch, formerly the superintendent of the Polk State School in Pennsylvania and now A. C. Rogers's successor at the Minnesota School for the Feebleminded noted:

> We don't consider sterilization for anyone who is to remain within an institution, but only for those who have reached a point where we hope they will get on successfully on parole.... We feel that before the child [sic] goes out on parole it is advisable to have a sterilization operation, not only from the eugenics point of view (these are mostly girls) but from the standpoint of their ability to get on, on parole, which is very much greater after a sterilization operation than it would be without sterilization. (American Association on Mental Deficiency 1934c)

At the 1938 annual meeting of the American Association on Mental Deficiency, G. B. Arnold (1938), a physician at the Virginia State Colony for Epileptics and Feeble-Minded, reported on Virginia's sterilization of its first 1,000 feebleminded clientele, 632 of whom had been paroled. Among these first sterilizations were 609 females and 391 males; and among these, 812 "came from families of the definitely low class—and by 'low class' we mean families whose heads are barely eking out an existence." Arnold reported only 139 patients from middle-class families and 8 from "families whose financial circumstances were definitely superior." Although sterilization might have lost its scientific respectability, it continued to serve the function of allowing a public institution like Virginia's to parole some of its lower class patients, particularly lower class female patients. Arnold put it bluntly: "We do not now sterilize a patient unless we feel that there is a good chance of his leaving the Colony."

Ironically, however, as the Great Depression made parole, discharge, and sterilization important options for superintendents, conditions in the community made discharging inmates difficult. When Bernstein opened his industrial colony for women in 1917, "organized labor was not entirely happy over the arrangement, but accepted it because local labor supply was insufficient to keep the mill operating to capacity" (Millias 1942). Labor shortages during the war provided few incentives for such opposition. By the 1930s, however, labor unions became increasingly intolerant of these enterprises.

Farm colonies, too, which were thriving in the 1920s, were by the 1930s mainly providing for the needs of the institution. Farmers in upstate New York were increasingly less likely to need extra hands. For that reason, the rate of farm paroles slowed after 1933. By that year, Bernstein began to compromise his original hope for parole. "Any boy or girl," he claimed to his colleagues, "that goes into a home and has a place to eat and sleep in a decent environment, even if there is no money, is better off than the boy or girl that stays in the institution" (American Association on Mental Deficiency 1934a). Women who had once lived in colonies and gone out to work in local industries or as domestic servants now remained in the colony, where they passed the day "knitting, sewing, embroidery, table projects and field excursions." As such, the colony became more of a place for training than a place to live and from which to go to work, thus increasingly resembling the institution. Well-behaving morons and high-grade imbeciles from the colonies, who once would have graduated to productive jobs in local communities, were now only a bit more likely than their lower grade counterparts to leave the institution.

As the Depression lingered, Bernstein continued to advocate for community placements, although even he admitted that such placements were now more likely to be with relatives. And even these placements were harder to come by. Mildred Thomason of the Minnesota State Board of Control reminded Bernstein, not without justification, that more and more families either did not want to take their children back into their homes or, because of the Depression, could not (American Association on Mental Deficiency 1934b). By 1942, Ward Millias (1942), Bernstein's assistant, claimed the only economically productive colonies were the domestic colonies, where women worked as servants in private homes. Even these colonies experienced a slowdown in demand. In response, Bernstein opened more colonies, not to serve as intermediate facilities but to relieve overcrowding at the institution.

Added to problems in the colonies were problems in the institution itself. Rome was having to accept greater numbers of "helpless and paralytic children and those who [could not] go to live in colonies because of their physical condition" and greater numbers of "borderline" delinquents (Herald, March 1937, 7; April 1937, 5). As early as 1930, Bernstein noted: "These hard times outside make it necessary that we admit a considerably larger number of boys and girls in order to relieve distress and dependency in families" (Herald, December 1930, 5). He complained of having to put beds in corridors and on floors of the institution (Herald, October 1930, 7). State welfare authorities increasingly called on him to take "high grade and borderline children of school age, small children who [could not] be cared for in communities" and "lower grades" needing total institutional care (Herald, January 1931, 7; January 1933, 5; February 1933, 5). After 1932, he opened several more "junior colonies" to accommodate the growing number of "young children of low grade of mentality" (Herald, June, 1932, 5). In 1932, Bernstein told the Rome community:

As work becomes less available outside, especially that of the labor class, more and more of our boys and girls who have been out on parole or have been discharged, are returning to the institution in distress, out of work or out of funds, and only in a few instances have we been able to find positions where they can at least remain with families even though they earn no money.

Under these conditions it is very difficult for our social welfare department to rehabilitate these boys, and we are sorry to say a number of them are developing serious delinquent tendencies, especially those who have been discharged. When they return here in the status of guests of the institution for a time . . . some of them practice their delinquent tendencies on other inmates and employees. We fear that it will be necessary to have these boys recommitted to the institution and placed in our lock-up department, where they can be controlled and kept out of trouble, until industrial conditions outside improve to the extent that they will be able to secure work. (*Herald*, November, 1932, 5)

In the midst of the slowdown in community employment for parolees, Bernstein faced continuing requests for the admission of new clientele. In September 1932, he reported two to four new admissions daily. By April 1933, in what proved to be the depths of the depression, Bernstein reported twenty-five applications for admission to Rome per month (*Herald*, April 1933). In exasperation, he decided to discharge some inmates to families in the community without going through the typical colony and parole procedures. Most of these were women who became nurses and family servants, living for room and board (*Herald*, September 1932, 3; R. Wilbur 1969, 29). As the decade wore on, however, even these placements became difficult.

The addition in 1933 of Civil Works Administration workers provided some relief for his attendant staff faced with growing institutional and colony over-crowding (*Herald*, January 1934, 5; February 1934, 2, 5; Riggs 1936, 75–76). The opening of the Wassaic State School in 1933 lowered his institution's population for a time, but, by the following year, it began to increase again. By 1935, it stood at its 1932 census. For the next thirty years, until 1966, the census increased annually (R. Wilbur 1969, 37).

By 1935, he acknowledged that the institution was serving mainly custodial patients and defective delinquents who, he insisted, needed "lock-up treatment to prevent them from performing their delinquencies and crimes and running away from the institution" (*Herald*, June 1935, 5). All other inmates were in colonies, which by 1935 numbered fifty-two and which had become essentially holding facili-ties as the institution filled with custodials and delinquents.

Letters from paroled and discharged inmates, which had been featured so prom-inently in the *Herald* before 1930, were now only occasionally printed. When they did appear, they were hardly as uplifting as they had once been. Angelina Belfiglin, a "discharged girl," wrote, for example, "I've been out of work for 10 weeks. The Cigar factory is shut down. It's a tough break—I've been trying to get a different job. I go out every morning for a job" (*Herald*, June 1933, 3).

In 1936, another issue provided a final blow to Bernstein's plan of colonies, parole, and discharge. The eight-hour day, a reform pushed by organized labor and the Roosevelt administration, came to the Rome facility. In October 1936, Bernstein complained to authorities in Albany that he did not have enough additional atten-dants for the three shifts. To make the new three-shift staff arrangements work, then, Bernstein and most other superintendents had to turn to a labor source well known to them all: the inmate. To supplement the attendant care needed for the new eight-hour day, Bernstein used "higher grade moron boys and girls to help over the least important hours" (*Herald,* October 1936). The need for additional help at the institution coupled with the economic depression "on the outside" made the vision of the Rome Plan increasingly less realized and realizable.

When Charles Bernstein died in 1942, the population of the Rome State School was 3,950 inmates, making it one of the largest facilities in the nation. It was no small irony that the champion of parole and community placement would die as the head of one of the nation's grand institutions. For a while after his death, Ward Millias, Bernstein's long-time assistant, led the institution, and most thought he was the logical successor to Bernstein. The state department of mental hygiene appointed James P. Kelleher, however, in an effort to gain its own control over the facility. Bernstein had acquired a reputation for "working over" the state legislature.[12] State officials believed (and, as it turned out, correctly) that Kelleher, who headed Rome until 1956, would operate the institution through the state board of mental hygiene and not as an extension of himself.

By 1943, in the midst of the military draft, the number of staff at Rome had fallen by one hundred. The next year it would be down by another one hundred while the institutional patient population continued to increase. In the face of staff shortages, Kelleher began to look with disfavor on the colonies. By the end of 1943, he had closed twelve of the fifty-one colonies still operating at Bernstein's death. At the time of Kelleher's retirement in 1956, only ten colonies remained, with a total population of 293 patients. In addition, during Kelleher's term there was no new construction at the Rome facility (indeed, none occurred until the early 1960s) (R. Wilbur 1969, 33–34). By 1956, 4,958 patients (293 of whom were in colonies) were crowded into what was essentially the same institution Bernstein had left at his death in 1942, when the population had been 3,940 (about 1,000 of whom were in colonies). All this meant that the focus was once again on the institution (P. Ferguson 1994, 83–162; see also Smith, Noll, and Wehmeyer 2013).

What happened at Rome happened in institution after institution in the United States during the Depression and war (albeit at Rome on a much larger scale). At the Southbury Training School in Connecticut, Ernest N. Roselle (1942), whom Seymour Sarason (1988, 136, 143), then a young psychologist at the training school, remembered as a progressive superintendent of a new and not-so-crowded institution, was nevertheless planning "the wider use of high-grade persons. . . to assist in the care of . . . low-grade and infirm patients." In 1933, Governor J. C. B. Ebringhaus of North Carolina acknowledged that the Caswell Training School had in the twenty years since its opening become "merely a custodial institution" (North Carolina State Archives, State Board of Public Welfare 1933). North Carolina had been one of the Southern states most influenced by the Rome Plan (e.g., Caswell Training School 1926; see also E. Brown and Genheimer 1969; Noll 1995, 145–146; Noll 2005). At the Alabama Home for Mental Defectives, the medical superintendent W. D. Partlow admitted Della Raye Rogers, her mother and aunt, along with her brother, Dovie, because their uncle in 1929 could no longer feed the family on the proceeds of share-cropping (Penley 2002). Throughout the nation, people like the Rogers family were admitted to institutions for the feebleminded to avoid starvation. In the face of the economic depression, colonies, parole, and discharge seemed out of the question.

At the Kansas Training School (formerly the Kansas State Asylum), B. A. Nash of the University of Kansas School of Education concluded, "This institution is a dumping ground for all sorts of undesirables or unfortunate persons who are sent without any expert evidence that the cases are sufficiently mentally-deficient to be institutionalized on those grounds. ... [T]here is nothing in the institution that is vocational in nature" (cited in J. Holman 1966). Parole and discharge, which had been instituted at the Kansas school in 1922, had stopped by 1940. In 1929, the Columbus State School in Ohio had hired a staff of trained social workers to handle the anticipated paroles and discharges. By 1933, the anticipation and the social workers were gone (Ohio Department of Public Welfare 1929, 1934). By 1935, the Lincoln State School and Colony had brought to a halt its experiment with community placement; its farm colonies began to look merely like a separate institution adjacent to the main institution. In a *Sample Book* presented to the state legislature in 1936, institutional authorities showed the self-contained work of the institution and the farm colonies (Lincoln State School and Colony 1935–36; see also note 10). There had never been much interest in community placement at the Illinois facility; now there was nearly none. In March 1941, as the economy improved and before the country's entry into war, Lincoln officials photographed conditions at the school. The photographs, showing leaking roofs, unrepaired walkways, badly needed tuck-pointing, and so forth, were meant to arouse public and legislative sympathy; the war would delay sympathy and repairs for several more years (Lincoln State School and Colony 1880–1941).

At Pennhurst State School in Pennsylvania, institutional officials were "reluctant to release some of [their] better worker patients since professional personnel to train others [was not] obtainable" (Angell 1944, 4). At the Utah State Training School, officials still allowed for parole but only if the parolee was sterilized. "Some of the children [*sic*] seem a little sorry about it," reported a conscientious objector working at the school, "but most of them are eager to get it over with because they are then given more opportunities to get out on their own" (Angell 1944, 4). At the Rosewood State Training School in Maryland, however, Gordan C. Zahn, a conscientious objector, noted: "The goal of every admission to Rosewood (except those which are obviously custodial in nature) should be parole. Yet in those three years [1944–46] the only paroles of Rosewood resulted from successful 'escapes' or from actual court actions instituted by interested parties. Since the great majority of children [*sic*] there are not blessed with sufficiently interested parties, the latter cases were few indeed" (Zahn 1946*b*, 4).[13] Sarason (1988, 147) noted that when he arrived at Southbury in 1942:

> In those days and for some years thereafter, commitment was via the probate courts, which meant that the state assumed the role of legal guardian. And legal guardianship meant that we at Southbury determined when and under what conditions a child [*sic*] could go home for visits, extended stays, or a work placement. In principle as well as in practice, it was similar to being sent to prison, that is, the state was in charge of your future. The words *parole* and *work placement* were somewhat euphemistic, because they referred to two (and only two) types

of situations: if you were female, you were placed as a maid in a private home; if you were male, you were put on someone's farm. There were very few placements, and in every instance the individual placed was a "familial defective," that is, coming from a "Kallikak, subcultural" background. No one from a "nice" middle-class family was ever placed other than in their own home, which meant they were rarely placed, because we and their families believed they were already in the best placement possible.

Summing up his experience at Southbury between 1942 and 1945, Sarason (1988, 168) remembered, "For a year after its opening, Southbury existed for its residents; after that, the residents existed for the organization."[14]

The practice of sterilizing mental defectives was also affected by change. Before 1940, states had sterilized insane patients and mental defectives at about the same rate. After 1940, sterilizing mentally deficient people became the more common practice. By 1946, the rate was almost two defectives for every one insane person sterilized (Gamble 1948). Some of this shift no doubt reflected the increased use of lobotomies, which in the 1940s became all the rage in the state hospitals (Valenstein 1986). The insane, it was increasingly believed, were unlikely to leave the institution, so sterilization seemed hardly urgent. Better to cut the head.

Between 1942 and 1947, institutions in twenty-seven states where sterilizations were authorized and practiced reported sterilizing 6,212 mentally deficient patients. In nearly every one of these states, the rate of sterilizations (as a part of the general population) had increased each year since 1935 (Gamble 1948; see also Ladd-Taylor 1997). With this increase in sterilization came a "new" rationale for sterilizations. In the postwar institutions, now housing more than 116,000 patients, or in the community into which a few were still being discharged, sterilization became once again a tool for countering the "hereditary nature of feeblemindedness and its more certain permanence" (Gamble 1948). Once again in the history of intellectual disability, the ends changed but the means lingered.[15]

CONCLUSION

Between the 1890s and World War II, medical superintendents changed their rationale for promoting the sterilization of mentally deficient people. Their *cognitive* justifications belied a more consistent *professional* agenda: the survival of their institutions in changing social and economic conditions. In its survival, the institution provided the superintendents with control and legitimacy. Aside from its benefit of restricting mentally disabled people from having children, sterilization became important in enlarging the authority of superintendents in ever-growing institutions. As a mechanism of control, then, sterilization had an institutional function quite apart from its explicit medical purpose.

As the Great Depression lingered and war loomed, superintendents were faced with inmates who were ready to be paroled but, without jobs, were not. At the same time, they faced increasing demands to take more and more mentally deficient people, often from families who were unable to cope with hard times. In the face of these realities, superintendents again saw in the sterilized higher grade inmate a new source of institutional labor. Unable to find work "on the outside," these inmates became critical to the care of lower functioning inmates. When war came and the armed services drafted attendants, inmates once eligible for parole were more than ever needed in the growing but understaffed facilities. Through much of the 1930s and all the 1940s, parole waned, although sterilization did not (Angell 1944; Gamble 1948).

If the sterilization of mentally deficient people became a means of social control affected by factors external and internal to the institution itself, what does this say for the history of controlling groups of deviants? Were superintendents the victims of forces they could not control, were they the purveyors of what David Rothman (1980) has called "convenience" in the face of "conscience," or were they agents in a process to rid society of social disruption and social waste? It is difficult to find in their words and actions a benign intent for sterilization. Some superintendents may have found the technical aspects of sterilization interesting, but almost all recognized in it the potential to control feeble minds. Yet it would be wrong to see their actions as conspiratorial. Although many of them were attracted to the eugenics scare, most saw in sterilization a less grandiose purpose. By constructing sterilization as a tool for institutional survival and control, superintendents made it a day-to-day part of the life and meaning of the institution. As such, the control became increasingly routine, ordinary, and hence self-regulatory. After all, the most effective social controls are often those that give the appearance of being day-to-day care.

NOTES

1. Using census data, Lerman (1982, 34–39) argues that as the rate of institutionalization in almshouses decreased between 1890 and 1923, the rate of institutionalization increased in insane asylums and institutions for feebleminded people. He claims that these census data suggest that there was merely a change of venue for the "dependent, delinquent, and defective." As such, responsibility for these groups shifted from a local, county responsibility (the almshouse) to state responsibility (the institution). My review of admissions records of the Illinois asylum (see Table 6.1) suggests that more applications to the Lincoln school came from parents, relatives, or local physicians or welfare authorities than from almshouse officials. This fact, however, does not contradict Lerman's observation that the public feebleminded institution shifted the locus of care and control of the feebleminded from local to state authorities.

2. W. H. C. Smith's Application Book #1 listed in meticulous detail the applications of 1,650 clients between 1897 and 1911. Smith noted the referral source for almost every application. These referrals came from superintendents of public institutions, social welfare agents, superintendents of other private facilities, advertisements in educational and medical periodicals, and the relatives of inmates, and as a result of Smith's prizewinning display at the 1904 World's Fair in Saint Louis (J. Trent 1998). The application books reveal the network of public and private facilities in the placement process.

In his perceptive analysis of deinstitutionalization, Paul Lerman (1982, 11) stated, "Prior to the passage of the Social Security Act of 1935, there were few proprietary institutions providing care and supervision to population groups comparable to those age groups residing in state-sponsored institutions. . . . There were few private, nonprofit facilities to rival the dominance of the public sector." Although Lerman is correct to note that it was only with federal assistance that the profit-making facilities began to have large numbers of "dependent" and "delinquent" groups, in the field of intellectual disability, the proprietary institution had an old (certainly pre-1935) and important history.

3. A few superintendents did stay in their jobs, however. B. O. Whitten, the first superintendent of the South Carolina Training School, for example, took charge of the facility in 1919 and retired in 1967 at the age of eighty (Whitten 1967).

4. Tyor and Bell (1984, 105–122) argue that institutional superintendents and social welfare authorities debated the issue of "segregation or sterilization." It is their position that professional and personal preferences led these groups to emphasize one of the two policies; that is, to emphasize either segregating feeble minds in institutions to prevent them from propagating or sterilizing them as a preferable way of meeting the same problem. Fox (1978, 27–34), focusing on the history of insanity in California between 1870 and 1930, claims that superintendents regarded sterilization as a way to safely discharge insane and feebleminded inmates to make room in institutions for more inmates. This policy, Fox claims, encouraged more local officials and relatives to admit inmates as a way to get them "safely" sterilized. Ironically, Fox perceptively recognizes, rather than diminishing institutional populations, this policy actually increased the size of institutions. He also sees this policy linked with the interest after 1910 in Mendelian heredity.

Tyor and Bell fail to recognize the changing purposes for sterilization between 1890 and 1930 and its complex and changing linkage to segregation. Fox links the interest in Mendelian heredity of the 1910s with the interest in sterilization as a means of institutional discharge of the 1920s. In so doing, he fails to see that the former interest waned in the 1920s, even as sterilization regained interest, especially after 1927. The linkage of heredity and sterilization was periodic and hardly as consistent as Fox implies. Superintendents and social welfare authorities supported and justified sterilization for three reasons between 1890 and 1930: to control behavior in the institution, to deal with their eugenic fears, and to discharge inmates to make room for new applicants. The linkage of sterilization with both segregation and heredity was complex and often affected by concerns internal to the institution itself.

5. In 1911, twelve years after the last desexualizations at the Kansas asylum, F. C. Cave (1911) looked back on the "efficacy" of the operations: "As to tractability there is no appreciable difference, children [sic] of all grades and 'conditions of servitude' being kind, affectionate, easily controlled and willing to work to the best of their ability, giving us far less trouble than the same number of normal children would." He added with equal approval: "Among the boys, three have become obese. One especially assuming the feminine type, high-pitched voice, development of breasts, loss of hair on face, change of bodily contour. . . . All sexual desires have been lost and they are impotent in every sense of the word." The best review of the extrainstitutional medical interest in and advocacy of sterilization is Philip R. Reilly's work (Reilly 1991, see especially 31–40; see also Radford 1991).

6. Reilly (1991) is too quick to conclude that superintendents and their allies were consistent in their support for or opposition to sterilization. Alexander Johnson,

for example, whom Reilly notes (on page 44) opposed sterilization in 1909, would a few years later warm to the procedure. Not all superintendents, as I noted, were consistent in their views of sterilization.

7. The court's decision would be blunted but not overturned by its 1942 ruling in *Skinner v. Oklahoma* (Nourse 2008). This decision restricted the states' ability to sterilize involuntarily convicted felons.

8. Whitney rejected Neil A. Dayton's (1931) study, which claimed that high death rates among mental defectives made their rapid propagation unlikely. He insisted that Dayton's sample had relied on imbeciles and idiots, who were not the problem. Morons were the mental defectives most likely to be breeders, and it was they who were likely to be in the community. Whitney would later be remembered for his extensive writings on dog obedience training (see "Whitney, Leon Fradley" 1969).

9. The secondary literature on eugenics has grown over the past fifty years. In addition to Craven and Kevles, see also Allen (1975), Black (2012), Castle (2002), Chase (1977), N. Deutsch (2009), Grinspoon (2013), M. Haller (1963), Hansen and King (2013), Kline (2001), Ladd-Taylor (1997, 2014), E. Larson (1995), Lombardo (2008), Ludmerer (1972), Pickens (1968), Rosen (2004), and J. Trent (2001). Additionally, Barker (1983, 1989), Dowbiggin (1997), Dyck (2013), Hasain (1996), Jackson (2000), Malacrida (2015), and McLaren (1986) have written on eugenics, sterilization, and intellectual disability in the pre–World War I and interwar years in England and Canada. Both note that sterilization and elements of the "menace of the feebleminded" continued among practitioners even after eugenics went out of favor in scientific circles.

10. This situation was also apparent at the Lincoln State School and Colony in Illinois. The farm colonies were located about two miles southeast of the institution's main "campus." Begun as small facilities to house "farm boys," by the 1930s, they had become a separate functioning institution. Eventually with its own hospital and recreational facilities, the farm colony (by 1940, institutional officials usually referred to the singular, colony) housed more than 2,000 of what by 1956 had become a total institutional population of 5,306. Although many of the inmates worked on the farm's 1,200 acres producing most of the food for the institution even into the 1960s, by 1940, many of the inmates living in the farm colony were not needed or not able to work the farm. After the Depression and war, the farm colony had become an extension of the institution itself—another way of coping with more than 5,000 disabled people. Returning trained workers would no longer be a serious mission of the farm colony at Lincoln or at other facilities.

In 1936, inmates produced the following crops: 113 tons of alfalfa, 970 bushels of wheat, 20 tons of oats and hay, 1,822 bushels of corn, 127 tons of straw, 450 tons of silage, 39 tons of pumpkins, and 44,286 bushels of garden crops. Added to these crops were 57,428 gallons of milk, 7,249 dozen eggs, and 19,551 pounds of beef, 2,452 of veal, 310 of goat meat, 172,555 of pork, 4,780 of poultry, and 6,451 of duck. In the institution, they also laundered 32 tons of clothing per week, sewed 58,131 garments, and mended 170,269 more. They made 3,892 new mattresses, 1,542 new pillows, 1,500 coat hangers, and 3,500 fly swatters and repaired 1,741 pairs of shoes.

In short, with inmate labor, the institution had become nearly self-contained. Community placement was not central; institutional sufficiency was (Lincoln State School and Colony 1935–36).

11. In his first annual report, for example, Bernstein insisted:

    The time has now arrived when it is a fully demonstrated fact that the term "unteachable idiots" should no longer be used in connection with this asylum, or in fact any other, it being surely an unwarranted stigma on the lives of those poor unfortunates to so characterize them when as a matter of fact not one percent, if any, of our inmates are truly unteachable, many of them able to read and write and over fifty percent have been taught to be useful. (quoted in Riggs 1936, 18–19)

12. Gunnar Dybwad (1990) remembered Charles Bernstein getting the attention of New York state legislators by placing women from colonies operated by his institution in the lobby of a prominent Albany hotel where legislators lived during legislative sessions. After legislators noticed these normal women for several days, Bernstein announced to the legislators that the women were inmates at Rome. Dybwad remembered this incident as an example of Bernstein's skill at "working over" the legislature, a skill mental hygiene officials did not want to deal with in his successor.

13. Nine years earlier, the psychiatrist Leo Kanner had seen the situation at Rosewood differently. Before his colleagues at the 1937 annual meeting of the American Psychiatric Association, Kanner (1938) renewed a theme not heard for more than two decades. Women released from the Rosewood School in Maryland, he claimed, were exploited as maids and were likely to become pregnant, spread venereal diseases, and inflict "grave harm and perils on themselves and the communities in which they live or lived" (Kanner 1938, 1025). Economic hard times, it appeared, had resurrected a once familiar theme: the fear of mental defectives in American communities. After a similar address before the Maryland Bar Association in April 1937, the *Baltimore Evening Sun* printed Kanner's caution in inch-high front-page headlines. By the time Zahn arrived at Rosewood, then, paroles had become a thing of the past.

14. In 1942, the same year that Sarason arrived at the Southbury institution, Henry Goddard (1942) defended his Kallikak study. As Sarason's statement suggests, Goddard's study had come under serious criticism, now even from a new generation of psychologists like Sarason (see also Reeves 1938).

15. Interest in sterilization among superintendents and academics continued through the 1960s. In 1950, at the annual meeting of the American Association on Mental Deficiency, for example, C. C. Hawke (1950) argued for the castration of mentally retarded offenders. In 1963, Herschel W. Nisonger (1963, 8), in his presidential address to the same association, claimed that "sterilization laws serve a useful purpose if applied wisely in specific cases." In 1974, a three-judge federal court in Alabama ruled (*Wyatt v. Aderholt*) that the state's eugenic sterilization law was unconstitutional and set standards and procedures to safeguard the constitutional rights of individuals in matters involving sterilization. In 1979, the Department of Health, Education and Welfare set standards for federal participation in funding sterilization (*Health Law Library Bulletin* 1979; see also Macklin and Macklin 1981). See also Chapter 8.

CHAPTER 7

༜

The Remaking of Intellectual Disability

Of War, Angels, Parents, and Politicians

BY WAR'S END

Shortly before her death in 1932, Mary Averell Harriman hired Margaret Bourke-White to take photographs of Letchworth Village. Harriman had been a trustee of the village since it opened in 1911, and one of her estates adjoined the facility. Nineteen thirty-two was a very different year from 1914, the year she had begun financing the Committee on Provision for the Feeble-Minded. In the depth of the Great Depression, the populations of the institutions were large, residents were sleeping two to a bed and in hallways, and the demand to admit more needy feeble minds was greater than ever. Yet funding was at best stable and at worst decreasing. As the Depression lingered and some states faced bankruptcy, public officials found few reasons to provide more resources to public facilities. The parole and discharge of capable inmates thus became an attractive way of making room for new clientele, especially low grades and juvenile defective-delinquents. Careful to parole only well-behaved inmates, superintendents like Letchworth's Charles Little were eager to demonstrate to politicians and the public that parole and discharge worked. The job of the up-and-coming Bourke-White, then, was to document the success of Letchworth's program.

Margaret Bourke-White knew little, if anything, about mental deficiency, and there is no indication she thought much of her Letchworth series. The photographs have not appeared in retrospective exhibits or printed editions of her work and are not mentioned in biographies of the photographer.[1] Yet they reflect both her particular style and the new vision superintendents were attempting to create (Figure 7.1, Figure 7.2). Most of the photographs are close-ups of patients, the name institutional officials now gave inmates, and are obviously posed. In several photographs, patients seem to be in uniforms, all looking alike, whereas earlier photographs had shown

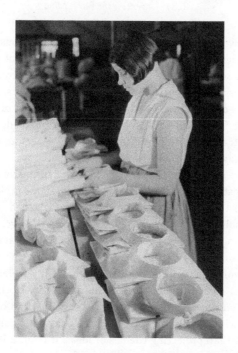

Figure 7.1:
In the Laundry, 1932. A photograph taken at Letchworth Village, New York, by Margaret Bourke-White. (Courtesy of Syracuse University Library, Special Collections Department, Margaret Bourke-White Papers)

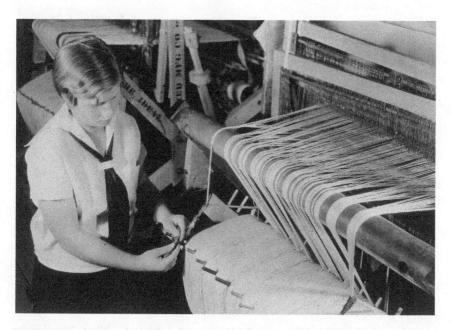

Figure 7.2:
Weaving, 1932. A photograph taken at Letchworth Village, New York, by Margaret Bourke-White. (Courtesy of Syracuse University Library, Special Collections Department, Margaret Bourke-White Papers)

inmates in their own Sunday-best clothes. The subjects are busy—doing laundry, ironing clothes, weaving, and studying—but look too neat and attractive to be really working. Their work seems contrived, real more in the meaning created by the photographer, not the reality of the work in the daily lives of the workers. None of the photos shows the "stigmata of degeneracy" so common in photographs of earlier times.

The patients at Letchworth Village looked well-groomed, crisp, and clean. Bourke-White portrayed children and teenagers any American community would welcome. These images were those Harriman and Little wanted to project to the outside world. There was still hope, they believed, that, properly supported, the nation's best public institution could continue to live up to the projection.[2]

In November 1941, shortly before the United States joined the new world war, Arnold Genthe published photographs of Letchworth Village, probably the last series of his long and distinguished career (Genthe 1944).[3] Taken nearly a decade after Harriman's death and five years after Little's, Genthe's photographs reflected an image of Letchworth quite different from Bourke-White's (Figure 7.3, Figure 7.4). In Genthe's images, most patients appeared in day-to-day clothing. Their appearances were hardly uniform. The work they did looked real and hard. In contrast to Bourke-White's precise portraits, Genthe's pictures have a snapshot quality, capturing moments more than projecting themes or ideas. If Bourke-White tried to project an image designed by Letchworth officials, Genthe attempted to capture the reality of Letchworth villagers as workers. There was little in Genthe's photographs

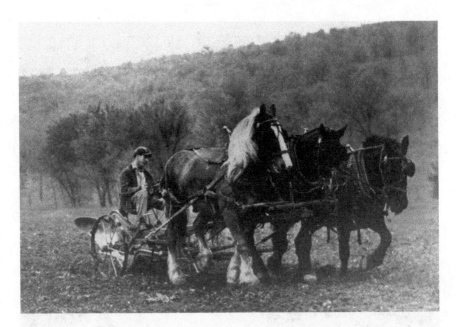

Figure 7.3:
Ready for a Deep Furrow, 1940. A photograph taken at Letchworth Village, New York, by Arnold Genthe. (From New York State, Department of Mental Hygiene, *Life at Letchworth Village*, 1948)

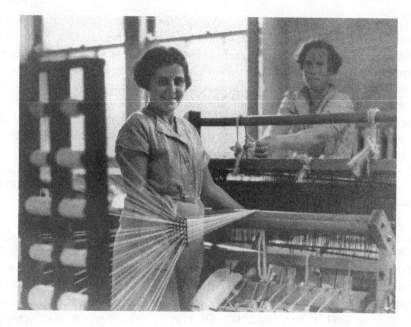

Figure 7.4:
At the Loom, 1940. A photograph taken at Letchworth Village, New York, by Arnold Genthe.
(From New York State, Department of Mental Hygiene, *Life at Letchworth Village*, 1948)

that suggested a world outside the institution. Genthe's patients were peasant-like, rooted in a community (albeit an institutional community) they were not likely to leave.

At the end of the 1940s, Irving Haberman did a third set of photographs of Letchworth Village. First appearing in the New York daily *PM* and reproduced in Albert Deutsch's *Shame of the States* (1948), Haberman's photographs departed from those of both Bourke-White and Genthe. Haberman's photographs were an exposé of the wretched conditions at Letchworth Village. Naked residents, unkempt and dirty, huddled in sterile dayrooms. Haberman's patients were helpless quasi-human beings, the victims of what Deutsch called "euthanasia through neglect." The focus and message of Haberman's photographs pushed the viewer not to the patient but to the inferno. Faces and activities were not important. Important was the hell made by the institution; important, too, was the implicit message that something needed to be done.

There was a certain irony in the attention paid to Letchworth Village in Deutsch's *Shame of the States*. Planned by some of America's leading architects and supported by several of its most generous philanthropists, the village regarded itself as the best public facility of its kind in the most progressive and bountiful state in the nation. In 1914, a committee of national advisers made up of Fernald, Rogers, Murdoch, and Johnstone—the preeminent authorities of the period—had made recommendations to Letchworth's board of managers (while the advisers were also meeting to form the Committee on Provision for the Feeble-Minded). Letchworth Village, they noted approvingly, had been planned to avoid "the bane of a large institution [to] insure the nearest approach to normal home life for the individual" (New York State, State Senate 1915, 11). The photographs of both Bourke-White and Genthe, in their own way, had projected this image. Deutsch, a New Yorker himself, knew that to point to the shame of Letchworth, the best institution of its sort, was to point to all other American institutions for mentally deficient people. Gone were the images of Bourke-White's teenager ready for parole and Genthe's simple, hard-working, if disheveled, laborer. Haberman showed victims condemned to America's best facility.

In 1972, Letchworth Village would for a fourth time be before a camera. Geraldo Rivera's television reports of Willowbrook State School and Letchworth Village gave not only New Yorkers but also a national audience a view of what Rivera (1972) called "the last great disgrace."

Exposés of public facilities for mentally ill and mentally deficient people appeared often after World War II. Some of America's leading reporters (Peter Lisagor of the *Chicago Daily News*, Mike Gorman then of the *Tulsa Daily Oklahoman*, and Al Ostrow of the *San Francisco News*, for example) gained recognition by exposing conditions in institutions around the nation. Much of the impetus for their investigations came from information first made available by conscientious objectors (COs). After 1941, more than 2,000 COs, primarily Quakers, Catholic Workers, Mennonites, and Brethren, worked as attendants in hospitals and training schools in nineteen states. Of these numbers, about 250 men served in fourteen training schools, with about 15 men in each school.[4] Throughout the war, public institutions experienced labor shortages because of the military call-up, and most, although not all, superintendents were glad to have men who were almost always better educated than ordinary attendants (Angell 1944; Grob 1991, 70–92; Sibley and Jacob 1952, 134–140, 160–164; Zahn 1946*a*, 1946*b*, 1946*c*).

Most COs worked in Civilian Public Service teams (known as CPS teams). Some kept diaries. Several began to compare observations and to meet informally to discuss the conditions they saw in state facilities and what they could do to make changes in them. Before the war's end, CPS teams around Philadelphia began to publish the *Psychiatric Aid*, a monthly magazine addressing issues of mental illness and deficiency. In it, they described run-down conditions in the public facilities and the inadequate and sometimes brutal treatment of patients. Most men worked in state hospitals and schools for several of the war years. Their observations could not be dismissed as casual or uninformed. Their notes and diaries chronicled beatings and tortures, deprivation and cruelty, even killings, but they primarily revealed benign neglect. Intent on making their findings known and reinforced by their common purpose, in 1946, the CPS men formed the National Mental Health Foundation (NMHF).

In January 1946, Channing B. Richardson (1946), a twenty-eight-year-old Quaker, published an article on his experiences at "a large state institution" in the *Christian Century*. He wrote:

> On this cold and wintry night there are 2,500 morons, imbeciles, and idiots asleep in the large brick buildings which surround me. For the past eleven months I have worked here, at one time with a group of 130 morons of school age and at another

time with 33 tubercular boys ranging from the lowest incontinent idiot to a moron who tinkers with radios. . . . Conditioned thoroughly by a pattern of violence over a period of years, these defectives have nothing to look back on and less to hope for. They know no beauty, no affection and no rewards. Accordingly they exhibit slight regard for consequences—even those "highgrades" who might think of consequences. In fact, one wonders whether daily corporeal punishment is not a type of fun or exercise for some of them. In many situations control is kept by using a working patient to intimidate the unwieldy group into keeping still.

Just as the inmates suffered from overcrowding and sterile routines, so, too, did the attendants:

One cannot work twelve hours a day in a stream of missed opportunities and amidst unhappiness without paying toll. Which or how much of the world's standards should be applied to those who will spend their lives in the institution? Is it necessary to appear to be on the verge of permanent anger to get results? (It surely seems to be, sometimes.) The practice of extreme patience, day after day, is wearing. . . . It is difficult to work ten to twelve hours a day, six days a week, living in a somber institutional room and eating a heavy institutional diet. To labor patiently in an emotionally tense situation and then to receive seventy or eighty dollars a month is not attractive to anyone, let alone a socially conscious person interested in the complicated problems of deficiency. This is the result of penny-pinching by state legislatures and ignorance among the people. That is where the blame lies when an ill trained or crude attendant harms a patient.[5]

In one of several letters responding to Richardson's article, Harmon Wilkinson (1946) of the newly founded NMHF noted the foundation had received reports from "a substantial number" of CPS workers in training schools. These reports, Wilkinson insisted, "do not present a very pretty picture." All indicated that education and recreation were inadequate. Indeed, most facilities were fully custodial with high grades providing much of the care for low grades. Each grade, then, had become part of the custodial transformation of state schools. Placement and parole had become unimportant. "In no instance," he wrote, "do our reports show sufficient assistance given to patients in receiving release and placement outside the institution."

The next year, the story of an anonymous CPS worker, "Don," confirmed Wilkinson's claim of blatant violence in institutions:

The names of the two visitors were familiar to Don. He had heard the supervisor talk about them as two of the "fine attendants we used to have before the war." Therefore, he showed them around the ward freely.

They teased and laughed at several patients, and then they asked to see "Stinkie." Don finally understood that they wanted to see the little feeble-minded boy who was kept in constant seclusion on the ward. He was an incorrigible little rascal who liked to spit on attendants and throw his food around and make as much trouble as he could.

"Hello, you little bastard," one of the visitors said. "Can you still spit?" The patient demonstrated that he could. Then the two men took great delight in pointing to scars for which they were responsible. "Look, his hair still hasn't grown out where I conked him with a broom. There's a remembrance from me he'll carry to his grave." And much more of the same.

As they left, they said, "Keep alive for us, Stinkie. As soon as the big money gives out at the war plant, we'll be back to play with you." (F. Wright 1947, 103)

Like Wilkinson, most CPS men noted that not all brutality came directly from attendants. Not infrequently, working patients given the authority from their attendants punished fellow inmates. In places like Letchworth Village, one-fourth of the paying jobs were vacant. Many attendants had been drafted and others found higher paying jobs in defense industries. Given this situation, patient labor had become essential to the operation of the institution. A conscientious objector at Pennhurst State Training School reported that institutional officials were reluctant to release "better worker patients" (Angell 1944). Harry C. Storrs, successor to Little at Letchworth Village, put it frankly: "If it wasn't for the help we get from many of the children [*sic*] themselves, we'd be sunk. The work of some of them is actually superior to that we get from some of our paid help" (cited in A. Deutsch 1948, 133). Gordon C. Zahn, a CPS worker at the Rosewood State Training School in Maryland, characterized the work of patients more bluntly: "Virtually all of the actual work involved in the operation of the institution is done by the children." He added, "In most cases patients assigned as 'helpers' to the specialized employees are stooges for these employees— doing the actual work while the others 'supervise' and collect the pay." When called upon to provide a rationale for this arrangement, Zahn noted, superintendents justified patient labor by claiming that high-grade patients "owe[d] their labor to the State to repay it for the cost of their care" (Zahn 1946a, 6). In this context, it is not surprising that patients, given the authority, became another source of cruelty.[6]

As it had been for much of its history, the public residential institution had become the instrument for controlling what Steven Spitzer (1975) has called "social junk" and, with the admission of more and more delinquents to the state schools, "social dynamite," too (Angell 1944; Zahn 1946c). Economic depression and war had not left the state school high on the agenda of either the public or policymakers. Although in general superintendents had received the CPS men enthusiastically, some had not, barely tolerating them for the needed labor they provided. And most were hardly supportive of the exposés the COs produced during and especially after the war (Angell 1944; Hutchinson 1946). The reports, however, were too consistent and too numerous to dismiss (see also Taylor 2009).

TELLING STORIES: THE PARENT-CONFESSIONAL GENRE OF THE 1950S

When she agreed to be a member of the board of directors of the newly created NMHF, Pearl S. Buck had already read its widely distributed pamphlet *Forgotten Children: The*

Story of Mental Deficiency (Krause and Stolzfus 1948). Considering herself a progressive, Buck took the reports of the CPS men seriously and, like many Americans, was horrified by them. Given the interest stirred by the pamphlet and the reports, Buck began her own story. In 1950, *The Child Who Never Grew* first appeared in *Ladies' Home Journal*, and, a few months later, it came out in a small volume by her longtime publisher, John Day Company (Buck 1950). *Readers' Digest* and *Time Magazine* also printed excerpts of the book. All royalties from the book, she stressed, would go to the Training School at Vineland, where her daughter, Carol, had lived since 1929. The book and magazine articles enjoyed widespread attention, and Buck received thousands of letters from parents. Although it is impossible to know to what extent the CPS reports may have influenced her, the timing of the story's release coupled with her membership on the NMHF's board of directors suggests that Buck had found an opportune moment to reveal her twenty-five-year secret.

Buck had not suspected that something might be wrong with her daughter until Carol was four. At first, Carol had developed normally. By her first birthday, however, she seemed to be behind. She began walking and talking later than other children. But she looked normal. Her Chinese nanny reassured Buck. Doctors, too, told her to be patient and wait. Still concerned, although not particularly worried, Buck took the opportunity of returning to the United States for graduate studies at Cornell to have Carol examined at the Mayo Clinic. There, in 1924, Buck remembered a doctor telling her: "I tell you, Madam, the child can never be normal. Do not deceive yourself. You will wear out your life and beggar your family unless you give up hope and face the truth. . . . Find a place where she can be happy and leave her there and live your own life" (Buck 1950, 11–23).

Buck returned with the child to China, however, where they remained for four years. Meanwhile, during that time, Buck had decided to become a writer and divorce Carol's father, Lossing Buck. In 1928, after a Reno divorce and a new marriage, Buck placed Carol at the Vineland Training School. A $2,000 loan from a New York patron helped cover the tuition at Vineland and allowed Buck to begin writing *The Good Earth*. Later, in *The Child Who Never Grew*, Buck, mentioning neither the loan, the divorce and remarriage, nor her book, described her decision to institutionalize Carol as one of allowing her daughter "to be with her own kind." As she had grown older, Buck stressed, Carol's normal peers had begun to reject her. Even though in China families always kept their disabled relatives, such a practice was not realistic for a twentieth-century American, not even for one living there (Buck 1950, 32–38; Harris 1969, 137–138, 334–335).

During her search for a place for Carol, Buck found that public facilities had "long waiting lists . . . were overcrowded and the children lived in strict routine." Echoing the observations of the CPS men, she added, "Oh, how my heart suffered for those big rooms of children sitting dully on benches, waiting, waiting!" At Vineland, however, she was impressed by E. R. Johnstone's gregarious personality. She felt reassured hearing the patients calling him "Uncle Ed." Most of all, she was taken by the school's motto: "Happiness first and all else follows."

Ten-year-old Carol, after her mother left her at Vineland, soon ran away, had to be restrained, and had trouble adapting to the new location. Buck, too, had trouble adapting. But eventually both mother and daughter adjusted to their new lives. "She is safe here," Buck wrote. "She has companionship. When she learns to fall in with the others in the small routines that are necessary in any big family, she will even enjoy the sense of being with the crowd" (Buck 1950, 42–49).

In 1932, Buck presented Vineland with $50,000, part of which paid for a cottage for Carol and other girls of her age and ability. Known as "Carol Cottage," the building was homelike, Buck believed, with its own playground and wading pool. In 1949, shortly before publication of *The Child Who Never Grew,* Vineland officials complained that visits to Buck's home disturbed Carol. They suggested that Buck stop them. Johnstone had tolerated the disturbances, but now Uncle Ed was dead. In response, Buck built a home just for Carol's stays, but eventually even her visits there ended. Although Buck continued to remain active on Vineland's board, Carol rarely left the institution after the early 1950s (Stirling 1983, 121, 218).

Buck, as a well-known literary figure and winner of the Nobel Prize for literature, offered an important confessional to other "bewildered and ashamed" parents. Anyone, even a famous person, could have a retarded child, she reassured them. Parents must not blame themselves. Instead they must face reality with "acceptance and endurance." Our children, she told parents, are forever children. They may acquire the bodies of adults, but mentally they will remain childlike. Rather than trying to find cures and treatments, parents had best accept their child's condition. To accept was to begin the important process of making the child's life pleasant and happy, of getting on with life, of ridding oneself of the emotional shame of having such a child (Buck 1950, 5–9; see also Brockley 2004).

Buck strongly advised parents to follow her own example by keeping "mentally retarded children"—a label now replacing "the mentally deficient"—at home through their early years. Yet, as these children grew older and began to experience the stress of peer rejection, parents must turn to the institution. In 1955, she wrote to one of the thousands of parents who communicated with her after the publication of her book, "I kept my child with me until she was ten years old. . . . [Then it] seemed essential that she have the companionship of her own kind and that she be put into an environment where she could spend her life happily and under special circumstances" (cited in Harris 1971, 177).

She downplayed the importance of heredity in mental deficiency. She had always been careful to claim no hereditary taint in her lineage. She had never thought her first husband very intelligent, and for that reason suspected Carol's condition lay with the Bucks. Years after the book's publication, she learned that phenylketonuria caused her daughter's disability. She seemed unburdened to know (Buck 1950, 7–8, 12; Stirling 1983, 72–73, 219–220).

With *The Child Who Never Grew,* Buck started a trend. The confessional genre continued in 1952, when Alfred A. Knopf published John P. Frank's *My Son's Story* (1952). Like Buck's book, Frank's received widespread public attention. *Time Magazine* covered his story, and excerpts of the book appeared in *Readers' Digest.* Frank was a twenty-nine-year-old professor of American constitutional law. A former clerk to Supreme Court Justice Hugo Black, he had begun his writing career with a 1949 biography of Black. In January 1947, Frank and his wife Lorraine had their first child,

John Peter. They had the normal expectations and anxieties of new parents about their firstborn. Like other parents of the postwar years, the Franks read books by Benjamin Spock and Arnold Gesell. They were concerned, although not alarmed, that Petey did not roll over when the books told them he should. Eventually, he began to have convulsions. Specialists confirmed their worst fears. Much of Petey's brain had atrophied. "He has no future," a doctor told Frank. "He will continue to have convulsions. He will never develop fully" (Frank 1952, 57). Taking the news as stoically as they could, the Franks planned for the future. Justices Black and Rutledge recommended institutional care and inquired about a suitable placement for the boy.

The physicians who had diagnosed his condition also recommended an institution. Most were blunt. "Mr. Frank, your impulse is going to be the normal one," claimed one doctor. "You will slowly absorb what I have told you, and when you have completely absorbed it, you won't believe it. You will look at the attractive youngster, and you won't believe that anything is very seriously wrong. More than that, you will suppose that whatever is the trouble can be cured" (Frank 1952, 58). Another doctor counseled, "Some time between the ages of four and six, if he can run around, he may be impossible for your wife to manage. He may be hitting and biting" (Frank 1952, 68). A friend warned, "It will end up as a job that Lorraine can't possibly handle. It will sap her life, and seriously injure yours. It will create a home atmosphere that will be impossible for future children. I have seen families in this situation before. Let me urge you to place your child in an institution that can take care of him" (Frank 1952, 86).

Soon Lorraine Frank became pregnant again, and her husband was convinced that their son should be put in an institution. Lorraine, he stressed, could not cope with both Petey and another child. Despite the inquiries and help from influential friends, the Franks remained frustrated. They were attracted to Catholic facilities, but all seemed to be full or did not take children as young as Petey. Lorraine was not as sure as her husband that Petey should be institutionalized. She began to read about cures. The issue before John Frank became one of convincing his wife to give up the boy. Help came from doctors and Lorraine's family. All counseled putting Petey away. One trusted doctor noted, "I've seen home care for badly retarded children tried every way there is to try it, and it always fails. . . . And think of the child to be born" (Frank 1952, 145–146).

Eventually Lorraine acquiesced, John found a suitable facility, and, in September 1948, Petey at the age of nineteen-and-one-half months left home. The parents were pleased with the care and attention given children at Saint Rita's Home in Wisconsin. They visited Petey several times each year. To everyone's surprise, he learned to walk and talk. By the time he was four, he addressed his mother as "sister." The nuns were a bit embarrassed (Frank 1952, 152–209).

If the stories of Buck and Frank represented the stoic, secular response of the 1950s American family in the face of intellectual disability, the confession of Dale Evans Rogers was its sacred equivalent. Rogers, better known as Dale Evans, was one of America's best-known women in the postwar years. Along with her Hollywood-cowboy husband, Roy Rogers, she was popular in movies, traveling shows, and records and was just beginning to extend her fame to television. On March 16, 1953, nearly three years after the publication of Buck's book and less than a year after Frank's, Rogers (1953) came out with *Angel Unaware*. The book cost one dollar. At year's end, only two other books that year had sold more copies, the *Revised Standard Version of the Bible* and the *Power of Positive Thinking*. Part of the success of *Angel Unaware* was due to Norman Vincent Peale's introduction and endorsement, part to Rogers' fame, and part to the prerelease attention given the book. From Louella Parsons's gossip column to Roy's January 1953 appearance on Ralph Edwards's television show "This Is Your Life" to dozens of articles in movie magazines, Americans were ready for Dale's story (Garrison 1956, 9–10, 71–82).

Although they both had had children by previous marriages and would later adopt children, Roy Rogers and Dale Evans Rogers had only one child together, Robin, born in August 1950. In the foreword to her book, Rogers wrote:

> This is the story of what a baby girl named Robin Elizabeth accomplished in trans-forming the lives of the Roy Rogers family.
>
> Our baby came into the world with an appalling handicap, as you will discover when you read her story.
>
> I believe with all my heart that God sent her on a two-year mission to our household, to strengthen us spiritually and to draw us closer together in the knowledge and love and fellowship of God.
>
> It has been said that tragedy and sorrow never leave us where they find us. In this instance, both Roy and I are grateful to God for the privilege of learning some great lessons of truth through His tiny messenger, Robin Elizabeth Rogers. (D. Rogers 1953, 7)

Unlike the straightforward narrative of Buck's and Frank's books, Rogers's was written from the perspective of Robin, the retarded and now dead child. In heaven, looking down on the events of the past two years, Robin told the story of her brief life and, in so doing, provided commentary on the meaning, purpose, and effects of that life on her family. Dale and Roy, Robin in heaven related, "weren't ashamed of their little 'borderline' Mongoloid! A lot of parents are, you know. They whisk them off somewhere to keep them hidden, so others won't know. That's partly because they want to shelter these children from the eyes of curious people, and partly it's because of their own pride" (D. Rogers 1953, 26). Robin reassured the reader that her condition was not the result of heredity: "This affliction was no respecter of persons" (D. Rogers 1953, 27).

While Robin was still alive, the Rogers, on the advice of doctors, told few people that Robin had Down syndrome. At the Southern Baptist Convention meeting in San Francisco in 1951, delegates prayed for her recovery, although they knew only that she had some grave affliction. Doctors gave the family mixed recommendations about putting the child in an institution, but most counseled putting her in one. Mumps and encephalitis, however, made the decision unnecessary. Almost two years to the day after her birth, Robin died. In her grief, Dale wrote her book, finding in Robin's life a divine purpose.

In September 1950, one month after Robin's birth, Dale had read Buck's *The Child Who Never Grew*, excerpted in *Readers' Digest*. It had been "almost too much for Dale. Instead of easing her own load, she had now taken on [an] extra burden" (Garrison 1956, 46–47). If Buck and Frank counseled stoic acceptance of tragedy, Evans told readers that they must find transcendent meaning in mental retardation. When she planned the dust jacket of her book, Dale placed a photo of Robin in its upper right-hand corner. From the lower left side of the jacket, Roy and Dale in western costumes look up, through the title, at their angelic daughter. Sent from paradise, the Rogers suggested, all special children should be kept at home. Angels have a purpose that is lost in an institution.

In the midst of the publicity surrounding the book's publication in 1952, the Los Angeles Exceptional Children's Foundation contacted Rogers. The primary parents' organization in Los Angeles, the foundation had two years earlier become part of the newly organized National Association for Retarded Children (NARC). Rogers decided to give royalties of the book to the new national organization. Delighted to receive its first and only major contribution, the NARC and its local chapter promoted the book. In 1953, Rogers made a long-playing record that the association distributed around the country. Money from sales of *Angel Unaware* and the notoriety resulting from NARC's association with Rogers launched the association as an important new actor in the history of intellectual disability.

The public disclosures by Buck, Frank, and Rogers were the most prominent and influential examples of a phenomenon that had begun after World War II and that continued to grow throughout the 1950s. Parents were confessing to the existence of mentally defective children in their families. Most followed Rogers's advice, but many did not, deciding instead to institutionalize their retarded child. In popular magazines of all sorts, parents reassured themselves as they reassured each other that leaving their child at an institution was the best course for the child and for the family. Most parents talked about the advantages of the institution, and, before the CPS exposés, many parents had linked these personal advantages to what they saw as a pleasant environment. "So it was that we decided in favor of a State hospital," wrote an anonymous father in a 1945 edition of the *Rotarian*. "Taking Mary Lou to it was a heartbreaking experience, but we were fortified with the conviction that in this move lay the sole hope for happiness for all four of us.... In this community, we saw also, there were no thoughtless neighbors gossiping about the unfortunates and jeering at them and their families" ("We Committed Our Child" 1945).

In *Better Homes and Gardens*, Judith Crist (1950), the future film critic, wrote about the family of Peter Wattris. Peter's parents, Crist stressed, were both college graduates. After an attack of whooping cough, Peter's development had slowed. Enrolling their son in a special school, the Wattrises looked forward to Peter "learn[ing] to be a carpenter's helper or a delivery boy or a farm hand." The Wattrises resisted institutionalizing Peter. Yet they remained concerned about possible rejection of him by people in their neighborhood and community. Crist noted that the siblings of retarded children were often emotionally scarred by the embarrassment of a feebleminded brother or sister.

Crist strongly supported institutionalization. Most retarded children were more at ease in an institution, she wrote, than in community settings, where they had to endure the stress of competition. In the institution, they competed with their own kind. The institution or the special school provided the best environment for a stressless and emotionally reassuring learning experience. The institution, in short, was the best place to turn retarded children into productive adults. Many, she emphasized, could even become self-supporting. "Graduates of special classes or institutional training find 20 percent of the world's work within their abilities," she noted. "They can be domestic workers, farm workers, factory workers; helpers to cooks, carpenters, painters, mechanics, and plumbers; countermen; porters; attendants; pantry maids; handy men; maintenance men—among hundreds of simple occupations that require a willing heart, a semi-skilled hand, and a conscientious mind."

In the popular *Coronet* magazine, Robert Robinson (1953) wrote about a family's struggles with their nine-year-old retarded son, Eddie. At first, they had taken Eddie from doctor to doctor. Coming to terms with their normal looking but certainly retarded child was difficult: "Our boy is an idiot. We accept that fact. But until that day four years ago when both of us faced it, we had no family life, were near divorce, and Joyce teetered on the terrifying edge of insanity." Eventually, a practical nurse in the home brought relief for the anxious parents, but the parents finally acknowledged, "Some day, we'll put him in an institution."[7]

As bad as the postwar institution might be, many parents and social welfare authorities saw in it the promise of relief for the postwar, middle-class American family beset by a handicapped child. Some parents, like Dale and Roy Rogers, remained unconvinced, but many others would look to the institution. Few physicians advised against institutionalization; indeed, most told parents they had few other sensible alternatives. For those who could afford private institutional care, all the better. But for those "on the way up" in postwar America, the public facility became an increasingly attractive alternative. Not since the 1860s had Middle America been so drawn to the state school.

CONSTRUCTING RETARDED CHILDREN

The years between 1945 and 1955 marked a period of irony in the care and control of intellectually disabled people. On the one hand, the postwar exposés, although relatively short-lived, drew the nation's attention to the run-down condition of institutions that had resulted from the Depression and war. Institutions were housing more and more disabled people with fewer and fewer resources. Those housed appeared to be more severely disabled than in the past. Capable patients were usually assumed to be delinquents (Angell 1944; Zahn 1946c). As CPS workers had pointed out and many superintendents had acknowledged, many of these delinquents were used to do the work once done by paid staff. Needed to fill labor shortages, more capable patients were less likely to leave the institution than were their equivalents a generation earlier.[8] In this context, brutality, exploitation, neglect, and routinized boredom were too often the rule, not the exception.

On the other hand, the confessional literature and the founding of the NARC reflected the growing integration of middle-class and well-to-do families into what through most of the twentieth century had been facilities for the lower class. Well-off parents were confessing to the institutionalization of their children. There should be no shame in placing a retarded child in a public facility, parents were telling each other. Coming to terms with the institution became an important, if tacit, function of the confessional literature and the new parents' associations.

Americans read that having a retarded child was nothing to be ashamed of and that heredity played only a small part. Although Americans read that many institutions were snake pits, retarded people in them were forgotten children, and neglect had reached the point of euthanasia, they also read that placing a child in an institution as Buck and the Franks had done was not a reprehensible thing to do. Indeed, a family's stability and emotional well-being likely depended on it. By 1955, public institutions for intellectually disabled people would once again include some of the well-off. By 1970, 75 percent of the public facilities housing intellectually disabled people had been built after 1950. This growth in both numbers of facilities and numbers of the institutionalized was made possible by a class rearrangement of the public institution. Although still primarily housing the children and relatives of the poor, not since the Civil War had institutions been so open to people who looked on themselves as middle class. How could overcrowded institutional warehouses like those described by Deutsch and conscientious objectors after World War II become sources for ensuring the stability of families with disabled children in the 1950s?

Parents formed local associations and, in 1950, a national association out of what they believed was a necessity. In 1948, there were 4,970 teachers of mentally retarded students in 10,308 local schools teaching 86,960 students, and 1,208 teachers in 5,926 residential schools teaching 21,460 (Mackie 1969, 14, 36–37, 48). Mackie estimated that only 15 percent of mentally disabled children living with parents or relatives were receiving special education. Most of these were in urban settings, and most were in special schools or classes segregated from other children. This segregation, however, did not preclude the integration of several disabilities in the special education class (Mackie 1969, 4–5, 37). The mentally retarded were frequently schooled with the mentally ill, the physically disabled, and juvenile delinquents. In other words, special education classes and schools, when they existed at all, had become the dumping grounds for many "problem children." In 1950, many parents with intellectually disabled youngsters could not find schools for their children. And many who could find schools or special classes found them inadequate.

The emergence of local associations of parents of retarded children also occurred in the midst of major changes in the postwar American family (Brockley 2004; K. Jones 1999, 174–230; May 1988). One of the most apparent changes occurred in marriage and birth rates, which had diminished during the Depression reflecting lower incomes, dislocation, housing shortages, and personal stress. Postwar optimism and the boom economy, however, changed both those trends. Filling the new suburban lives of the American family after the war were children, and plenty of them. As Elaine Tyler May (1988, 135–161) has pointed out, the baby boom of the postwar years was not merely a demographic wonder but also an ideology permeating American culture. Essential to this "reproductive consensus," as May calls it, was not only having lots of children but having healthy and normal children. As adult fulfillment in the 1950s became more and more a matter of successful parenting, parents who had retarded children were not just a little suspect.

Depression and war had had other, more subtle, effects on the American family. Many American fathers had become severed from their families either through having to migrate for jobs or because of military service. Sometimes their stints away from home lasted several months, sometimes several years, sometimes forever. Not just a working-class phenomenon, the Depression and war meant that more of the middle and professional classes would not be at home. The idea of home, too, had become more amorphous. Once, many Americans had identified themselves with particular houses in particular neighborhoods in particular communities. These personal markers, of course, had usually included extended family members, many of whom were part of familiar work settings and intimate neighborhood schools. Extended families, which had been in decline since the nineteenth century, became even less common after the war.

In some interesting ways, other events of the postwar years exaggerated these changes. The growing fear of the Soviet bloc and the Korean War kept many American families in military- and war-related industries. These families, like their predecessors a decade earlier, had to be mobile. War industries and their many suppliers required a work force able to move to new locations quickly and without fuss. Also, a burgeoning economy fueling the reconstruction of Europe and Japan meant more money and more consumption for Americans. In their automobiles, moving from city to city, and from suburb to suburb, American families had greater opportunities and greater consumer options. In front of their new television sets, they found a source of private and predictable entertainment. In new cities, in new neighborhoods, in new schools, in new work settings, Americans discovered in the television a common American vision. This vision, of course, reinforced the new consumer interest, the new consumer "freedom," and the new link between entertainment, labor-saving devices, consumption, and individualism. The desire to consume in increasingly self-contained suburbs meant that increasingly more well-off Americans were willing to accept unpleasant aspects of their ever-isolated family lives and to look for new ways of reconciling what they believed was inevitable (Brockley 2004; Creadick 2010, 118–149; Freeman 2012, 113–142; Jezer 1982, 176–234).

Fundamental changes in the American family coupled with the confessional literature of famous and ordinary people led to the growth of voluntary associations of parents of retarded children. They had different motives and needs. Some parents were concerned with finding community services or the right institution, some worried about guardianship, others were just coming to terms with what their family doctor had told them was a hopeless situation. But their differences bespoke what was common to all of them. As a group, families with retarded members could demonstrate their normality far better than such families of previous generations. They would not be Kallikaks; rather, they would be ordinary postwar families. Throughout the nation, from Seattle, Los Angeles, Little Rock, Minneapolis, and

Cleveland, to Montgomery, Trenton, New York, and Boston, local parents and relatives of retarded children formed groups to support each other and to get services for their children. They met other parents who, like themselves, had placed a child in a public or private institution. They placed ads or wrote letters to their local newspapers. And, as mentioned earlier, they began reading in popular magazines and books about parents like themselves (Brockley 2004; G. Dybwad 1990; R. Dybwad 1990a, 1990b; Hornick 2012, 72–83, K. Jones 2004; Schwartzenberg 2005).

When several local groups met in Minneapolis in late September 1950 to form a national association, they provided what would become for the first time in the American history of intellectual disability a voice for parents and relatives. In only a few years, the NARC would become one of the most powerful human services lobbies in the nation (Felicetti 1975, 111–116; McCullagh 1988). With few exceptions, the members were middle- and upper-class parents (Castles 2004; G. Dybwad 1990; R. Dybwad 1990a; K. Jones 2004; Kollings 1962; Lund 1959; Pumphrey, 1990; Schwartzenberg 2005).

By 1952, there were 119 local chapters of the association; by 1958, 550. Many local and state chapters became large enough to hire their own executive director. Soon they were working with local and state officials. At the national office, funded by royalties from *Angel Unaware*, NARC's first executive director, Salvatore G. DiMichael, initiated a national public awareness campaign. By the mid-1950s, the national association had distributed thousands of pamphlets to civic groups, physicians, and legislators. In October 1954, it persuaded President Eisenhower to proclaim the second week of November "National Retarded Children's Week." Also that year, the association organized radio and television spots about retardation. Pearl Buck, Supreme Court Chief Justice Earl Warren, and Oveta Culp Hobby, the secretary of the Department of Health, Education, and Welfare, broadcasted to Americans a new message about retardation: retarded children could be helped; people need not fear retarded children; with proper education and support, many retarded children could develop their potential; and, by implication, having a retarded child was nothing to be ashamed of (G. Dybwad 1990) (Figure 7.5).[9]

The burgeoning of parents' groups in the 1950s exaggerated a picture of the victimized parent that had its origins in the exposés of the postwar years. As Helen Herrick (1959) noted, NARC parents in their first decade shaped the agenda of retardation around themselves and their children as victims. But as "angry lobbyists," they also became a powerful source of change, causing concern among professionals who had so long dominated the field of mental deficiency. Organized into the NARC, parents could more easily express the love-hate relationship they developed with residential institutions and with the medical profession that they saw dominating those institutions (see also R. Dybwad 1990a, 1990b).

As victims, parents needed help for a tragic situation. "One of the most heartbreaking situations in American life," Deutsch (1948, 123) wrote, "arises in families burdened with the care of low-grade mental defectives at home because they can't get them placed in proper institutions." Echoing the concern of most physicians of the period, Deutsch (who was not a physician) added, "The inability of thousands

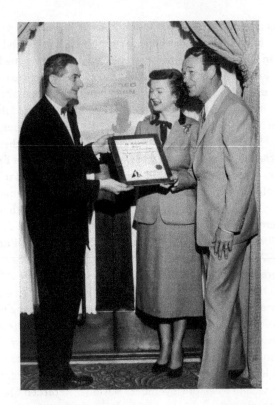

Figure 7.5:
National Association for Retarded Children's executive director, Gunnar Dybwad, presents Distinguished Service Award to Dale Evans Rogers and Roy Rogers, 1959. (from the author's collection) [Previous figures may be found after p. 224 in the 1994 edition of *Inventing the Feeble Mind*.]

of families to get their children admitted to institutions has taken a great toll of family breakdown" (see also Deutsch 1950; Levinson 1952, 15–17; Spock 1961, 1–18). Medical experts writing in popular magazines and books insisted that parents not feel guilty about their retarded children; instead, they advised parents who could not cope to put their retarded children away and forget about them (e.g., Holt 1955; Levinson 1952, 38–39; Spock 1957, 590–593). In a time when professional (and especially medical) advice was never so revered, parents took the counsel seriously (May 1988, 26–27, 187–192). Decades later, across the United States, adults learned about institutionalized brothers and sisters whom they never knew existed or whom they scarcely remembered.[10]

In response, some states, for example, New York, began to lift their earlier prohibition against admitting infants and toddlers to state facilities. At Letchworth Village, a new "Babies Building" opened in 1948. Other states in the 1950s and 1960s began to liberalize their admission policies, allowing large numbers of small children to become the newest members of the "institutional family" (Committee on Education of the AAMD 1951; Goldstein 1959; Kurtz 1967; Tarjan et al. 1961). As parents and local physicians pressured more states to open more facilities to take younger and often severely disabled children, states in the 1950s and 1960s responded by opening new facilities (American Association on Mental Deficiency 1965). Although the populations of the state psychiatric hospitals peaked in 1955, the populations of state schools continued to grow until 1968.[11] Pressure from an increasingly well-organized NARC, many of whose members had children in state facilities or anticipated the day when their children would be in such facilities, sustained the growth and development of institutions.

If they remained supportive of the public facility, believing that in their support they were preserving the stability and well-being of their own families, many members of NARC also kept a jaundiced eye on the institution. For these parents, having services in their own communities was more pressing. Usually the most settled among them, these parents started and enlarged special education classes in local schools or, when public officials refused to begin such classes, established their own schools. Some, too, set up sheltered workshops for their growing children. Many had not followed the advice of their physician; they had kept their children at home. If asked, most acknowledged the likelihood that eventually their child would join the ranks of the institutionalized. But as long as they lived, these parents proudly insisted, they would keep their child at home. At every meeting of the NARC, "retarded children can be helped" continued to be the parents' rallying cry.

The growth of special education classes attested (at least in part) to the NARC's political and administrative success. The 86,980 mentally retarded children in these classes in 1948 rose to 223,594 in 1958, to 393,237 in 1963, and to 495,000 by 1966. Whereas the general school population during this period rose by 70 percent, the overall special education population increased by 500 percent (Mackie 1969). In 1948, there were 4,970 teachers for the mentally retarded; by 1966, there were 29,200 teachers. (Despite this growth, Mackie estimated that 50 percent of retarded children in 1966 were getting no education, and 50 percent of local school systems had no special education programs.)

In their quest to call attention to their youngsters, parents had insisted that their children receive specialized education. Most were convinced that retarded children could not learn in the regular classroom because of the intellectual gap between normal and retarded children. The risk of emotionally scarring the intellectually disabled child precluded regular schooling. Parents wanted services especially suited for special children. By 1963, less than 10 percent of retarded public school children spent any time in regular classes (Mackie 1969). Thus, in their struggle to expand community services to supplement state institutions, parents reinforced a vision of special education that went back to the beginning of the century. Like their counterparts earlier in the century, special children in local schools would learn together, segregated from their chronological peers. Like them, too, special children would prepare for an uncertain future. Rhetorically, they were developing their potential, but potential for what? Their parents, like the professionals before them, were uneasy about providing an answer.

THE BEST, THE BRIGHTEST, AND THE RETARDED

From the time he was elected to Congress in 1946 until his rise to the presidency in 1961, John F. Kennedy had supported mental health legislation but had hardly been a leader on its behalf. Other politicians, like Alabama's Lister Hill in the Senate and Rhode Island's John Fogerty in the House, had taken up the cause of mental health in the late 1940s and 1950s. Joining them was a growing and influential mental health lobby. Made up of psychiatrists like Robert H. Felix and the Menninger brothers, and advocates like Mike Gorman and Albert Deutsch, the lobby supported legislation during the period—from the creation of the National Institute of Mental Health (NIMH) in 1946, to the 1955 establishment of the Mental Health Study Act, to the nearly 700 percent increase in funding during the Eisenhower years (Braddock 1987, 14–18; Foley and Sharfstein 1983, 17–38; Grob 1991, 44–92, 157–238; Torrey 1988, 77–87). These psychiatrists and their mental health allies did not entirely ignore intellectual disability; rather, they treated it as what Howard Potter (1965) called "the Cinderella of psychiatry" (see also Felicetti 1975, 68–74; Grob 1991, 213, 219, 349 [note 16]).

Several reasons account for this treatment. One was the mental health lobby's postwar opposition, which would last for another decade, to the state hospital and its survival. The community mental health center was to be a new source of treatment for the mentally ill. The intellectually disabled might receive services in communities as well, but the mental health lobby was neither concerned with closing the state schools nor sure that such closing was necessary and proper. When it was involved at all, the mental health lobby, like parents of retarded children, was more concerned that state institutions for intellectually disabled people be improved and made more readily available for those waiting to be admitted. Closing the state schools was not on their agenda, but neither was active support for them.

The coming of Camelot to Washington in 1961 kindled the aspirations of many Americans. Advocates of services for mentally retarded citizens were no exception. Shortly after assuming his new office, Kennedy appointed a presidential panel on mental retardation. Making up the panel were NIMH representatives and leaders from the American Association on Mental Deficiency. Notably absent were representatives from parents' groups. Only Elizabeth Boggs, a parent and NARC member, was appointed to advocate for the interests of consumers. As an academic, Boggs was assumed by the professionals to share their perspective, not that of what most privately considered an interfering parent. Notably present on the panel were several educators and psychologists, whose professions by 1960 represented 60 percent of the membership of the American Association on Mental Deficiency. Although the panel included psychiatrists, the nonmedical professionals were staking their claim for the future (Berkowitz 1980; G. Dybwad 1990; Felicetti 1975, 68–74; Milligan 1961).

The split between the psychiatrists and the behavioral scientists in the field of mental retardation had its origin long before the 1960s. The earliest medical superintendents of state schools had been interested in education and had felt no need to justify or reconcile this interest with their professional aspirations. As early as the

1870s, however, medicine and education had begun to diverge as superintendents began to treat multihandicapped and so-called uneducable idiots while leaving to educators the training of simple idiots.

By 1915, Goddard's psychometrics and the national recognition of the Johnstone and Johnson brothers-in-law established the legitimacy of psychologists, social workers, and educators not only as service providers but also as researchers and social reformers. Intelligence testing, a skill many psychiatrists acquired, nevertheless became primarily the psychologist's tool. Added to this tool would be the psychologist's growing confidence in behaviorism. Psychiatrists by the end of the Eisenhower years had become predominantly psychodynamic and increasingly focused on treatment outside the institution. Those who remained in institutions (in both state hospitals and state schools) were likely to be administrators (Grob 1991, 60–62,102–114). In the state schools, psychoanalysis had never made much sense; almost all psychodynamically oriented psychiatrists saw the retarded as hardly receptive to psychodynamic insight. Indeed, most psychiatrists (inside or outside state schools) were quick to say, albeit privately, that the mentally retarded were boring. In the state school, psychiatrists who were not administrating usually did little more than prescribe medications, order restraints for recalcitrant residents, and arrange transfers to the state hospital for clients whose mental illness began to appear more prominent than their retardation. Psychiatry's dominant tool after the war, the psychodynamic-analytical method, therefore, never became workable in state schools.

When *the Diagnostic and Statistical Manual: Mental Disorders* (DSM1) appeared in 1952, psychiatry's ambivalence about mental deficiency became apparent. In its report, the American Psychiatric Association's Committee on Nomenclature and Statistics formulated diagnostic categories of intellectual disability by IQ levels. Although insisting that "other factors" also must be used to determine mental deficiency, the committee remained vague about any nonpsychometric factors. Whether they acknowledged it or not, even psychiatrists were using another profession's tools, categories, and language as their own (American Psychiatric Association 1952, 23–24).

Another tool soon emerged, however, to compete with the dominant psychometric model in state facilities: behaviorism. Although behaviorists had had some interest in the training of intellectually disabled people even as early as the 1930s, behavior modification did not become an important (and eventually dominant) training approach in the state schools until after 1960. As a concept and set of procedures first formulated by psychologists, behavior modification would remain associated with their interest in empirical, laboratory research (Berkson and Landesman-Dwyer 1977; L. Watson 1970). By 1960, then, the tools and roles of medicine and the behavioral sciences were becoming clearly delineated and only occasionally confused in the context of state schools (J. Trent 1982, 179–225).

These roles were also reinforced by changes in the location and funding for research. Even in the early 1950s, research published in the *American Journal of Mental Deficiency* (AJMD), the only source focusing exclusively on intellectual disability, was carried out principally in state residential facilities and primarily by researchers working in the institution itself. As NIMH funding increased in the 1950s and new sources developed in the 1960s, the residential facility headed by psychiatrists continued to lose its influence. By the middle 1960s, research reported in the *AJMD* was principally carried out in universities and increasingly reflected the emphasis on behaviorism, a trend that continued into the 1970s. In losing control over the location and focus of research, psychiatric superintendents began to lose control of the thinking about intellectual disability. This loss was even more apparent in the change of editors and editorial board members of the *AJMD* (Table 7.1, Table 7.2). Between its founding in 1876 and 1948, medical superintendents had dominated the editorial decisions of the journal. After 1947, no physicians were ever again the senior editor of the *AJMD*, and, by the 1970s, only a few were associate editors. Psychiatrists might still control the administration of the state schools, but they would become hard-pressed after the 1960s to influence the thinking about mental retardation.

In this context, then, it is not surprising that the Kennedys had mixed feelings about how to direct their most important philanthropic project: the Joseph P. Kennedy, Jr. Foundation. All members of the family had participated in its founding in 1946 to honor its deceased eldest son, although Eunice Kennedy Shriver was to take the most visible interest in its work. Mental retardation, to be sure, would be its principal focus. About that there was no question. But how would the Kennedy family's largess shape the field of mental retardation? Parents' groups were emerging and receiving funding from celebrities like Dale Evans Rogers. But the parents were consumers and participants. The Kennedys before September 1962 were not willing to identify themselves in this way. Nor were they interested in seeing their money go to mere advocates. A major foundation should be scientific and authoritative, applying its energy to basic research. In looking for advice, they found that authorities in mental retardation were state superintendents, a few of whom had developed ties to universities, especially after NIMH funding became available in 1946. Among the most productive was George Tarjan, a physician and superintendent of the Pacific State Hospital in California. According to Tarjan, the emerging mental health lobby in particular and psychiatry in general cared little for mental

Table 7.1. PROFESSIONS OF EDITORS OF THE *AMERICAN JOURNAL OF MENTAL DEFICIENCY*, 1972–76

Profession	Number of Editors	(% of Total)
Psychology	75	(63)
Medicine	16	(13)
Education	14	(12)
Social Work/ Sociology	5	(4)
Other	9	(8)
Total	119	(100)

Table 7.2. PROFESSIONS OF SENIOR EDITORS
OF THE *AMERICAN JOURNAL OF MENTAL
DEFICIENCY*, 1876–1990

Name	Dates	Profession
Isaac N. Kerlin	1876–189 1	Physician
A. C. Rogers	1891–1916	Physician
Fred Kuhlmann[a]	1916–1917	Psychologist
M. J. Murdoch	1917–1921	Physician
Benjamin J. Baker	1921–1925	Physician
Howard W. Potter	1925–1931	Physician
Groves B. Smith	1931–1936	Physician
E. Arthur Whitney	1936–1939	Physician
Edward J. Humphreys	1939–1948	Physician
Richard H. Hungerford	1948–1959	Educator
William Sloan	1959–1969	Psychologist
H. Carl Haywood	1969–1979	Psychologist
Nancy Robinson	1979–1987	Psychologist
Earl C. Butterfield	1987–1990	Psychologist

Note: The journal has had several names over its history.
[a]Kuhlmann, a psychologist where Rogers was superintendent,
became editor of the journal for about one year after Rogers'
death

retardation. If the Kennedys wanted to fund research in a serious manner, they must fund medical research not linked with the mental health establishment. Soon the Kennedy foundation was supporting university-based research on the causes of mental retardation and, interestingly enough, on basic behavioral and scientific treatment of the condition. Joining Tarjan as principal adviser to the Kennedy foundation was Robert Cooke, a pediatrician and father of two intellectually disabled children (Berkowitz 1980; Foley and Sharfstein 1983, 44–57).

Their reason for focusing their efforts away from both the emerging parents' groups and the mental health lobby and on the university was not entirely a matter of philanthropic efficiency. Rosemary Kennedy, the family's first daughter and third child, had been born in the midst of the 1919 flu epidemic. As she grew, she appeared slow, what in the 1920s people called backward, possibly a result of exposure to the flu. She learned to read and write, although more slowly than her peers, to socialize with the family; in short, to get on as a Kennedy. But she was different. In her young adult years, the family began to notice changes in her behavior. From being lovable and gentle, Rosemary became increasingly more withdrawn and hostile. In the summer of 1941, after she attacked her maternal grandfather, the then aged John "Honey Fitz" Fitzgerald, her father, Joseph Kennedy, followed the advice of doctors who suggested a new and effective treatment, prefrontal lobotomy. That fall, doctors at Saint Elizabeth's Hospital in Washington, DC, performed the operation. The outcome of the procedure was not quite what the family had anticipated. Before long it was apparent that the once mildly retarded Rosemary Kennedy had become more severely disabled. What the flu virus had impaired, the surgeon's knife had destroyed. Although they had never before permanently institutionalized her, the Kennedys placed their daughter in a private facility in Wisconsin, where she lived until her death in 2005 at the age of eight-six (Collier and Horowitz 1984, 67–69, 114–116; Goodwin 1987, 639–644; K. Larson 2015; O'Brien 2004; T. Shriver 2014).

Although other parents had for more than a decade been confessing their family's disability and forming associations to do things about their situation, the Kennedys were reluctant to reveal their story as much because of Rosemary's lobotomy as because of her purported retardation. When they did decide to disclose their own family secret, in September 1962, they did so as "hope for retarded children" and "a fight against mental retardation." Parents need not be ashamed of mental retardation, Eunice Kennedy Shriver wrote in a *Saturday Evening Post* article that she had reviewed carefully with the White House. Retardation can befall any family, even a famous one. What was important was to understand that retardation could be understood and prevented and that retarded children could be helped (E. Shriver 1962). A nation that could make the Soviets blink could fight mental retardation.

Given the Kennedy family's ongoing relationship with researchers and medical specialists, it is not surprising that when John Kennedy formed his panel on mental retardation, giving to his sister Eunice a prominent place in its deliberations, he appointed only professionals. These professionals were soon telling Eunice Kennedy Shriver that proposed federal funding for mental retardation had to be separated from funding for mental illness. Psychiatrists and the mental health lobby should no longer control funding for mental retardation (Felicetti 1975, 68–74; Foley and Sharfstein 1983, 44; Grob 1991, 219; see also Morrissey and Goldman 1980).

In 1963, Congress acted on the committee's recommendation. New legislation ensured that funding for mental retardation would come out of the National Institute on Child Health and Human Development (NICHHD) created in the previous Congress and administered by the National Institute of Health, not by NIMH. Established to provide research and training funds, the NICHHD projected in its very name the direction set by a new breed of researchers groomed on Kennedy foundation support and committed to the Kennedy interest in scientific research. Mental retardation, they stressed, should be considered a health and human development problem, one that could be tackled scientifically. Researchers trained in mental retardation should be committed to the scientific ethos. Thus the fight would be a medical fight, a psychological fight, a scientific fight, but neither a psychiatric one nor a consumer one.

Consequently, the influence of the state school declined even further. Once the locus of virtually all research, the public institution after 1963 lost control of the necessary funding. Soon institutions were important only for their readily available and easily accessible research subjects. Universities, which now had the research dollars and the attention of the First Family, had become the locus of research into mental deficiency. For the first time in the history of intellectual disability in the

United States, universities were seriously interested in state institutions. Many established faculty liaison positions, others opened laboratories on the grounds of the schools. Most started student internships, especially in the behavioral sciences. Others set up demonstration projects to test a new drug, treatment, or program (often using problematic ethical standards).[12] Occasionally, an institutional superintendent, now often called a director, took part in or even led research projects. But most continued to do what they had always done: manage the institution. In their administrative role, they sustained what joy they might receive from the job. The glamour, the recognition, the direct contact with governors and legislators, were for the most part diminished, if not gone. Their focus was totally, even obsessively, the institution.

The new hero in mental retardation was the university researcher. In December 1962, the Joseph P. Kennedy, Jr., Foundation held its first International Awards dinner in Washington, DC. It was quite an affair. The master of ceremonies was Adlai E. Stevenson, United States ambassador to the United Nations. Welcoming the guests was Sargent Shriver, the foundation's executive director; Judy Garland sang. President Kennedy himself presented the awards. All the winners were university scientists, but none associated with psychiatry or mental health. They were Ivar A. Foelling for his work on phenylketonuria, Murray L. Barr and Joe Hin Tjio for their work on genetics, and Jerome Lejeune for his discovery of chromosomal abnormality in Down syndrome. Joining the four hard-science award winners were Samuel A. Kirk for his work in special education and the NARC for its "role in awakening the nation to the problems of mental retardation and for proving, through a diversity of means, that the retarded can be helped" (on Kirk, see Danforth 2009, 137–203). The ceremonies concluded with several clips from *A Child Is Waiting*, the just completed but not yet released film produced by Stanley Kramer and directed by John Cassavetes. The film starred Burt Lancaster, Judy Garland, Bruce Richey, and Cassavetes' wife, Gena Rowlands. It was a night of stars—theatrical, political, and scientific.

Cassavetes' film suggested the mood developing in the newly emerging matrix of interests involved in mental retardation. As he had demonstrated in other films, Cassavetes was interested in genuine, spontaneous, and unsentimental emotions. Filmed at the Pacific State Hospital in Pomona, California (where George Tarjan, one of the Kennedy's principal advisers on mental retardation, was superintendent), *A Child Is Waiting* used mentally retarded children living at the hospital. Judy Garland played an inexperienced but well-meaning teacher, and Burt Lancaster, a concerned but firm superintendent (and incidentally a psychologist, not a psychiatrist). When young Reuben Widdencombe, a newly admitted patient played by Bruce Richey (an actor, not a hospital resident), gains Garland's attention and concern, Lancaster insists that Reuben must first adapt to being at the institution. Certainly he can learn and develop, Lancaster tells Garland, but only after he has accepted the reality of his new situation. When Cassavetes brings Reuben's mother, played by Gena Rowlands, into the action, he refuses to cast her in a sentimental way. As a parent of a retarded boy, she is portrayed as unable to accept the fact that her son is retarded, but for Cassavetes her lack of acceptance is understandable. The film leaves us feeling the emotions of patient, parent, teacher, and superintendent—all parts of the unresolved dilemma, as Cassavetes saw it, of mental retardation.

Cassavetes' vision reflected and became another wrinkle in an expanding perspective of mental retardation. Retarded children could be helped, but help was a technical matter that could succeed only after all actors in the life of the child accepted the reality of retardation. Of course, this "reality" was both causative and effective: mental retardation was real, but real in ways defined by those who were insisting on its reality. By linking help to both technology and acceptance, professionals and parents were beginning an uneasy accommodation.

THE WAXING AND WANING OF INSTITUTIONS

Between 1950 and 1970, state authorities built, refurbished, and added to more public facilities than in any other period of their American history. Prior to 1964, when funds from the Mental Retardation Facilities and Community Mental Health Centers Construction Act became available, states had principally used Hill-Burton Act moneys to expand the number and size of their state schools (Braddock 1987, 17). To be sure, these new projects were, more often than not, less grandiose than their nineteenth- and early twentieth-century counterparts. Of the newer facilities, most were planned to house smaller numbers than the older facilities, although it could not have escaped the historically sensitive that the older facilities had originally been planned for small numbers. Most of the new institutions and additions to old ones displayed contemporary architectural styles. Usually single-storied, with horizontal windows, plain lines, and little if any ornamentation, most new buildings and additions nevertheless kept some familiar features. In most, there were the common tile walls, easy to keep clean and hard to break. In many, the floor plans imitated those first devised for the nineteenth-century "cottage." Usually a large dayroom separated two or more dormitory rooms, each of which housed two or three dozen residents (as the inmates were generally called by the 1960s). Sometimes a game room and sitting rooms were added to the cottage. Most, too, had self-contained dining rooms; in some of these there were tables and chairs; in others, a long metal table with round, attached seats that pulled out for sitting and pulled in for easy cleaning.

Some of the institutions of the 1960s had amenities that their earlier counterparts lacked. Most built swimming pools, and many had skating rinks, nature walks, and miniature golf. Almost all had up-to-date playground equipment. Many had a chapel, often donated by sympathetic citizenry and often furnished with sophisticated acoustical equipment. The new Western Carolina Center in Morganton, North Carolina, even included a golf course.

Accompanying these architectural changes were other changes in these new facilities that were both ironic and self-destructive. The first transformation was in the numbers. Between 1946 and 1967, the populations of institutions for intellectually disabled people rose from 116,828 to 193,188, an increase of 65 percent and nearly twice the rate of increase in the general population. Each year, two thousand to five thousand new residents joined America's intellectual disability institutional population. States built new facilities to accommodate the new demand, which the very construction had, of course, helped to create. Public Law 88–164, the Mental Retardation Facilities and Community Mental Health Centers Construction Act of 1963, authorized $67,500,000 between 1964 and 1968 "for grants for construction of public and other nonprofit facilities for the mentally retarded." These new federal funds only encouraged new institutions for more residents. Indeed, between 1964 and 1965, the first year dollars were available from the new federal legislation, the nation's intellectual disability institutional population saw its largest increase ever, from 179,599 to 187,273.

The federal dollars (from both Hill-Burton and Public Law 88–164) paid for construction; they did not pay for upkeep and maintenance. As they had since the nineteenth century, the states had the responsibility to maintain what had become ever-growing institutions of intellectually disabled people under their care. By the last half of the 1960s, more and more states were finding that more and more disabled people in more and more public facilities were a drain on state budgets.

A second change was in the characteristics of the populations. During the 1950s and 1960s, small children and more severely disabled children and adults replaced juvenile delinquents. This change had a dual effect. To be sure, "defective delinquents" had been the concern of institutional officials since the 1880s. During the Depression and World War II, institutions had taken so many teenagers and young adults labeled delinquent that most superintendents were annoyed by their presence. In some facilities, officials built "lock-up" buildings on the grounds of the state institution to accommodate the demand. At the Lincoln State School and Colony, one building was known as "the prison." Most offenders, institutional authorities believed, made useful workers when they worked and stayed out of trouble, but enough of them would do neither, so institutional officials were constantly complaining. The 1950s interest in juvenile delinquency and the subsequent building of new detention centers for delinquents meant that, by the 1960s, institutions for the intellectually disabled had fewer residents labeled delinquents under their care. As this population diminished (although it was never entirely eliminated), the state facilities for the intellectually disabled were taking on greater numbers of severely disabled people while losing the free labor provided by delinquents. By 1967, the states began to feel the costs of this change.

Thus, as increasingly more clientele in the 1960s were likely to be even more disabled than their counterparts in earlier decades, the new equipment so prominently displayed at the newest (and even at older) institutions began to stand as a reminder of the growing irony of services. Pools, nature walks, chapels, and golf courses meant little to severely disabled residents who rarely left their "cottages."

As the institutions filled in the 1950s and 1960s, some skepticism left over from the postwar exposés lingered. Parents who were, on the one hand, advocating for more humane institutions where care for their children could be guaranteed after the parents' deaths were also seeing conditions they did not like. Postwar prosperity had not come to the public institution. The effects of new buildings and finer furnishings were more often than not soon undone by overcrowding. As they became more involved in learning about the operations of the institutions, parents began to ask questions of institutional officials and legislators. Also, stories once only known within the tight circle of institutional employees began to surface.

In 1958, *Life* magazine ran the story of Mayo Buckner (Wallace 1958). The boldly printed title of the article read, "A Lifetime Thrown Away by a Mistake 59 Years Ago: Mental Homes Wrongly Hold Thousands Like Mayo Buckner." Born in 1890 to an Iowa family, Buckner was the family's second son. There was little indication why his mother placed him in the Iowa Home for Feeble-Minded Children shortly after his eighth birthday. He was a shy child and had a peculiar habit of rolling his eyes. This habit reminded his mother of Blind Boone, the popular Missouri minstrel, who had frightened her while pregnant with Mayo. On the day she admitted Mayo to the Iowa facility, institutional officials labeled him a "medium grade imbecile." At first, Buckner took annual two-week vacations with his family. In 1910, George Mogridge, the superintendent of the Iowa Home, wrote Buckner's mother, "I am glad to know that Mayo is enjoying his vacation. I might say, however, as a result of my observations, that long visits by boys of Mayo's age are sometimes not in the best interests of the child.... I have found that the many things they see in the outside world whet their appetite for such things, and they are often discontented when they return to me." Two years later at vacation time, Mogridge wrote again to Mrs. Buckner: "Mayo has for some little time been working with our printer and seems to enjoy this work quite well. It seems to me, in view of this fact, that a short visit would be preferable to an extended one. There are quite a good many little jobs of printing to be done" (Wallace 1958).

Good in the print shop and a gifted clarinetist in the institution's band, Buckner had become a valuable part of the Iowa facility. In 1957, Alfred Sasser, the newly appointed thirty-three-year-old superintendent at the Iowa institution, had Buckner tested. His IQ was 120. In the institution for fifty-nine of his sixty-seven years, Buckner, the *Life* article noted, was only one of more than fifty inmates at the institution whose IQs were normal. Indeed, several inmates had intelligence levels higher than many of the institution's employees. The article claimed that among the 130,000 inmates in the nation's ninety public institutions at least 5,000 were not retarded (Wallace 1958).[13]

As word began to reach the public about conditions in state institutions, so, too, did the media begin to portray intellectually disabled adults as capable of normal lives. Eunice Kennedy Shriver's 1962 *Saturday Evening Post* article, while stressing help for retarded children, noted that retarded adults, too, could learn and, if the conditions were right, could live outside the institution. Other articles in popular print stressed similar themes (e.g., Hansen 1961; Oettinger 1963; Strait 1962; "Struggle to Mend Children's Minds" 1964; Woodring 1962).

Hollywood also joined in promoting the new vision. In 1962, Olivia de Havilland and Rossano Brazzi starred in *Light in the Piazza*. On a trip to Italy with her mother, Clara Johnson, an intellectually disabled and beautiful American, falls in love with an Italian man. Her mother, played by de Havilland, knows her daughter has been disabled since early childhood after being kicked by a pony. Her father opposes the romance, so much so that he threatens to institutionalize Clara on the family's return to the United States. Mrs. Johnson senses the young couple's true feelings. Knowing that the wealth provided by both well-to-do families will allow for servants and tutors for future offspring, she facilitates her daughter's plans for marriage. The parents of the young man approve of Clara and appear unconcerned by her innocent, childlike behavior. When the father and son, and mother and daughter, go to fill out necessary marriage forms, the father, it appears, notices Clara's passport, which lists her as "retarded." Abruptly, he leaves the building. Everything seems lost. To the mother's, daughter's, and audience's relief, however, the young man's father confesses that he had become disturbed when he saw from Clara's passport that she was older than her prospective beau. Then, as it turns out, the father has not correctly remembered his own son's age. The parents patch things up, the two families reconcile, and the couple marries. For Hollywood in 1962, happiness and security are possible for a beautiful intellectually disabled woman, albeit one with money. It is noteworthy, too, that the disabled "member of the wedding" was female. A "retarded" man marrying a woman who was not disabled would likely have evoked very different sympathies.

A growing literature that focused on the mental hospital, but which began to be applied to intellectual disability, joined the articles in the popular press and films. Erving Goffman's *Asylums* appeared in 1961. Funded by the NIMH, Goffman spent a year in Saint Elizabeth's Hospital in Washington, DC, where he observed the daily patient–staff interactions. Out of these observations, he argued that mental hospitals operated as "total institutions." As such, they stripped mental patients of their individuality and provoked deviant reactions from them. Labeled deviants, institutionalized patients only reacted with more hostility, thereby confirming the label. Eventually, most institutionalized patients so thoroughly absorbed the label that the coercion and humiliation associated with total institutionalization became more a matter of routine than of necessity. According to Goffman, the essence of mental illness was not essential; rather, mental illness lay in an institutionally ascribed process of labeling.

Two other books critical of psychiatry and the treatment of the mentally ill also appeared that year: Thomas Szasz's *The Myth of Mental Illness* (1961) and Gerald Caplan's *An Approach to Community Mental Health* (1961). Along with Goffman's *Asylums*, both books questioned the reality of mental illness, suggesting that the manipulation of mental illness often involved labels more convenient for the labeler than for those labeled. And all suggested (albeit in very different ways) that the mental hospital was beyond improvement. In 1962, these themes were echoed in Ken Kesey's *One Flew over the Cuckoo's Nest* (1962) and in 1967 in Philippe de Broca's film *King of Hearts*. Maybe, both suggested, the real oppressors are the so-called sane. The mad know more about sharing, cooperation, and joy than do the rest of warring, manipulative, greedy, and power-driven humanity (see also Grob 1991, 283–292).

The first salvo pointing to dehumanization in institutions for intellectually disabled people came with Robert F. Kennedy's September 1965 attack on conditions in the Rome and Willowbrook State Schools in New York. Although a US senator with little direct influence over state lawmakers and the Republican governor Nelson

A. Rockefeller, who were concentrating state energy and dollars on the Albany Mall Project, Kennedy addressed a joint session of the New York State legislature. He told the lawmakers that mentally retarded people in their state's public institutions were being denied equal access to education and "deprived of their civil liberties by being forced to live amidst brutality and human excrement and intestinal disease" (Rivera 1972, 52–56; "Where Toys Are Locked Away" 1965).

Kennedy's address had been preceded by research done by Robert Edgerton, a California sociologist, in the early 1960s (Edgerton and Sabagh 1962; MacAndrew and Edgerton 1964). Edgerton and his colleagues had observed intellectually disabled people at the Pacific State Hospital. They saw the institution as a place "constitut[ing] a staggering visual, auditory, and olfactory assault on the presupposedly invariant character of the natural normal world of everyday life" (MacAndrew and Edgerton 1964, 314). The same conclusion, only more brutal and graphic, appeared in Burton Blatt and Fred Kaplan's *Christmas in Purgatory* (1966). Reproduced the next year in *Look* magazine, the photographic essay brought the largest amount of reader response in the magazine's history (Blatt 1973; Blatt and Mangel 1967). What Albert Q. Maisel's 1946 *Life* magazine article had done to shock the nation about conditions in mental hospitals, Blatt and Mangel's *Look* article did for state schools for intellectually disabled people twenty years later. Neglect, filth, and pervasive boredom, all characteristics of "Christmas in Purgatory," brought the nation once again in touch with a state-operated hell.

Under attack in New York, the public institution for the intellectually disabled soon found itself also assailed in other parts of the country. In January 1967, Ronald W. Reagan, the newly elected California governor, ordered all state agencies to eliminate 10 percent of what he characterized as "fat" from their budgets. More specifically, he insisted that state hospitals and institutions for the retarded cut their budgets by $17 million. This cut, Reagan insisted, would eliminate 3,700 state jobs, close fourteen state-operated outpatient clinics, and begin a process of community-based care, with communities taking greater responsibility for the guardianship of their "mental patients." Angered by reaction to his proposals, Reagan remarked that state hospitals (and prisons) constituted the "biggest hotel chain in the state" (Kerby 1967).

Nine months later, Niels Erik Bank-Mikkelsen, the director of the Danish national services for intellectual disability, visited the Sonoma State Hospital, a large institution for the intellectually disabled in California. Even before Reagan's proposed cuts had fully taken effect, Bank-Mikkelsen found conditions in the institution dreadful. He told a reporter: "I couldn't believe my eyes. It was worse than any institution I have seen in visits to a dozen foreign countries. . . . In our country, we would not be allowed to treat cattle like that." What he had found were wards of naked adults sleeping on cement floors often in their own excrement or wandering in open day-rooms. Not uncommon were "head bangers." Many residents were heavily medicated, existing in a pharmacological daze, a daze exacerbated by the constant shouting and screaming around them. In its defense, the California commissioner of health and welfare insisted that the state's treatment of the retarded was "the most advanced in the nation." Bank-Mikkelsen feared he might be right ("Question of Priorities" 1967).

While Rockefeller and Reagan were trying with some success to reduce spending in New York and California, George Wallace, the governor of Alabama and soon to be candidate for the presidency, began cutting funds for mental health and mental retardation in his state.[14] After the death of his wife, Governor Lurleen Wallace, in 1968 and his return to the governor's mansion nearly three years later, Wallace was determined to make the University of Alabama's Medical School in Birmingham one of the best in the nation. In order to concentrate money there, he continued a policy of small and, by all accounts, inadequate appropriations for Alabama's state hospitals and schools. At the time, Alabama ranked last among the fifty states in per capita funding for mental health services, so the reductions appeared especially dire. As had been the case in New York and California, loss of jobs for state workers looked imminent (Cavalier and McCarver 1981; Lerman 1982, 159–164).

In Illinois, Mary Downey, a program director and forty-year employee of the Lincoln State School, complained that although the institution was less crowded than twenty years earlier, wards were more unkempt and patient care was much worse. Two-thirds of the residents were labeled severely or profoundly retarded, but there were "fewer working students." The loss of this important source of labor was exacerbated by Governor Richard Ogilvie's proposal to lay off paid staff at the Lincoln and Dixon State Schools, the largest facilities in Illinois, while also decreasing the population of higher functioning residents in both institutions. What scared employees most was the threatened loss of two important sources of care— patient and other paid workers. Protests from parents and officials delayed, for a time, the shift in policy (J. Watson 1970a, 1970c).

On March 17, 1970, the Springfield [Mass.] *Union* published the first of a six-part series with the front-page headline, "The Tragedy of Belchertown" (Shanks 1970). The articles told the story of the overcrowded and, indeed, brutal conditions at the Belchertown State School in western Massachusetts. Residents were tied to benches and beds, many were naked, toilets were broken and overflowing, there no privacy, and days passed with few activities and even fewer staff. Years of underfunding only compounded years of overcrowding. The next year, Benjamin Ricci, a parent who had first placed his son Bobby at the institution in 1953, published *Crimes against Humanity* and became a leader of a parents' group that began to draw attention to state-supported neglect and abuse. Eventually, the exposé would call attention to persistent mistreatment at all Massachusetts residential facilities (Hornick 2012, 69–72, 84–103).

Two years earlier, members of the Pennsylvania Association for Retarded Children (PARC) became increasingly uneasy that the legislature and Governor William Scranton were ignoring the recommendations of their Public Law 88–156 state report. In the fall of that year, Gunnar Dybwad, a consultant for the association, told members of PARC's executive committee the only solution to the state's indifference was court action. At first, Dybwad remembered, they resisted. Parents had spent nearly two decades building working relationships with state officials, and they feared a lawsuit would jeopardize their gains. At PARC's 1969 convention in the following spring, John Haggarty, the executive director, reported on conditions at Pennhurst State School. He showed a slide of a boy who had died of burns under questionable circumstances at the facility. The slide had its intended effect. The association sued the state that year (G. Dybwad 1990).

A lawsuit was also on the minds of employees at Partlow State School in Alabama. With frustration still high over the dismissal of professional staff in Alabama's institutions and with fears of new layoffs, in 1970, the employees had lawyers begin efforts that led the next year to a class-action suit against the Alabama Department of Mental Health. Along with the Pennhurst suit in Pennsylvania, *Wyatt v. Stickney*, argued before federal Judge Frank M. Johnson, Jr. in Alabama, became an important legal action in what was the beginning of nearly a decade of litigations. By 1973, from legal actions to prohibit involuntary servitude in intellectual disability institutions (which had the effect of depriving institutions of their traditional and cheapest source of labor) to suits guaranteeing equal educational opportunities in public schools, advocates for intellectually disabled citizens were heading in the direction of closing public institutions and eliminating self-contained special public schools and classes (Bass 1993, 277–303; Cavalier and McCarver 1981).

When Geraldo Rivera (1972) exposed conditions at the Willowbrook State School on Long Island and Letchworth Village in January 1972, the New York station that aired the footage received more calls than ever before in its history. Its "Willowbrook: The Last Great Disgrace," airing at prime time in early February, attracted 2.5 million viewers, the highest rating of any local news special in the history of American television. About this time, the Associated Press, the Universal Press, the *New York Times*, the *Village Voice*, and national television talk shows picked up the story. What New Yorkers first and then other Americans learned was that Willowbrook and Letchworth were not unlike Nazi death camps. At Willowbrook, Rivera told his viewers, 100 percent of all residents contracted hepatitis within six months of entering the institution. Most of the severely disabled residents were naked or only partially clothed. Many, too, lay on dayroom floors in their own feces. The smells at both institutions were unbearable. To build the $1.5 billion Albany Mall Project, Governor Rockefeller and the legislature had forced the Department of Mental Hygiene to freeze hiring. Between 1968 and November 1970, Willowbrook had lost 912 of its 3,383 employees, most of whom were direct patient-care staff. And "to trim the waste and fat from the mental hygiene budget," Willowbrook was scheduled to lose another 300 employees. Rivera found Letchworth even worse. Once the premier New York and even American institution, Letchworth Village had become "a deeper circle in the inferno." Rivera later wrote:

> Virtually every patient in building Tau was undressed and there was shit everywhere; it looked and smelled like a poorly kept kennel. It was so bad I was afraid that people watching television, emotionally drained from a week of Willowbrook, would either not look at it or not believe it.
>
> The residents of Tau were young girls. Many of them had physical deformities; most were literally smeared with feces—their roommates', their own. They looked like children who had been out making mudpies. My stomach still turns just thinking about it.

But they were, after all, just little girls. And those little girls—just like your sister or daughter—wanted to be held and loved. When we walked into the wards, they came toward us. I wanted to hold them, but it was too frightening. They were like lepers, and I was afraid they would somehow infect me. (Rivera 1972, 78, 80)

In 1967, the institution had seemed improvable. Even in their *Look* article in 1967, Blatt and Mangel had found "hope" in the institution, showing photographs of Seaside Regional Center, a new and apparently progressive institution in Connecticut. But for different reasons grounded in different ideological rationales, states in the late 1960s failed to significantly increase (and in some cases began to reduce) funding for institutions for their intellectually disabled citizens. This failure occurred after already two decades of little or no funding increases but constant dumping of new clientele into institutions. New federal dollars had not been matched by state dollars. With the exposés that continued to emerge in the late 1960s and early 1970s, the state school joined the state hospital as increasingly out of favor. Thus, although there was never unanimity, by 1972 more and more parents and advocates seemed to be echoing Rivera's sentiment, "We've got to close that goddamned place down" (Rivera 1972, 147; see also Goode et al. 2013; Rothman and Rothman 1984; J. Watson 1970*a–e*).[15]

As civil libertarians, parents, and public officials in the 1970s began to look unfavorably on public residential institutions, they also began to question special schools and special classes. Both Project Head Start, enacted as part of the Economic Opportunity Act of 1964, and the Elementary and Secondary Education Act (ESEA) enacted the next year emphasized educational opportunities for disadvantaged children. Basic to both pieces of legislation was the assumption that federal dollars effused into local school programs would meet the needs of special populations—needs not met by either local or state educational programs. Intellectually disabled children were not specifically the focus of either federal program, but both programs opened the door to new questions about how to educate children with unique needs.

These questions, as noted earlier, had already been brewing. Labeling theorists, civil libertarians, and artists were portraying segregated institutions as dehumanizing. The special school and the special classroom were segregated facilities, too; it was not surprising, then, that they came under similar attack. Ironically, the attack on special education came not just from proponents of change, but also from opponents. Most prominent among the latter were academics skeptical of the claims made for the outcomes projected for the new federal legislation. Indeed, the new federal initiative had evoked heated debates over the relationship of intelligence to race, class, and heredity. Arthur R. Jensen (1969, 1972), William Shockley (1972), and Richard C. Herrnstein(1971, 1973), the most prominent critics of the Great Society's educational programs, argued (not only in professional journals but also to the educated public) that federal aid to public schools for the educationally disadvantaged was likely a waste of resources. Even the most well-intended educators, they claimed, could not modify the intelligence of children, certainly not in proportion to the expectations suggested by the legislation.

These Jeremiahs aroused a wave of opposition in the professional and popular media (e.g., Chomsky 1972; Jencks, 1969; Jencks and Bane 1973; Kamin 1974; Lewontin 1970). Their critics, primarily sociologists, began to formulate arguments for the expansion of educational services for intellectually disabled children and for the development of those services in the context of what became known as mainstreaming. Several studies on the effects of labeling and IQ on public school children bolstered their arguments, countering the claims of the new-day hereditarians (e.g., Beeghley and Butler 1974; Edgerton and Edgerton 1973; Mercer 1972b, 1973, 1974). Sociologist Jane Mercer's 1972 article "IQ: The Lethal Label" in the popular Psychology Today presented to the public the thrust of the labeling theorists' response (Mercer 1972a). According to Mercer, many schoolchildren became mentally retarded because school officials ascribed the mentally retarded label to them because of factors related to race and class. Their "mental retardation" had little to do with mental capacity. Placed in special education programs, these children behaved in ways that merely fulfilled the ascribed label. After they left school and returned home for the day, however, they demonstrated that they could function quite well in day-to-day community life. They had become what Mercer called "six-hour retarded children" (Mercer 1973, 89). Their "retardation" was a product of their time in school. Programs created ostensibly to treat deficiency were, in fact, creating and sustaining deficiency.

Into this questioning of the effects of federal legislation on the one hand and special education on the other, two federal court rulings pushed educational services toward desegregation and mainstreaming. In 1972, Judge Joseph Waddy, in Mills v. Board of Education of the District of Columbia (1972), ordered the Washington, DC school board to provide appropriate public education to all of its children and to create procedures guaranteeing due process for children suspended from school or placed in special education classes. This case was the first to guarantee intellectually disabled children a constitutional right to public education. In a similar case the same year, Pennsylvania Association for Retarded Children v. Commonwealth of Pennsylvania (1971, 1972), the federal court declared that the exclusionary provisions of Pennsylvania's compulsory school attendance laws were unconstitutional. Without due process, authorities in Pennsylvania could not exclude children from its schools, and, by extension, other states with compulsory attendance laws were similarly affected (Abeson 1977; Herr 1983).

In the midst of court rulings calling for the inclusion of disabled children in public schools, calls for mainstreaming, and the realization that state residential institutions were no longer going to be an important option for such children, Congress in 1975 passed the Education for All Handicapped Children Act (Public Law 94–142). Between 1976 and 1980, federal funding resulting from this act increased from $100 million to more than $800 million. Between 1981 and 1985, the rate of increase was less dramatic; however, by 1985, the federal funding stood at $1.1 billion (Braddock 1987, 38–39). Interestingly, the total number of intellectually disabled children served by the program decreased from 838,083 in school year 1977 to 653,010 in 1984. The primary reason for this change was a redefinition of labels. Encouraged by prevailing trends and the federal legislation, school officials redesignated "mildly retarded children," or "educable retarded children," as "children with learning disabilities" (Braddock 1987, 39). Since 1976, the moneys also have provided ways to keep children out of state facilities, most of which since that time no longer admit children and accept few adults.

INTO PUBLIC PLACES

They were strange bedfellows—local and state officials eager to cut costs and advocates eager to close inhumane state facilities and to eliminate local segregated special education programs. The community model so prominent among mental health supporters was beginning to be talked about in meetings of the Association for Retarded Citizens, the latest name for this principal advocacy group (once the National Association for Retarded Children). State officials, too, were speaking, if cautiously, about mainstreaming, normalization, and community placement. Even the staid and orthodox American Association on Mental Deficiency began to entertain the new ideas. In states like California, where the governor's cutbacks made the policy a necessity, mental health authorities were placing residents outside of state facilities. Most went where discharged residents had always gone—to the home of parents or relatives. The county home was now almost exclusively a place for the elderly. Without relatives, where would retarded people go?

Changes made to Medicaid and Supplemental Security Income in the early and mid-1970s to simplify the depopulation of the state mental hospitals, along with the enactment of Public Law 94-142, soon provided answers. To be sure, some states, for example, Nebraska, had already begun to experiment with extrainstitutional services, but most states had done little before the early 1970s. By allowing for a new source of community placement for mentally retarded people, the intermediate care facility (ICF), federal officials created community housing for many intellectually disabled people whom institutional officials only a few years earlier would never have considered proper candidates for discharge. Added to these community facilities were an array of other community-based residences: family-care homes, child and adult foster-care homes, group homes, supervised apartment living programs, and nursing homes (not of the intermediate care variety). Along with these programs, Public Law 94-142 provided a way of keeping retarded children in schools and thereby out of institutions.

As early as 1972, twenty-eight states had changed their Medicaid plans to allow for ICFs for intellectually disabled people, better known as the ICF/MRs (Braddock 1987, 22). By 1976, most states were using Medicaid funding to plan for the deinstitutionalization of incarcerated retarded adults. In less than a decade, facilities that had seemed indispensable were being viewed as antiquated.

Within this developing picture of deinstitutionalization evolved an important paradigm: normalization. First imported in the mid-1960s from Scandinavia by Gunnar and Rosemary Dybwad through their work with the International League of Societies for the Mentally Handicapped, normalization was elevated to a principle in 1972 in Wolf Wolfensberger's influential book, *The Principle of Normalization in Human Services.*[16] Already known as a champion of new thinking about mental retardation, by 1970, Wolfensberger had begun an apostolic campaign to denounce state schools and to establish the community as the sole locus of services for disabled citizens (Kugel and Wolfensberger 1969; Wolfensberger 1972). In frequent public appearances before professional and parent groups, Wolfensberger, who around the time began to wear only black clothing, set a tone not unlike that of Isaac N. Kerlin, Josephine Shaw Lowell, Henry H. Goddard, and other earlier crusaders. If the moral intensity of his message was like theirs, the message itself was quite different.

Like many others during the period, Wolfensberger was influenced by Erving Goffman's theory of deviance. A psychologist, Wolfensberger had worked between 1964 and 1971 at the Nebraska Psychiatric Institute in Omaha, where he had been involved in that state's pioneering program of deinstitutionalization. Struck firsthand by Goffman's portrayal of the dehumanizing effects of the total institution and affected by his own escape as a child from the Nazi Holocaust, Wolfensberger began to construct a rationale for taking the national vision of care away from the institution and, indeed, for changing the very vision of care.

According to Wolfensberger, mentally retarded people were deviant not as the result of their own choosing but because their "observed quality" was viewed "as negatively value-charged" (Wolfensberger 1972, 13). Many well-meaning policymakers and service providers, while attempting to serve the best interests of mentally retarded people, actually only called attention to their deviances. Large state residential institutions, specialized school programs, and sheltered workshops—all drew attention to the uniquely devalued qualities of retarded people. Retarded people, of course, absorbed these devalued qualities as they took on role expectations that, in turn, only reinforced the same devalued qualities. Soon images of the retarded person as, for example, eternally childlike or subhuman were viewed as natural.

While drawing on Goffman's views on deviance and labeling, Wolfensberger also turned to another sociological tradition, structural functionalism, to formulate a way of breaking through the effects of labeling. Unlike Goffman, who believed that the closing of mental hospitals would only "raise a [public] clamor for new ones," Wolfensberger envisioned a method to end the labeling process and the dehumanization associated with the total institution (on Goffman, see Stein 1991). Labeled deviant, mentally retarded people assumed roles that violated social norms. To change those roles and the expectations associated with them, service providers must do two things, Wolfensberger insisted: work with mentally retarded people to help them assume socially valued behaviors and integrate them into culturally normative settings. Integration, a functionalist alternative to Goffman's pessimistic outlook, became for Wolfensberger a moral means to an even grander end.

To integrate mentally retarded citizens into daily life, Wolfensberger claimed, human services providers had to commit themselves not only to the principle of normalization but also to the fine-tuning of normal social institutions to "provide the framework for a cathedral of human dignity" (Wolfensberger 1972, 73). Dignity, as the moral end of normalization and integration, of course, could never happen in the deviancy-maintaining public institution. Only in normal communities could mentally retarded people learn behaviors that would lead to social acceptance, a wiping away of negative labels, and full participation in the mainstream of American life.

During this period, Wolfensberger and his associate, Linda Glenn, developed a system for measuring the compliance of service systems with this new goal. In obsessive detail about nearly every imaginable aspect of community life, the Program Analysis of Service Systems (PASS) assessed how well services succeeded in reaching Wolfensberger's vision of normalization, social integration, and dignity (Wolfensberger and Glenn 1975). The focus of change, Wolfensberger and Glenn insisted, must be both the retarded person and the community. By 1980, thousands of service providers around the country had attended intensive PASS workshops to experience what Wolfensberger called the "ideology of normalization." And even more had read *The Principle of Normalization in Human Services.*[17]

What Wolfensberger provided in the decade of the 1970s was an important intellectual rationale, a moral grounding, and indefatigable energy to a policy—deinstitutionalization—already waiting to happen. What he added was a detailed, if formalistic, vision of the beloved community—a community where ordinary citizens would no longer either fear or pity intellectually disabled citizens, where disabled people could live and die as the rest of us live and die.

In this confluence—one, of state officials eager to shift responsibilities for services to the federal level; two, of civil libertarians ready to close inhumane institutions and segregated special classes; and three, of a vision of normalization that provided a rationale and method for opening communities to disabled people—the deinstitutionalization of intellectually disabled people from public facilities was rapid and continuous. In 1967, there were 193,188 residents in public intellectual disability institutions; in 1988, 91,440. The Lincoln State School and Colony, for example, housed more than 5,000 residents in its peak years in the late 1950s; by 1990, the Lincoln Developmental Center had acquired a new name while losing 4,500 of its population. Letchworth Village, whose population peaked at more than 4,000 in the mid-1960s, was down to 630 by 1990, while the total intellectual disability institutional population in New York dropped from more than 20,000 to 7,000 (Corcoran 1991). Between 1970 and 1990, forty-four institutions for intellectually disabled citizens in twenty states closed (or were scheduled to close) or were converted to other facilities (usually prisons). Many of these facilities were the oldest institutions, but some, like Bowen in Illinois, Woodhaven in Pennsylvania, and Waterbury in Connecticut, were built after 1963 (Braddock et al. 1990). Where did intellectually disabled people go during these decades?

The answer calls into question two widely held views about "progress toward deinstitutionalization" (see Table 7.3).[18] First, almost all parents, professionals, and public officials involved in services for intellectually disabled citizens would agree that depopulation of public residential facilities and the growth of community-based services led to the demise of the inhumane institution. Almost all would also agree that with changes in public (and principally federal) funding, increasingly more intellectually disabled people are under the watchful eye of local public

Table 7.3. RESIDENTIAL FACILITIES FOR PEOPLE
WITH INTELLECTUAL DISABILITY, UNITED STATES, 1988
AND 2009

Type of Facility	No. of Citizens in 1988 and 2009	
Congregate facilities (16+ beds)	1988	2009
Institutions	91,440	32,909
Large private facilities	46,351[a]	26,695
Private nursing homes	50,606	29,608
Total	188,397	89,212
Small facilities (<16 beds)		
Public ICF/MRs	3,335	
Private ICF/MRs	23,949	
Public & Private ICF/MRs		34,498
Other residences[b]	98,252	177,358
Total	125,557	211,856
Total clients in residential facilities	313,954	301,068

[a]These facilities included approximately 32,000 clients in large ICF/MRs
(intermediate care facilities for people with intellectual disability) and 14,000 in
large non-ICF/MRs. Only 2,000 of these citizens were in publicly operated facilities.
[b]These facilities included family care homes, group homes, foster care, and other
specialized living arrangements.

agencies. The data during these decades suggested something quite different. Of the
nearly 314,000 people in community residential facilities, more than 188,000 were
in congregate facilities of sixteen beds or more. These facilities included traditional
(albeit now smaller) institutions, nursing homes, and large private non-nursing do-
miciles. Additionally, as Braddock (1987, 184) has reported, three-fourths of fiscal
year 1985 federal ICF/MR dollars, the principal resource for deinstitutionalization,
provided for institutional, not community, placements. This "institutional bias," as
Braddock has called it, along with the flattening of federal support for intellectual
disability services during the Reagan and Bush presidencies, meant that federal
dollars for community-based services for more than a decade remained, at best,
constant. These constant dollars, of course, had to support growing numbers of
clientele who are more disabled than their counterparts placed out of public facilities a decade earlier.

Second, the data between 1970 and 2009 also suggested that, rather than being
under the direct control of local public agencies, most residential facilities are operated by private and often for-profit individuals or companies. Although some private nonprofit operators housed intellectually disabled people, especially in group
homes, in most states, nursing homes, ICF/MR facilities, and large non-nursing
homes exist to make profit. Although there remains great variability among states,
in most cases, large private institutions merely replaced large public institutions
(see also Lerman 1982, 12–13, 60, 212–216).

CONCLUSION

Between 1880 and 1950, intellectual disability had largely been seen as a problem of lower class teenagers and adults. Not infrequently, that group was regarded as a threat to the social order. During the heyday of the eugenics scare (1908–20), Americans began to see poor, immigrant, and working-class intellectually disabled teenagers and adults as the nation's primary "menace." The growth of the confessional literature of well-to-do and middle-class parents would change this perception. After the early 1950s, Americans were increasingly likely to see intellectually disabled people as perpetual children.

Ironically, as this image grew, the number of residential institutions housing intellectually disabled people also grew. Indeed, between 1950 and 1968, institutions for intellectually disabled people expanded at a faster rate than in any other period of their American history. Thus, in the midst of the popularizing of the "retarded child," the incarceration of intellectually disabled people (children and adults) increased as middle- and upper-class Americans found it respectable and even therapeutic to institutionalize their retarded children. What the "menace of the feebleminded" in the first quarter of the century had only partially accomplished, the infantilizing of intellectually disabled people in the 1950s finally achieved. In the name of family stability, all classes of Americans could now turn to the institution to house all ages of these disabled people. The parents' confessional literature sustained this new popular image of intellectual disability and of the residential institution.

The growth of the public institutions, however, contained the seeds of their destruction. Exposés of the war years left little doubt in the minds of many concerned Americans that state schools had become places of "forgotten children," where neglect and abuse were common. As the number of facilities multiplied and their populations grew in the 1950s and 1960s, doubts continued to linger. Were institutions that segregated residents from day-to-day life the best places for so many intellectually disabled Americans? Added to these doubts were the ever-rising costs of state institutions. State officials began to ask: Could states afford to bankroll more and more growth? As the doubts persisted, changes in federal policy eagerly supported by most of the states shifted the focus of the care and training from the institution to communities. Beginning in the late 1960s, states quickly depopulated their state schools.

This change proved to be a financial boon to the states. After expending state funds to upgrade their institutions in the 1970s, which included massive reductions in institutional populations, the states used federal dollars to keep the (now much smaller) institutions going. Also, funds from Public Law 94-142 ensured the education of all disabled children at, primarily, federal expense. For many states, federal support came just in time; few appeared willing to finance the continued rates of institutional growth, especially in the face of court-ordered prohibitions of the involuntary servitude of higher functioning residents.

The communities that received the intellectually disabled people also received federal assistance to make their new lives work. Just as local governments, beginning in the 1840s, had shifted the locus of care to states, states by the 1970s had shifted the funding of community care to the federal government. Local and state governments continued to operate services, but Washington paid for them and thus Washington could set the agenda.

This agenda has not been without its own contradictions and inconsistencies. Although the federal government has championed community-based services, it has not always put its money where its mouth is. In the 1970s and 1980s, a great many federal dollars continued to go to institutional services now housing only a tiny portion of the nation's population of intellectually disabled citizens, and, in the decade of the 1980s, the funding of community-based services at best held its own. Despite the enormous number of intellectually disabled citizens who received services in communities, there continued to be an "institutional bias" (Braddock 1987, 183–184). Likewise, with the coming of Ronald Reagan to the White House and his commitment to the "new federalism," states were given greater authority to use federal funding as they choose. In contrast to the vision of the Kennedy and Johnson years to use federal dollars to standardize services among the states, the Reagan agenda during the 1980s and extending into the 1990s did not diminish wide variations in the service provisions of the states. These variations were both qualitative and quantitative (Braddock et al. 1990, 18–21).

By the end of the 1980s, there were reasons for both hope and concern. On the hopeful side, few intellectually disabled people any longer lived in the "back wards" of large state-operated institutions. In communities, many intellectually disabled people were part of innovative learning, occupational, and living arrangements. Public schools, which had only two decades ago regularly excluded disabled children, were no longer apt to do so. Since 1975, "individualized educational plans" mandated by federal legislation (principally Public Law 94-142) ensured that these children were more likely than before to get an education geared to their specific needs. Even severely and profoundly intellectually disabled children and adults, who only little more than a decade ago were treated as hopeless "vegetables," were proving that they could develop, learn, and work. Even more capable intellectually disabled citizens held full-time jobs, had families, and paid taxes—and wrecked cars, had extramarital affairs, and got audited by the IRS (Edgerton and Bercovici 1976; Janicki, Krauss, and Seltzer 1988; Kingsley and Levitz 2007; Perske 1980). As the popular television program of the decade starring Chris Burke, a man with Down syndrome, puts it, "life goes on." The Americans with Disabilities Act, federal legislation that took effect in 1992, also proved to make it harder for employers, service providers, and various social institutions to discriminate against disabled citizens.

For others, things did not look so hopeful. In some community "workshops," intellectually disabled people played games and did perpetual "training" because the workshop could not find paying work for them. Some public schools that had emphasized mainstreaming for nearly two decades still segregated intellectually disabled children, transporting them to schools in easily identified special-education buses and vans. "Sped" (special ed) jokes replaced the "little moron" jokes of an earlier era, and the rhetoric of "you idiot, you moron, you imbecile, and that's so retarded" grew over the past decade, especially in American television culture.[19] In addition, intellectually disabled people seem to appear more and more frequently in prisons, the only state institutions to grow in the 1980s (see, for example, Ben-Moshe 2013; Perske 1991; Wolfensberger 1987). Several people identified as intellectually disabled awaited death sentences in these facilities. (While Bill Clinton, the governor of Arkansas, campaigned for the presidency in New Hampshire in January 1992, reporters appeared more interested in his purported extramarital affairs than in "his personal okay [in January 1992] for the execution of an imbecile Arkansas murderer." Indeed, the national media hardly mentioned it [see Hitchens 1992, 45].) Finally, in congregate ICF/MRs, some intellectually disabled people found themselves merely reinstitutionalized, often in urban and rural wastelands away from easily accessible services, faced with routinized activities, and denied opportunities for all but the most innocuous choices. In short, there were, along with hopeful signs, reasons for concern.

As they did in the 1840s, intellectually disabled people who had money, supportive relatives, and understanding neighbors and employers did well in American communities. As they did in the 1840s, intellectually disabled people who did not have those things, did not. For some, the community had become the beloved community; for others, the lonely crowd.

NOTES

1. Margaret Bourke-White's papers and photographs are at Syracuse University. To my knowledge, the Letchworth photographs were only printed in some of the annual reports of Letchworh Village (e.g., New York State, Department of Mental Hygiene 1937, 1948).
2. It is ironic, given the content of Bourke-White's 1932 photograph's of inmates at Letchworth Village, that seven years later she would marry the novelist, Erskine Caldwell, whose novels, *Tobacco Road* (1932) and *God's Little Acre* (1933) became an important literary example of support for eugenics and the involuntary sterilization of the poor (Keely 2002; Lancaster 2007).
3. The Arnold Genthe Collection, most of which is uncatalogued, is in the Library of Congress. Besides the *US Camera* publication, Genthe's photographs of Letchworth Village can be seen in the annual reports of 1948. See note 1 above.
4. According to the National Service Board for Religious Objectors ("CPS Camps and Units" 1944), there were about 250 Civilian Public Service men working in the following training schools as of 30 June 1944:

Location	No. of Men
American Friends Service Committee	90
New Jersey State Training School	16
Delaware State Colony	14
Pennhurst State Training School, Pa.	29
Maine Training School	16
District of Columbia Training School, Laurel, Md.	15

Mennonite Central Committee	71
Vineland Training School, N.J.	16
Exeter Training School, R.I.	15
Southern Wisconsin Colony	25
Utah State Training School	15
Brethren Service Committee	70
Mansfield State Training School, Conn.	15
Western State Custodial School, Wash.	30
Lynchburg State Colony, Va.	25
Association of Catholic COs	21
Rosewood State Training School, Md.	21
American Baptist Home Mission Society	1
Skillman Village, N.J.	1

A Mennonite CPS unit was added after July 1944 at the Woodbine Colony for Feeble-Minded Men in New York.

5. Letters to the editor of the *Christian Century* corroborated Richardson's description and analysis (e.g., "Conditions in Mental Hospitals" 1946).

6. Grob (1991, 8-9) describes similar staff shortages and overcrowding in psychiatric facilities during the war years. Although he notes the work of CPS men in these facilities, Grob avoids their reports about brutality.

7. Other family stories of the decade included "A Mountain Moves" (1954), Bruckner (1954), Gramm (1951), Piccola (1955), M. McDonald (1956), Schreiber (1955). For a perspective on the parents' movement primarily in the 1970s and 1980s, see R. Dybwad 1990*b* and Wehmeyer and Schalock 2013.

8. Edith M. Stern (1948, 64) in the popular *Woman's Home Companion* quoted several superintendents who told her they kept high-grade inmates in the institution simply for their labor. "I'm sure over twenty percent of the high-grades now in state training schools could get out and get along if they weren't so useful," claimed one unnamed superintendent. According to another, "We couldn't run the place without the working children [*sic*]!" Yet another claimed, "I'd have to hire ten men to do the work of the farm boys." Referring to female-inmate housekeepers, the wife of a superintendent told Stern, "I like to keep them as long as I can."

9. It was during this period that Congress also held hearings on mental health; President Eisenhower, Secretary Hobby, and others spoke out about health and mental health issues; and Congress established the Commission on Mental Health. Although mental retardation and mental health lobbies were both organizing at the time, the former, made up primarily of parents and relatives, kept a distance from the latter, which was, for the most part, composed of professionals.

10. For example, on November 28, 2010, CBS News televised "Where's Molly?" the story of cameraman Jeff Daly's reunion with his sister Molly after a forty-seven year separation. Daly's parents had placed Molly in Oregon's Fairview State Institution in the 1950s. See: http://www.cbsnews.com/news/wheres-molly/

11. Foley and Sharfstein (1983, 95–96) point out that the deinstitutionalization of state hospitals "as deliberate public policy" did not begin until the late 1960s and early 1970s, that is, at about the same time that such policy developed for state facilities for intellectually disabled people. The decline that began in 1955 in the

state hospitals was the result of the introduction of new psychotropic drugs. Lerman (1982, 2–3) notes, however, that although one-day census counts of hospital populations peaked in the mid-1950s, annual admissions actually increased between 1955 and 1972, implying greater turnover. In 1972 state officials began to use Supplemental Security Income funding for deinstitutionalization. For Lerman, federal programs and "welfare policy" changes, more than drugs, shaped the course of deinstitutionalization (see also Butterfield 1976).

12. Three examples of questionable ethical standards in research carried out at public residential institutions include Albert Sabin's polio serum trials at the Sonoma State Home in California and the New Jersey State Colony for Feebleminded Men, Jonas Salk's 1952 polio vaccine trials at the Polk State School in Pennsylvania, and Jay S. Birnbrauer's 1968 electric shock punishment experiments carried out at Murdoch Center in North Carolina (Birnbrauer 1968; Brockley 2004, 156; DiAntonio 2005, 55).

13. Nearly all American institutions for intellectually disabled people had stories about residents who were not intellectually disabled (by any definition). These stories were especially common in the older facilities. For example, in 1936 family members placed Gladys Burr in the Norwich State Hospital after institutional authorities labeled her mentally defective despite the fact that IQ tests showed that, even by 1936 standards, she was not disabled. After forty-two years in the facility, she was released in 1978. In 1985, she won a $235,000 settlement from the state of Connecticut ("Gladys Burr" 1989). A resident of the Caswell Training School for the Feeble-Minded was not so fortunate. Shortly before World War I, relatives placed her in the North Carolina institution. A daughter of a well-to-do eastern North Carolina planter, she had given birth to a "negro child" shortly before her entrance to the Caswell Training School. What else but feeblemindedness could explain this disgrace? People eager to admit her to the training school concluded. Though never disabled, she died in 1976 at another facility, Murdoch Center, where she had been transferred after World War II. She was eighty-five years old (Murdoch Center Resident 1976).

14. George Wallace served as governor of Alabama from 1963 to 1967. In 1967, his wife, Lurleen, succeeded him. By all accounts, George Wallace remained head of state until her death.

15. Given Geraldo Rivera's reputation since the Willowbrook exposés, his first public claim to fame, it could be argued that his picture of Willowbrook and Letchworth contained a certain amount of hyperbole. This may be true. But my experience working as an attendant in a public institution in 1973 confirms Rivera's report. If anything, what I saw daily was even worse than what he found. For a study from the "insider perspective" of eleven institutions in 1970 and 1971, see Biklen 1977. Biklen's and his students' observations parallel Rivera's findings (see also Braginsky and Braginsky 1971).

16. Other influential writings on normalization during the late 1960s and early 1970s include Bank-Mikkelsen 1969; G. Dybwad 1964, 1969, 1973; Mullins 1971; Nirje 1970; Perske 1972; Roos 1970; Vanier 1971.

17. In 1983, Wolfensberger proposed replacing the word normalization with what he called social role valorization (Wolfensberger 1983). In so doing, he hoped to answer critics who were beginning to regard his version of normalization as manipulative. Although he claimed to respect the diversity that intellectually disabled people might bring to everyday life, his change of terminology did not convince some doubters.

CHAPTER 8

༄

Intellectual Disability and
the Dilemma of Doubt

HENRY DARGER AND JUDITH SCOTT

On April 12, 1973, Nathan Lerner, a Chicago photographer, unlocked the door of the one-and-a-half room apartment of his tenant, Henry Darger (Figure 8.1). Accompanying Lerner was another of his renters, David Berglund. Darger lay sick in St. Mary's Home, a Catholic nursing facility on Chicago's Near Northside. The facility was operated by the Little Sisters of the Poor. It was Darger's eighty-first birthday; the next day he would die. Anticipating the death, Lerner and Berglund entered Darger's apartment to clear out the thousands of magazines, newspapers, pamphlets, and books that Darger had accumulated since he first rented the rooms in 1930. There were piles upon piles of paper. At first, the men had every reason to throw the items into the apartment's trash cans. Yet after removing several loads of Darger's hoard, they came upon something that they had hardly anticipated. There among the heaps of paper was a manuscript—an amazing, if bizarre novel of more than 15,000 pages. Further discoveries revealed a trove of fascinating illustrations. Most were watercolors and pencil drawings, but others were tracings and collages. Darger had carefully attached much of his art to the pages of bound volumes. Lerner, an artist himself, soon saw that his tenant had created something quite extraordinary: an incredibly long novel illustrated with intriguing works of art (Figure 8.1).

By the time of Lerner's death twenty years later, historians, critics, and collectors of "outsider art"—art done by untrained artists—were well aware of Henry Darger's work. With the publication of John MacGregor's book, *Henry Darger: The Realms of the Unreal* in 2002, the fame of his watercolors, drawings, collages, and writings spread to an even wider audience. Additional studies of Darger's work,

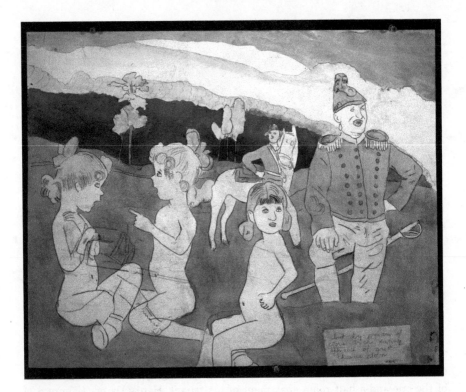

Figure 8.1:
Art of Henry Darger "By Means of a Clever Trick" (Courtesy of the estate of Henry Darger, Art Resource, New York, NY)

along with North American, Asian, and European exhibits in important galleries and museums worldwide, only added to the artist's reputation and to the public's curiosity (Biesenbach 2014; Elledge 2013; MacGregor 2002; M. Trent 2012).

For a man who, through sixty years of his adult life, did only three things—work as a janitor, attend daily Catholic Mass and confession, and create the longest novel in the English language—Darger, the reclusive hoarder, had after his death become famous. That Darger had spent four years of his adolescence (1904–08) as an inmate at the Illinois Asylum for Feeble-Minded Children only added to his status as a most peculiar outsider artist. Indeed, his feeblemindedness has complicated criticism of his art and writings; yet, his feeblemindedness has also obscured claims for the man's brilliance. How could a man who, in his early adolescence, had received the feebleminded label and had spent four years in a residential institution become a talented artist and the writer of a lengthy novel? What does the 1904 diagnosis of feeblemindedness that Darger received say about the constructions and the constructors of intellectual disability? Is the disability merely a condition defined by authorities and ascribed by those same authorities to unusual, eccentric, or otherwise nonconforming people like Darger?[1]

If Darger's so-called feeblemindedness challenges the essential nature of intellectual disability, the disability of Judith Scott seems to create an even greater question about the nature of intellectual disability and of intelligence itself. Judith and her twin sister Joyce were born to a middle-class family in Cincinnati, Ohio, in 1943. Early family photographs show the girls lying side-by-side in a perambulator, playing together on a floor filled with toys, and sleeping together. Like all twins, they developed a close bond. Yet, the girls had two important differences—one known by their parents and one unknown. Physicians had confirmed that Judith had Down syndrome, but the same physicians, along with Cincinnati school authorities, had failed to detect the deafness that the girl had acquired after a bout of scarlet fever. Joyce developed normal speech for a preschooler, but Judith failed to speak. In 1950, when the twins were seven years old, the Scotts, following the advice of several medical specialists and their Protestant minister, placed Judith in the Columbus States School, Ohio's oldest institution for intellectually disabled people. As they had advised tens of thousands of other North American families, both local and institutional authorities told the family to forget about their mentally deficient daughter. With their Down syndrome family member now one hundred miles away, the family back in Cincinnati was able to do just that.

In 1985, against the advice of her mother, Joyce Scott, now an adult and living in northern California, visited her sister, whom she had rarely seen during the previous thirty-five years. The visit led Joyce to become Judith's legal guardian, remove her from the large Ohio residential state facility, and bring her to live with her in California. The next year, Joyce made arrangements for Judith to attend the Creative Growth Art Center in Oakland. Unusual in its day, the Center provided space, materials, and instruction that allowed adults with intellectual and developmental disabilities to create art work, but with the freedom to develop art in creative and unique ways (Scott 2016).

During her first two years at the Center, Judith seemed to care little for drawing and painting. She attended the Center daily, but showed no interest in doing art until the fiber artist Sylvia Seventy came for a workshop. Quite suddenly and apparently inspired by Seventy, Judith began to construct fabric sculptures by wrapping fibers—string, yarn, cloth, even plastic tubing—around and among ordinary objects found in the studios of the Center. The sculptures were sometimes small enough to hold in the artist's hands, but other times so large as to nearly fill a room. Frequently, the fibers incorporated objects hidden in the interiors of the wrappings, as if to be known to the artist, but not to the viewer. For five days each week for eighteen years, until her death in 2005, Judith Scott, created these remarkable sculptures (Figure 8.2).

While Henry Darger would receive fame only in death, Judith Scott became known in her lifetime. At first, her works were shown in conjunction with other art produced by the artists at the Oakland Center. Eventually, however, her fabric sculptures began to appear in one-person shows, in California and, soon thereafter, around the nation. In the last years of her life and since her death, her works have appeared in international galleries and museums. Some of her works are in the

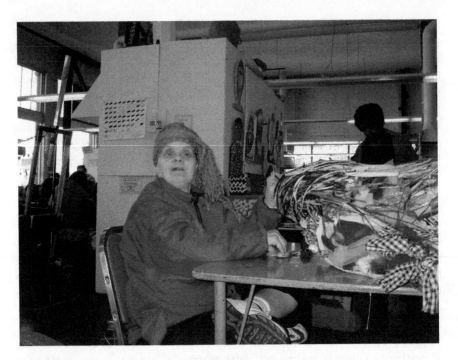

Figure 8.2:
Judith Scott at work on her fabric sculpture (Courtesy of Lilia Scott)

permanent collections of museums in the United States and in several European countries (Morris and Higgs 2014; Sellen 2008).

Just as art historians puzzled over Darger's art and unusual life story, so, too, have they found Judith Scott's creativity fascinating and, given her long institutionalization, baffling. Henry Darger, one may suppose, received the label of feebleminded because he was a poor (and probably unusual) child. His mother had died when he was an infant, and his father was physically disabled and sickly. When his father could no longer care for him, and with no relatives or friends to turn to, city welfare authorities, upon the advice of a physician, turned to a readily available public facility to shelter the boy. In addition to Darger's poverty, the Chicago physician who examined him reported that Darger was a "self-abuser."[2] Poverty and masturbation, not intellectual disability, were surely the twelve-year-old boy's conditions. Darger's four-year residency at the Illinois Asylum for Feeble-Minded Children was merely an inappropriate placement. Certainly, many have concluded, Darger was not really feebleminded.

But then there is Scott, a woman with an indisputably real condition: namely, Down syndrome. For more than fifty years, scientists have observed the extra genetic material, usually on chromosome 21, characteristic of Down syndrome. Scott's intellectual disability, complicated by her deafness, was surely not a mere label. Down syndrome is material, but Scott has produced work of arts—unforgettably moving fabric sculptures—that would seem impossible for her to have accomplished given the ordinary descriptions ascribed to her condition. Her sculptures—nearly one hundred of them—are hardly flukes of a one-time occurrence of an otherwise naturally weak-minded person. How can such works come from a feeble mind?

DEFINING INTELLECTUAL DISABILITY

In 1992, the American Association on Mental Retardation (AAMR), the fourth name that the interdisciplinary association had given itself since its founding in 1876, presented to its membership a new definition of mental retardation (Luckasson et al. 1992). The new definition was a product of the association's Committee on Terminology and Classification. There had been several definitions and many labels over the years. The new definition created some immediate controversy, but it would take a few years for the definition's shift in outlook to arouse the ire of more than a few of the association's members. At stake was a definition, but also at stake was the control of that definition. As the association's latest definition went, so, too, would the American Psychiatric Association likely adopt the definition for the next edition of its *Diagnostic and Statistical Manual* and with the new definition would potentially come new criteria for publicly funded social programs and assistance.

During the early decades of the twentieth century, the AAMR's predecessor organization, the American Association for the Study of the Feeble-Minded, had placed intelligence and the capacity of professional psychologists to measure intelligence at the heart of its definition of mental retardation. For eighty years, intelligence tests had scored intelligence, and such testing had its origin in detecting feeble-mindedness and measuring its severity. Also by the 1970s and 1980s, intelligence testing, a tool of psychology, had completed a shift begun in the 1910s from mental retardation as a concern of medicine (and particularly psychiatry) to mental retardation as a concern of psychology. Although the 1992 definition retained a place for intelligence and its measurement, the new AAMR definition for the first time shifted an ancillary element of previous definitions to the most prominent part of the new definition. Mental retardation, the association now claimed, "refers to substantial limitations in present functioning. It is characterized by significantly subaverage intellectual functioning, existing concurrently with related limitations in two or more of the following applicable adaptive skill areas: communication, self-care, home living, social skills, community use, self-direction, health and safety, functional academics, leisure and work. Mental retardation manifests before age 18." The association added, "Significantly sub-average intellectual functioning means an IQ score of 70 to 75 or below on a standardized individual intelligence test. Related limitations refers to adaptive skill limitations that are related more to functional applications than [to] other circumstances such as cultural diversity or sensory impairment" (Luckasson et al. 1992, 1).

This previous concern, given new prominence, was functioning—and not just abstract functioning, but functioning in several specified contexts of everyday life. For the first time in its history, the AAMR definers suggested that mental retardation was not merely a condition that people have, but it was also a circumstance pliable by the conditions of the environments in which people live. Thus, mental retardation was primarily the result of barriers to necessary functions. This change was more than sleight of hand and the AAMR membership committed to the primacy of intelligence testing knew it. To define mental retardation not simply as an absence of measurable general intelligence was to abandon years of a reliable, if (as some believed) a hardly valid, tool in the arsenal of one of the association's oldest and most dominant disciplines, psychology. Unlike the association's three previous definitions (Heber, 1961; Grossman, 1973, 1983), the new definition made no mention of "general intelligence." After 1992, it would seem, intelligence took a back seat to environmental barriers. The change in definition—a change that, with some modification, was reaffirmed and strengthened in yet another new definition in 2002 and has thus stood for more than twenty years—was made possible by the Committee on Terminology and Classification's membership. Rather than being led by cognitive psychologists, the Committee's first authors were an attorney and a pediatrician. Neither had a professional commitment to what one observer called the "defectology-approach" (Greenspan 1995, 684–685). This independence allowed the committee to ground the new definition of mental retardation away from an individual's deficit of intelligence. Instead, the committee centered the definition in the environment's failure to provide necessary accommodations to allow an individual to function in ordinary living situations (Luckasson et al. 2002; Wehmeyer et al. 2008). Barriers to day-to-day functioning rather than the severity of so-called lack of general intelligence would now distinguish mental retardation, or what the association in 2005 decided to call intellectual disability—a label that, in 2010, through Rosa's Law, would remove "mental retardation" from all federal codes and regulations and compel the states to do likewise (Bersani 2007*b*).

The resistance of psychologists loyal to previous definitions of mental retardation, now called intellectual disability, reached a crescendo in a 2006 volume of essays, *What Is Mental Retardation? Ideas for an Evolving Disability in the 21st Century* (Switzsky and Greenspan 2006). The year before the book's appearance, the AAMR had once again changed its own name, on this occasion to the American Association on Intellectual and Developmental Disabilities (AAIDD). It was the fifth name the association had given itself since 1876. With "intellectual and developmental disabilities" replacing mental retardation in the association's title, the book's appearance shortly after the name change begged the question: Why argue for a defunct definition of an abandoned label?

The answer lay in the composition of the volume's contributors. Among them were twenty males (77 percent) and six females (23 percent). Each of the authors came from ethnic backgrounds that most people would label white. Nine of the authors, including both of the editors, were retired and one was deceased (38 percent). Most of the remaining contributors were, as the English say, of a certain age. Two of the authors were physicians (8 percent), one was a member of the clergy (4 percent), and six identified themselves with special education (23 percent). All the remaining 17 authors, by far the largest number, were psychologists (65 percent). Only four (15 percent) of the authors played a part in the 1992 or 2002 definitions, or in both. Twenty-two (85 percent) did not participate. Among the four definition contributors, two were physicians and two were psychologists. Thus, among the seventeen psychologists who contributed to *What Is Mental Retardation*, fifteen psychologists (88 percent) criticized the 1992 and 2002 definitional documents, in the creation of which they played no part.

Entirely white, mostly male, mostly senior, mostly psychologists, and mostly noncontributors to the 1992 and 2002 AAMR definitions—what else did these psychologists have in common? Among the seventeen, all at the time were (or had been) members of the AAIDD, usually over their entire careers. Several of the book's contributors had served as officers of the association, and several had also been members and served in leadership positions of the American Psychological Association's Division 33, now called Intellectual and Developmental Disabilities. Most of the fifteen men and two women remembered the Association when it was the AAMR and even the American Association on Mental Deficiency (AAMD, the organization's third incarnation). Several contributors began their careers when "mentally defective, mental defect, mental deficiency, and mongoloid" were familiar labels, and several could remember when distinctions between "high grades" and "low grades" were commonly made.

Most contributors could recall a time when large residential institutions were numerous, not exceptional. Indeed, not a few of these psychologists began their careers when institutional inmates provided readily available subjects for dissertations and professional publications. In the days before institutional review boards and written informed consent from subjects, these researchers looked back to the places like Murdoch Center in North Carolina, Clover Bottom Center in Tennessee, Partlow State School in Alabama, Vineland Training School in New Jersey, Fernald State School in Massachusetts, and Lincoln State School in Illinois where inmates enjoyed time away from institutional boredom on the one hand or labor on the institution's farm on the other to participate as subjects in a researcher's latest project. Only a few of the group enthusiastically embraced deinstitutionalization in the 1970s and 1980s; most remained publicly neutral, if privately uneasy. As the championing of civil rights, normalization, least-restricted environments, and finally self-advocacy began to shift the focus of services away from intelligence and pathology toward community resources and socialization, several of the members of this group began to express concern about directions in the field. It is not surprising, then, that most members of this group argued (in different ways and using different tones) the position that the 1992 AAMR definition and its substantial reaffirmation in 2002 departed from reality, from evidential history, even from professional competence.

Without an exception, the definitional critics grounded their evaluations on neither judgments nor interpretations, but on what they believed were universally apparent findings. These findings were in every case tied to general intelligence. Timeless, disembodied, transcultural, and universal—intelligence became the group's primary interest because it served, in the case of intellectual and developmental disabilities (a.k.a. mental retardation), as the central tool for defining the otherwise historical, embodied, culturally bound, and parochial thing known by many names. Apart from the demand of judgmental and interpretative passions, intelligence to these purveyors of general intelligence represented a cool indifference. Nevertheless, if intelligence represented a cool indifference, the defense of the IQ as the fundamental basis for defining intelligence became the "privileges of salesmen to defend" (Barbetta et al. 2014, 64).

The 1992 and 2002 definitions suggested that measuring general intelligence was not its own end. The information that the testing of intelligence provides was only an aid in the process of one human being interacting within his or her context. The process and movement of people in their multilayered, diverse systems and contextual environments made ludicrous, for the 1992 and 2002 definers, the atomistic reduction of human beings to tests that fix intelligence to unmovable intervals of a stable construct. Following the tradition of educator John Dewey and psychologist William James, the 1992 and 2002 definitions regarded intelligence as an ongoing process, its measurement as only a tool, and its efficacy as the tool's usefulness in making the process work—work, of course, for both the individual tested and for the context. The claim for fixed intelligence, apart from its context, became useful for little more than social stratification. When that IQ-driven stratification becomes social policy applied to intellectual and developmental disabilities (e.g. "the prevention of mental retardation"), it becomes little more than latter-day eugenics (J. Trent 2008).

INSTITUTIONS AND COMMUNITIES

At their peak in 1967, large public institutions in the United States created to house children and adults with intellectual disability had a total population of nearly 200,000 residents. Another 30,000 labeled "retarded" populated the nation's various public psychiatric facilities. By 2004. that number had decreased to 41,214 residents. In 2008, the population had further declined to 32,909. By 2012, the states reported only 22,099 residents in 147 facilities of sixteen inmates or larger.[3]

The number of those facilities in the 1964 stood at 354; by 2012, 207 institutions had closed or been converted to other purposes. Nine states plan to close fourteen additional large facilities by 2020, thus bringing the number to 133 institutions in the United States. Among these 221 closures, thirteen states and the District of Columbia have completely eliminated all congregate institutions for intellectually disabled people, thereby no longer housing any of their citizens in such facilities (Braddock 2007; Braddock et al. 2015; Ferguson, Ferguson, and Wehmeyer, 2013; S. Larson et al. 2014; National Council of Disability 2009).

A study from the University of Minnesota's Residential Information Systems Project estimates that in 2012 there were 4,677,319 people with intellectual disabilities living in the United States. Of this number, about 24 percent or 1,138,121 received long-term financial support and services through various federal, state, and local programs and agencies. Of the population receiving such support, 634,988 people (56 percent), many of whom are children, get their assistance in a family member's home, and 207,128 individuals (18 percent) received assistance while living in a small group setting. Another 122,665 individuals (11 percent) of this population used their assistance to own or rent their home. A fourth group of 85,384 people (8 percent) live in an intermediate care facility for people with intellectual and developmental disabilities, known as an ICF/IDD, and 58,753 (5 percent) live in a foster care or host home. Only 28,064 (2 percent) live in large congregate institutional or large nursing facilities. These data show that the trend away from institutionalization begun in the late 1960s has continued for more than fifty years. There are those who predict the public residential institution's inevitable demise; yet, in several states, despite the trend, the institutions have transformed themselves from facilities that hold the unwanted to facilities that house the unwelcomed (Braddock et al. 2015; S. Larson et al. 2014).

Some of those unwelcomed intellectually disabled people are adults who, in addition to cognitive disability, have other developmental, sensory, or psychiatric impairments. Their multiple disabilities have complicated their adjustment to ordinary community living—living that for older adults likely developed in a large institution, or for younger adults, in the home of their parents. Other members of the unwelcomed are individuals whose intellectual disability is severe enough to require ongoing and complex assistance. In settings where institutional authorities or family members negotiated the conditions of daily activities and human interaction, some of these adults have found challenges to functioning outside the institution or the family home. Some adults have failed to adapt easily to the interpersonal demands of independent home life, work settings, and civic activities. In several states, the large institutions have become places for these sometimes disruptive or distracted adults to return for behavioral modification treatment. Relying on the practices of operant conditioning and usually ignoring the perspectives of the recalcitrant adult, behavior modifiers (still congregated in large public institutions) treat behaviors that have prevented smooth community adjustments. Usually, the focus of these institutional sojourns is solely the individual's behavior, which, more often than not, is the sole focus of the change. As such, the focus of change is always the individual and his or her bad behavior. This singular attention supplants the possibility that the individual's inappropriate behavior may be quite appropriate given the maladaptive conditions of her or his environment. In the institutional setting, the community's failure to provide accommodation for the individual's disabilities is hardly ever acknowledged, much less recognized. The singular focus of the behavior modifiers' task is to alter behavior, thus ensuring that the environmental conditions that precipitated the recalcitrant behavior are overlooked. Institutions have become settings to change individual behaviors but hardly ever to change administrative, organizational, or community behaviors.

A second function of twentieth-first-century public institutions, now populated by far fewer residents, is the employment they provide for people living in what are often small-town or rural communities where many of these facilities are located. In some communities, the loss of jobs for attendants and other staff has been offset by the conversion of the state school to an alternative facility, most often to a prison. In other communities where state public employees have stable and strong unions, institutions have remained open. In some states, communities with institutions have used powerful politicians to sustain the facility. In many of these institutions, state management depends upon federal Medicaid payments to fund the services provided. Ironically, as institutional populations have decreased, the number of staff has increased, so that per resident costs have never been higher. Where deinstitutionalization has worked well, state officials have integrated unions and local politicians into the planning for institutional diminution and closure, along with planning for the transfer of funding and jobs for new community-based services.

In other locations, states have retained institutions where there are well-organized and influential parents groups. These parents have usually had their children in the state school for decades. Their adult children are more often than not severely and profoundly disabled, with medical problems that often leave them fragile. At Massachusetts's Fernald Developmental Center, the state's oldest (and also one of the nation's oldest) institutions, parents and relatives successfully frustrated the efforts of state authorities to close the facility's nearly empty residential cottages. Until 2014, neither a decades-old court order nor some of the most potentially valuable real estate in Metropolitan Boston coveted by developers had shaken the resolve of the relatives of the few residents to keep the Center open. And no Massachusetts elected official showed the fortitude to defy the families. At the time, the facility had only thirteen residents at an annual cost of about $1 million per resident. On November 13, 2014, the institution, once housing more than 2,500 residents, finally closed. The next month, the city of Waltham, Massachusetts purchased its 186-acre campus from the state ("City Takes Ownership of Fernald Property" 2014).

In New York, deinstitutionalization took an even more curious route. Faced with strong advocates, a new community-based service philosophy, and judicial mandates, New York in the early 1990s moved to a goal of closing all the state's mental retardation institutions by 2000. Institutional closure would be an undertaking that would involve several interest groups. Central to the process were the service needs of newly deinstitutionalized residents, most of whom required multiple types of assistance for their complex disabilities. Unlike most other states, New York had large numbers of community facilities—usually group homes—that were operated by parents' organizations. These organizations had achieved influence and power among state elected officials.

Deinstitutionalization in New York raised several questions. Could residents be integrated into existing services operated by parents and other agencies? How many and what kinds of new facilities should be built, and could those facilities avoid the institutional structures of the past? Could the closure of rural institutions mesh with the greater community needs of urban New York? How might the state integrate public employees who worked in the state's institutions into the network of small community agencies? And, most importantly, how would New York pay for the conversion?

In 1995, shortly after he took office, Republican governor George Pataki stopped what had been the state's four-year commitment to total institutional closure. "This was a remarkable reversal of what had seemed to be an inevitable process" (Castellani 2005, 241). Anticipating that the new governor would be favorably disposed toward their interests, private providers positioned themselves for greater influence and, hence, for greater benefits from the new course of institutional clo-sure. Specialized service providers saw opportunities to provide new community services to the "frail elderly, behaviorally problematic, or criminally involved" (Castellani 2005, 259). By the late 1990s, there seemed to be few voices of op-position to the Pataki administration's reversal. Federal Medicaid funding, now relieving the state of fiscal responsibilities, provided generous revenues to public agencies and private providers alike. These revenues, which seemed to satisfy ev-eryone, muted the institutionalization-versus-deinstitutionalization debate of the earlier decade. Yet, ironically, the workers in community-based facilities, now oper-ated not by the state but by private owners, were paid less and had fewer benefits than their predecessors working in the public institutions. What was true of staff pay in New York was even truer in most other states (Bogenschutz et al. 2014). As Paul Castellani argues, what had once been "snake pit" institutions like Willowbrook State School have become a mixture of private and public, community-based and institutional "cash cows." As of 2010, New York continues to have more than 2,000 inmates in its public institutions, and the quality of its community-based services remained inconsistent (Castellani 2005; Lakin et al. 2010).

After more than forty years of consistent state deinstitutionalization, most intellectually disabled people now live, go to school, work, play, and participate in many organizations in every American community. Each school day in public schools across the nation, intellectually disabled children likely attend at least a few classes with nondisabled children. In some schools, this integration extends to most classes. Disabled children may have teaching assistants or, on occasion, student peers who help disabled students with learning tasks. In other schools, in-tellectually disabled students find themselves integrated into a few classes but not into most. Although some mainstreaming (as this integration is often called) may be more inclusive in some schools than in others, there is no question that a new generation of nondisabled public school children have received education with dis-abled children. Even forty years ago, this integration would have been unthinkable. Past generations of children experienced disability—always away from school—as unusual, peculiar, and even frightening experiences. Today, disability for many American public school students is ordinary and hardly atypical. As such, a new generation of students—disabled and nondisabled—has begun to regard disability as an everyday part of many people's lives.[4]

If intellectually disabled children are more likely to find themselves integrated in American schools than ever before, the racial disparity in the labeling of children receiving special education services has hardly changed since the 1960s. African American children especially continue to be disproportionately assigned to spe-cial classes and programs. African Americans represent 33 percent of students identified as intellectually disabled, yet they make up only 17 percent of the na-tion's school population. As such, school officials are twice as likely to label African American students as being intellectually disabled as they are to ascribe the label to white students. Also, African American students in special education programs are more likely to be in restrictive, segregated programs and less likely to be in settings where they receive at least some instruction with nondisabled students. Although the Individuals with Disabilities Education Act reauthorizations of 1997 and 2004 stressed both the prevention of the mislabeling of racial minorities and the avoidance of disproportionate dropout rates among minorities labeled with disabilities, many school systems appear to ignore the reauthorizations' emphasis (Skiba et al. 2008, 265–270).

With its successes and flaws, educational mainstreaming has paralleled a change in the proportion of intellectually disabled students in school populations. This change has come about because of the rediscovery of autism. Beginning in the 1980s, psychologists and special educators began to pay attention to autism. Although the psychiatrist Leo Kanner (1943) had first noted the condition in 1943, medical authorities regarded autism as incurable and untreatable. Many children with autism (both before and after Kanner's identification) were routinely placed in public mental retardation institutions. In those settings, they languished in institutional "back wards," where they received no services, educational or otherwise. Amid sterile conditions, only broken by the endless noise of a lone television set and the incoherent cries and noises of low-functioning residents, these children's autism soon transformed into a profound psychosis, one deeper than the most impenetrable schizophrenia. In the worst of all possible settings, the institutionalized children and adults with autism lived from day to day, sitting on long wooden benches, some ceaselessly rocking or spinning, others banging their heads against tiled walls, and still others playing with their genitalia.

First identified as a developmental disability by the Development Disabilities Services and Facilities Construction Act of 1975 (P.L. 94–103), autism as a developmental disability was linked with, but also separated from, mental retardation. With federal funding now available for research on autism and with new programs directed to people with autism, the response of institutional segregation no longer seemed necessary. Quite suddenly, state authorities suspended the institutional integration of most autistic children with intellectually disabled people. At the same time, the new recognition of autism opened community school services to children with autism. With the new recognition, fewer children were labeled intellectually disabled, while growing numbers of children began to receive the autism label. From 1999 to 2008, for example, the number of developmentally disabled children receiving educational services increased from 885,696 students in 1999 to 1,078,053 students in 2008. The changed represented a growth of nearly 22 percent, while the growth rate of the general school-aged population increased by only 5 percent. Interestingly, however, the portion of children labeled intellectually disabled decreased from 597,594 in 1999 to 475,713 in 2008. Thus, in a ten-year period, the number of intellectually disabled students dropped by more than 20 percent. During the same ten-year period, the children labeled autistic increased from 64,148 in 1999 to 292,638 in 2008, an increase of nearly 350 percent. This diminution of intellectual disability in the school population was, in large part, the outcome of the growth in the number of children labeled autistic (S. Larson and Lakin 2010; see also Bagatell 2010; Eyal 2013). There are more autistic children today, at least in part, because label shifting has occurred since the 1980s.

If the place of intellectually disabled children in communities has undergone changes over the past three decades, what has become of intellectually disabled adults in those same communities—of adults once confined to institutions as well as adults who never lived in institutions? My friend, Edward, is an example of a person who lived for more than a decade in a large public institution in North Carolina. In that state's early efforts to deinstitutionalize some of its intellectually disabled inmates, institutional officials in 1976 placed Edward in a four-person group home in a nearby urban community. Ten years earlier, county public assistance officials had confined Edward and his sister, Lois,[5] in a large public institution when their single mother appeared too poor and too dispirited to care for her oldest and middle child, leaving only her infant daughter to her care. A few years after he entered the facility, institutional officials surgically sterilized Edward. They did so under the authority of the state's Board of Eugenics, made up of medical and social welfare officials along with other private citizens.

When I first met him, Edward was about eighteen years old, could read and write, and was considered one of the institution's "high grade" residents. It was not long after I came to know Edward that I began to wonder why he was considered mentally retarded. Institutional caregivers also had the same curiosity about Edward's institutional confinement, but, as was the custom in the early 1970s, no one suggested that he return to his mother's community. He might not be "stupid," but he was ignorant of worldly matters, and his mother was dirt poor. In 1976, institutional officials paroled Edward to the group home where, at the time, I was employed by a local community agency. Eventually, Edward found steady employment, left the group home for an apartment, bought a car, married a woman, and started living the American Dream, albeit an economically precarious version of that mythical dream.

Thousands of people who were once involuntarily placed in large public institutions have, like Edward, done well in community settings. They have done well when social services officials have carefully planned their transition from the institution to a community and have secured public funding to sustain their new placement. For people living in a group home or an apartment residence, this care includes adequate housing with privacy, consisting at least of a room of one's own and of places to put one's possessions away from other people. It also includes commonly agreed upon rules and expectations for meal preparation, house cleaning, and other chores, along with agreed upon common space and time for visitors.

Living in communities also requires work for people whose capabilities encourage employers to hire them. Searching for jobs is usually facilitated by a social worker, an occupational therapist, or a job coach. When intellectually disabled people find employment, they must also find transportation. Some may learn to drive an automobile and even own a car, but most will rely on public transportation. Such reliance requires training in using buses, trains, or subway systems that can be a challenge for any citizen. At the job, disabled people must learn necessary job skills for performing expected tasks, but also they must learn the unwritten customs of being an employee. This last learning may be especially difficult for people who have lived much of their lives in sheltered or incarcerated settings.

All workers with disabilities face roadblocks to employment in the United States; intellectually disabled workers face especially onerous barriers. In 2010, the ARC (formally known as the Association for Retarded Citizens, and before that as the Association for Retarded Children), the principal voluntary association advocating for rights and services for intellectually disabled Americans, surveyed people with the disability and their families about several issues, one of which was employment. Surveys from more than 5,000 respondents indicated that only 15 percent of people with intellectual disability were employed in "integrated, competitive employment." Some of these wage earners were full-time workers; others worked less than full-time. Other studies confirm this finding and also indicate that another 20 percent are doing unpaid community activities. By far the largest number of intellectually disabled workers, 65 percent, labor in so-called facility-based jobs, what a decade earlier were likely called sheltered workshops. Of this final group, only 28 percent receive wages (ARC 2012, National Core Indicators 2012). Where there is integrated employment, older intellectually disabled workers are likely to be loyal, long-term employees, but their success depends on careful on-the-job training. Without this initial training, job recidivism is high, especially among young adults who have received inconsistent or no job training (Rusch and Dattilo 2012).

The sheltered workshop, the mainstay of employment for intellectually disabled adults, had its origin in the United States with the 1938 Fair Labor Standards Act.[6] Passed by Congress in response to the widespread unemployment brought about by the Great Depression, the federal legislation allowed employers to hire disabled workers at subminimum hourly earnings of up to 75 percent of the prevailing minimum wage. Going even further, the act also allowed employers in noncompetitive or "sheltered" work settings for severely disabled people to set no subminimum wage limit. Instead, wages, if ever provided, would be based solely on the worker's productivity. As such, a disabled worker in a sheltered workshop could receive wages not based on hourly work, but rather on items produced. If disabled workers produced little, they would receive low, or even no, wages.

The principal rationale for these subminimum wages in work settings "sheltered" from the competitive market was so-called vocational rehabilitation. Linked with occupational therapy, vocational rehabilitation had its origins in the readjustment and reeducation of disabled veterans. Its goal was vocational, but its methods were rehabilitative. In large part, then, work became a matter of healing, education, training, learning, and adapting. For the disabled war veteran, especially after World War II, this rehabilitation usually meant learning news ways of adaptation, access, and environmental interaction. But it also meant acquiring skills and knowledge for work. For adults with intellectual disability in the postwar period, work typically took place on the institutional farm or institutional workshop. But for those adults who remained in communities, the "sheltered workshop" was a place where "vocation" usually became perpetual rehabilitation.

After World War II and continuing into the 1960s, sheltered workshops opened throughout the United States. Often associated with a parents' organization like the Association for Retarded Children or voluntary associations like local Exchange Clubs, these facilities often became places of perpetual training. In them, workers did "piece work" exercises often in repetitive and perfunctory ways, producing little and earning less. With the movement to deinstitutionalization in the 1970s, critics of institutions increasingly began to regard sheltered workshops as little more than small institutions that happened to be located in communities. The institutional ambiance included child-like events, like visits from Santa Claus at Christmas time, Easter egg hunts in the spring, and playground equipment on the workshop's grounds. Staff usually referred to adult workers as boys and girls. In short, childish events and activities, along with staff attitudes, supplanted adult actions and expectations. If integration into American communities meant work in sheltered workshops, the integration appeared compromised by settings that were too "sheltered" to be genuine community-based employment. By the late 1970s, criticism of sheltered workshops became ubiquitous among critics of institutions—the sheltered workshop came to be seen as merely another institution.

To deal with the criticisms, many sheltered workshop, beginning in the late 1970s, changed their name, usually to a title including the words "industries" or "production." In Durham, North Carolina, for example, the Durham Exchange Club Sheltered Workshop became the Durham Exchange Club Industries. In Watertown, New York, the sheltered workshop became Production Unlimited. Other sheltered workshops dealt with criticisms by introducing Wolf Wolfensberger's principles of normalization to their staff. Since most staff by the 1980s had been acculturated to infantilizing their workers (even when they were not fully aware of doing so), they received the idea of introducing normal adult behaviors and expectations into the sheltered workshop setting with doubts and resistance. After all, they claimed, everyone knows that intellectually disabled workers are little more than child-like adults. Was not the expectation of adult behaviors a cruel way of treating these workers? Still other reformers introduced the practice of a token economy to educate workers in the behaviors of "self-management." Operant conditioning through the use of tokens provided workers rewards for appropriate "self-management" skills. The practice became widespread in the nation's sheltered workshop network in the 1970s and 1980s, but, as it did so, it also drew the criticism of parents, some staff, and workers themselves (Rusch and Dattilo 2012). Workers and their advocates reacted to what professionals failed to perceive; namely, the irony of using behavior modification's "self-management interventions" to promote self-determination.

Thus, despite the name changes, the attempts to re-educate staff, and the "self-management" token economies, sheltered workshop proponents found themselves in low regard by the end of the 1980s. Increasingly, advocates began to claim that workshops were exploiting their workers, and Congress's 1986 amendment to the Fair Labor Standards Act, allowing workshops to set wages at any minimum level that workshops wished, made the exploitation even easier to accomplish. Advocates and lawmakers were clearly at odds over the issue of work and wages. With the 1990 passage of the Americans with Disabilities Act (ADA), lawmakers provided advocates for integrated work settings a boost, albeit a small boost. The act made it illegal to deny employment to disabled workers merely on the basis of their disability. In 1999, they received a stronger boost. In that year, the US Supreme Court in its *Olmstead v. L. C. and E. W.* decision found that public officials could not segregate disabled people in institutional settings when professionals judged communities a better location for treatment and services. It noted that, "confinement in an institution severely diminishes the everyday life activities of individuals, including family relations, social contacts, work options, economic independence, educational advancement, and cultural enrichment" (*Olmstead v. L. C. and E. W.*, 1999). Work settings, by implication, had to be "everyday life activities." Sheltered workshops appeared more institutional than community-based, and they were hardly "work options."

By 2007, there were about 136,000 adults in workshop in forty-two states. It would be a decade after the *Olmstead* ruling before the Civil Rights Division of the US Justice Department began to enforce the decision for sheltered workshops. In 2009 also, President Barak Obama declared "The Year of Community Living," thus giving the Department Justice not only a policy mandate, but also a clear commitment to enforce inclusion. With both in hand, the department initiated legal actions against specific workshops and against community and state public agencies that supported these facilities.

The most significant of these actions was the Justice Department's 2014 litigation in *United States v. Rhode Island*. The case involved Providence, Rhode Island's use of sheltered workshops for many of its disabled high school students. The department claimed that "Rhode Island violated Title II of the Americans with Disabilities Act, by unjustifiably isolating persons with intellectual and developmental disabilities in sheltered workshops and facility-based day programs." It also found that the state failed "to provide state services in the most integrated setting appropriate to their needs and by putting Rhode Island high school students with intellectual and developmental disabilities at serious risk of segregation by failing to inform them of or provide them with state services that would allow them to work in an integrated workplace." On April 9, 2014, US District Court Judge Ronald R. Lugueux approved a consent decree between the state and the Justice Department that the court would supervise for ten years. The decree mandated that Rhode Island authorities develop a comprehensive plan to ensure appropriate employment and educational programming for intellectually disabled workers under its jurisdiction, and it required the Justice Department to monitor the state for compliance (Hoffman 2013; *United States v. Rhode Island*, 2014).

Despite these changes, subminimum-wage sheltered work settings like those of Goodwill Industries and subminimum-wage work initiatives at for-profit businesses like Applebee's restaurants and Barnes and Noble booksellers continue to pay most disabled workers less than half the prevailing minimum wage. These low-wage salaries stand in sharp contrast to the six- and seven-figure annual salaries of many local Goodwill executives (S. Adams 2013; Diament 2012).

For the full integration of intellectually disabled people into American communities—in schools, in houses and apartments, in workplaces—the rights that these citizens have acquired over the past forty years must be maintained. Advocates sustain these rights through legislation and regulations, all of which provide generic protection from discrimination. Beginning in the early 1990s, advocates recognized that the protection of rights required not only generic protection, but also individual safeguards. In 1974, in Salem, Oregon, the People First movement had its beginning. Its goal was advocacy carried out by people with intellectual disability. At a conference in Estes Park, Colorado, in September 1990, professionals discussed a newly emerging concept—self-advocacy. Around the nation, groups had experimented with teaching self-advocacy skills to people with intellectual disability. The Estes Park conference raised the issue of forming a national organization of self-advocates. The next year, in Nashville, Tennessee, advocates created "Self Advocates Becoming Empowered" (Dybwad and Bersani 1996; Ferguson, Ferguson, and Wehmeyer, 2013, 238). By 2012, there were about 1,200 self-advocacy groups in every state in the nation (Caldwell, Arnold, and Rizzolo, 2012).

Has the self-advocacy movement fulfilled its goal? Have people with intellectual disability learned the skills of advocating for themselves as they traverse the day-to-day challenges of living? In settings where training in self-advocacy skills is readily available and trainers have not only taught skills but have also learned from disabled participants about their own strengths and weaknesses, self-advocacy has proved effective. In Oregon, for example, where People First was launched, the Human Services Research Institute works with self-advocates to produce the bi-annual journal, *The Riot!* (2015). Edited by a staff of self-advocates and their allies, the journal provides information, ideas, opinions, stories, and a "love advice" column, all related to self-advocacy. The institute also provides technical assistance, literature, and items for people with intellectual disability. Thus, where local and regional self-advocacy organizations have received institutional support from a community voluntary association like the Human Services Research Institute, self-advocacy has thrived. In every flourishing case, the community-institutional support for self-advocacy provides organizational structure without supplanting the source of the advocacy—intellectually disabled people themselves.

SINS OF THE FATHERS: THE FERNALD SCIENCE CLUB AND STERILIZATIONS IN NORTH CAROLINA

The Fernald Science Club

On December 26, 1993, a front-page headline in the *Boston Globe* read, "Radiation Used on Retarded: Postwar Experiments Done at Fernald School" (1993). At the time, the Fernald Developmental Center (formerly Fernald State School), a Massachusetts institution founded by Samuel G. Howe in 1848 and named for its longtime medical superintendent Walter E. Fernald, had become a mere remnant of its once 2,500-inmate population. The article (and others that followed it) and the national attention that the revelation received took the American public back to the 1950s, to a time when the Fernald State School was approaching its population apogee. At the beginning of that decade, the institution's superintendent was psychiatrist Malcolm Farrell. An active member of both the American Psychiatric Association and the American Association on Mental Deficiency, Farrell was known for both his off-campus political skills at the Massachusetts State House and his inattention to the details of day-to-day life at the institution. His associate and the director of the school's Southard Laboratory was Clemens E. Benda. Like Farrell, Benda was a psychiatrist. His education in prewar Germany had emphasized neurology, and, like Farrell, he was an active member of the psychiatric and mental deficiency associations. Benda had immigrated to the United States in 1936. By the late 1940s, he had come to believe that most feeblemindedness was caused by malfunctioning glands—especially the pituitary and thyroid glands (D'Antonio 2005, 52–54).

In 1888, the Fernald State School had moved from South Boston twelve miles west to Waltham. At the time, Waltham was a factory town where workers made watches and textiles. As metropolitan Boston grew, the institution found itself increasingly surrounded by urban density, and the area's commuter rail system included the Waverley station located near the school. That rail system and the nearby station made the institution conveniently accessible to area universities.

Beginning during the superintendence of Fernald, the school's inmates became a source of research material for physicians at the Harvard Medical School. Most of this research had involved the pathological evaluation of autopsied brains of inmates. In 1918 and again in 1921, Fernald, along with E. E. Southard, a neuropsychiatrist at both the Harvard Medical School and the nearby Boston State Hospital (and for whom the research laboratory at the state school would be named after his death in 1920), and Annie E. Taft, a physician also at the Harvard Medical School and the custodian of its Neuropathological Collection, published their findings in two lavishly illustrated volumes entitled *Waverley Researches in the Pathology of the Feeble-Minded* (1918 and 1921). Like Fernald, Southard and Taft were caught up in the scientific curiosity of the eugenics movement, and, like him, they were interested in freeing feeblemindedness from the grip held at the time by psychological testers and bringing it back into the purview of medicine.

So, when Benda began his work in the 1940s, a tradition had already existed between research carried out using Fernald State School inmates (albeit dead inmates) by the school's physicians and Harvard University. To that tradition Benda added the Massachusetts Institute of Technology (MIT). In 1949, he and fellow scientists at MIT began a research project partially funded by the Quaker Oats Company. The purpose of the project was to measure the effect of phytic acid, a chemical found in nuts, seeds, legumes, and grains like oats, on the body's absorption of calcium in milk. To arrive at a measure, the scientists fed a group of boys at the school oat and farina cereal with and without phytic acid, and they compared the absorption of calcium by measuring and comparing the calcium levels in the boys' feces, urine, and blood. Benda called the group of boys who participated in the research the "Science Club."

Neither the boys nor their parents knew that the milk that they were ingesting for the research contained radioactive calcium. Benda told the boys—most of whom were "high grades"—that they were in a special project. To convince the boys of their distinctive status, he provided special gifts and outings for the Science Club participants. Informing the parents through individual letters, Benda claimed the importance of the research, but he failed to mention the matter of the radioactive calcium. What we know today as "informed consent" to participants and parents was, in the early 1950s, considered unnecessary and unimportant. The research continued until 1955, eventually also involving Harvard University and the US Atomic Energy Commission (D'Antonio 2005, 53–58, 238–255).

Most of the participants, whom Michael D'Antonio called "the state boys," had spent time at the institution more for their poverty and status as orphans than for their supposed low intelligence. In November 1957, several of the boys, now teenagers, rebelled against the institution's inhumane conditions. They rioted, occupying cottages and driving out attendants and other staff. They piled up mattresses and newspapers and set them on fire. They smashed windows, they tore sinks and toilets from their fittings, they broke light fixtures and tile walls, and they burned institutional records. It would take nearly ten hours to bring the siege to an end. It was a rare moment in which people labeled mentally defective rebelled so successfully against their incarcerators (D'Antonio 2005, 120–145).

Eventually, several of these young men left the institution. Most found jobs; some got married and had families. When the revelations about the radioactive experiments and the "Science Club" came to light at the end of 1993, members of the club contacted each other and one of them, Fred Boyce, traveled to Washington to testify before a Congressional Committee about the Fernald inmates' participation in the research. Nearly two years later, in October 1995—in the midst of the nation's obsession with the trial and acquittal of O. J. Simpson—President Bill Clinton issued an apology to the men who had participated as boys in the Science Club experiments. The Simpson acquittal ensured that little press attention was devoted to the apology. Later still, the Quaker Oats Company and MIT agreed to pay the men $1.2 million, or about $60,000 for each living participant (D'Antonio 2005, 120–145, 256–272).

Sterilizations in North Carolina

Nine years later, on December 9, 2002, the *Winston-Salem Journal* began the publication of a five-part series, "Against Their Will: North Carolina's Sterilization Programs" (Begos et al. 2013). The articles reported the creation and work of the state's Eugenics Board (later made a Commission). Between 1929 and 1974, the Board used the authority provided by the state's General Assembly to approve the involuntary sterilizations of more than 7,600 North Carolinians. Most of these citizens were poor, uneducated, and never represented by legal counsel. More women than men were sterilized. Before 1947, more whites than blacks were sterilized; by the 1950s, the reverse was true (Cahn 1998, 173, 179; Ladd-Taylor 2014; E. Larson 1995, 104–160). Some of the sterilized were living in one of the state's residential institutions. Some of the institutionalized were in psychiatric hospitals, but most were in state facilities for intellectually disabled people. Other sterilized citizens were merely living in local communities. The newspaper's findings created a stir throughout the state because it shed light on a state-sponsored practice that had remained publically muted into the 1960s.[7] Even after the North Carolina General Assembly ended the Eugenics Commission in 1974, it passed legislation in 1977 that allowed the state's District Court judges to order sterilizations for mentally retarded and mentally ill people without their consent (Glenna et al. 2007;Morrison 1965; Thomas 1998).

On February 13, 2003, North Carolina Governor Michael F. Easley, a Democrat in the second year of his second four-year term as the state's chief executive, issued a formal apology to the individuals whom the state had involuntarily sterilized. The articles in the *Winston-Salem Journal* had by that time circulated among other news channels across the state. For the first time, ordinary citizens of the state knew the history and consequences of legal, but questionably ethical, eugenic sterilizations. And citizens of the state learned about the cabal of medical, judicial, and social welfare officials, along with local and institutional officials who had perpetuated the Eugenics Commission for nearly five decades.

Four months later, the North Carolina General Assembly, under pressure generated by the recent revelations, repealed its 1977 state statute (North Carolina General Assembly 1977, 2003). With greater public awareness of the eugenic sterilization program, journalists and private citizens began to discuss legislation to provide reparations to sterilized victims. Some people suggested special funds for health costs; others advocated for a memorial structure, now that many of the involuntarily sterilized were dead. In 2010, under prodding from Governor Beverley Perdue, the General Assembly set aside a $250,000 for a foundation to study compensation for victims. In January 2012, the North Carolina Justice for Sterilization Victims Foundation issued its report, recommending a $50,000 compensation to each victim. The following year, the General Assembly appropriated funds for the compensation. The procedures for contacting and verifying the past sterilizations of living victims, most of whom were elderly, has proved difficult. Patrick L. McCory, the state's Republican governor since 2012, has shown no zeal for facilitating the verification process. As one victim put the situation, "I believe they're waiting for us to die" (Begos et al. 2013, 220).

In some respects North Carolina's nearly fifty-year practice of state-sanctioned and state-sponsored eugenic sterilizations mirrored sterilization programs carried out by other states, but, in other respects, it departed from those programs (Black 2003; Carey 1998; Castles 2002; Kline 2001; Ladd-Taylor1997, 2014; Schoen 2005; Vogel 1995). Like other states in the early decades of the twentieth century, the Tar Heel state had academics and social welfare authorities who believed that eugenics provided an efficient way to solve many, maybe most, social problems. As noted in previous chapters, early champions of eugenics argued that social problems were usually the result of feeblemindedness. The prostitute prostitutes herself because she is feebleminded. The petty thief thieves because he is feebleminded. The hobo and the vagrant are homeless because they are feebleminded. These social problems seemed inextricable and unsolvable; yet the claims of eugenics seemed to offer a new, simple, and progressive way to accomplish something that had once seemed impossible: the end of social problems through the elimination of the source of those problems, feeblemindedness. In North Carolina, as in other states, the debate over ending feeblemindedness was not over eugenics but over the best methods for applying eugenic principles. As such, the question became: Is the best method for ending the reproduction of feebleminded people, and thus for eliminating the social problems that they create, segregation or sterilization? In North Carolina, as in several other states, the answer became both. Some feeble minds should be segregated from the general population to keep them from reproducing, and some feeble minds should be sterilized, in either case to prevent them from producing more of their own kind.

In North Carolina, the principles and promise of eugenics had an especially effective champion in the biologist William Louis Poteat. Born in Caswell County, North Carolina in 1856, Poteat could remember a time when the field workers on his parents' tobacco plantation were their slaves. By the early years of the twentieth century, the extended Poteat family, including William, his brother Edwin, his sister Ida, and later their children, were known as an urbane and thoroughly Baptist family of educators. In 1878, eldest son "Billy" Poteat became a tutor of biology at Wake Forest College, and, in 1905, he assumed the presidency of the college, then located in the small town of Wake Forest, twenty miles northeast of the state capital, Raleigh. After becoming president, he continued to teach biology; indeed, teaching all of the biology course offerings until the college hired a second biologist 1920. When he resigned the presidency in 1927, he resumed his full-time appointment in the Biology Department, remaining there until his death in 1938 (Cocke 1948).

Poteat's faith in Darwinian evolution was no less strong than was his faith in the Baptist teachings of his Christian upbringing. He found no incompatibility between the two. His brother Edwin, a Baptist minister and president of Furman College in South Carolina, had married Harriet Gordon, the daughter of the most prominent evangelical and premillennialist of the period, the Baptist Boston minister, Adoniram Judson Gordon. The Poteats, however, were postmillennialists. Like many other Protestant clergy in the first quarter of the twentieth century, they saw in eugenics the promise of making the world righteous in order to bring about the Kingdom of God. What was unique about William Poteat's advocacy of eugenics was not theological, but rather that he made that advocacy in the South (Rosen 2004, 4, 17–22).

From this outlook, Poteat educated a generation of Wake Forest College students on what he claimed was the harmony of evolution, eugenics, and Christian faith. Some credited Poteat's students, later elected to the General Assembly, for preventing public school teaching restrictions on evolutionary theory and thus a Scopes-like "monkey" trial in North Carolina. Just as he effectively educated students not to fear Darwin's claims, he also skillfully persuaded the state's churches and denominational organizations to remain open to these claims. Speaking frequently to these groups, Poteat used his humor, Southern charm, and intelligence to lead many North Carolina churchgoers and church leaders to (at least) tolerate Darwin, even if they neither understood Darwin's theory nor fully appreciated its implications (Hall 2000, 51–102).

In 1925, he delivered the McNair Lectures, "Can Man Be a Christian To-Day?" at the University of North Carolina to "present a scholarly and forceful refutation of the fanatical attacks upon science" (Poteat 1925). At the time, fundamentalists, both inside the state and outside it, had viciously criticized Poteat's defense of evolution. In his lecture, he described ways that Christians could reconcile their faith with the new findings of science, arguing that the most appropriate way required Christians to "revise [their] conception of the origin and purpose of the Bible and so retain [their] reverence before its Divine authority without embarrassment before the assured results of science" (Poteat 1925, 696). In short, Poteat argued that the realm of faith and the work of science, although occasionally overlapping, were two important, but still separate spheres (Hall 2000, 149–150).

It was in this context that Poteat, as a champion of faith and science, argued for applying the principles of eugenics to the restriction of human reproduction. In 1921, he spoke to the Southern Baptist Education Association, "There can be no doubt that we are ready for the application of negative eugenics, that is, restrictive mating for the elimination of the obviously unfit." He added, "The feebleminded, the insane, the epileptic, the inebriate, the congenital defective of any type, and the victim of contagious diseases ought to be denied the opportunity of perpetuating their kind to the inevitable deterioration of the race" (Begos et al. 2013, 65–66; Hall 2000, 100–101).

By the end of the decade, the state had authorized eugenic sterilizations for "the mentally diseased, feeble minded, or epileptic." The General Assembly considered the legislation at the height of Poteat's defense of Darwin before civic and church groups. As an integral part of that defense was Poteat's advocacy of negative eugenics. His public speaking and writing about eugenics warmed legislators and the public alike to "restrictive mating." In the previous decade, the state had created the Caswell Training School for the Feeble-Minded at Kinston, where fertile feeble minds could be segregated from breeding with the opposite sex. But the 1929 legislation sanctioned a new means of control by allowing for sterilization. In doing so, it authorized officials at all North Carolina penal and charitable institutions to sterilize any inmate whose asexualization would benefit the individual and the public good. Going a step further, it opened sterilization to the state's 100 counties by giving local county commissioners the authority to approve sterilizations for any mentally defective person after receiving a petition from the person's next of kin or legal guardian. The county commissioners' approval was to be reviewed by the state's Commissioner of Public Welfare, the secretary of the State Board of Health, and, finally, by the chief medical officer of two of the state's institutions for the insane or feebleminded. But soon, county authorities routinely ignored this review by simply disregarding it.

During and after its passage, the 1929 legislation received Poteat's enthusiastic support. During the time, his defense of Darwin was only surpassed by his advocacy of eugenics. But the legislation soon proved to be too cumbersome and, among the counties, too inconsistently applied. To deal with these problems, the General Assembly in 1933 created the North Carolina Eugenics Board.[8] The board consisted of five members: the state's Commissioner of Public Welfare, the secretary of the State Board of Health, a medical officer of one of the institutions for the insane or feebleminded (chosen by the other members), the chief medical officer of the

Dorothea Dix Hospital for the Insane in Raleigh, and the state's attorney general. Charged with making decisions about sterilization, the board conducted hearings on cases brought before it from institutional or county officials. Each petition required a social history from a physician that indicated the insane, feebleminded, or epileptic person's medical and social history, as well as a physician's assessment of the likelihood of the person reproducing. In 1937, the General Assembly modified the legislation to allow the superintendents of the state hospitals for the insane and feebleminded to admit temporarily any feebleminded, mentally diseased, or epileptic person for the sole purpose of sterilizing them. The Eugenics Board approved all sterilizations, and many sterilizations became surgeries thereafter performed in institutions, even if the sterilized person immediately returned to her or his community (Castles 2002).

In 1942, the United States Supreme Court's decision in *Skinner v. Oklahoma* restricted the states from eugenically sterilizing convicted felons. In doing so, the Court had narrowed the broad authority to sterilize several categories of the socially deviant that it had given the states in its 1927 decision, *Buck v. Bell*. Nevertheless, the decision, coming in the midst of the national awareness of the recent Nazi mass sterilizations, changed nothing about the involuntary sterilization of feebleminded people either incarcerated in public institutions or living in local communities (Nourse 2008).

Still, it would not be until after World War II that North Carolina, unlike other states, would transform involuntary sterilizations into a frequent, if still publicly inconspicuous, procedure. Three years before William Louis Poteat became the president of Wake Forest College, the college opened a two-year medical school. In 1941, after a bequest from the estate of Reynolds Tobacco Company President Bowman Gray, the college moved its medical school to Winston-Salem. That same year, the new Bowman Gray School of Medicine established the nation's first medical school department of genetics and appointed as its first director Dr. William Allan. Allan's view about practical eugenics was from the beginning clear, "It seems to me that the only way to attain the goal of positive eugenics is to actually practice negative eugenics—the prevention of the birth of the mentally and physically unfit." Joining Allan was Dr. C. Nash Herndon, who, upon Allan's unexpected death in 1943, found himself in the new role of the genetics department's head. The interest in and advocacy for eugenics initiated by Poteat would find even greater legitimacy at Wake Forest College in Herndon's work at the college's medical school (Begos et al. 2013, 35).

Like Allan, Herndon was a committed supporter of both eugenics and eugenic sterilization. He was an active member of the American Eugenics Society, becoming its president from 1953 to 1955. He also served as president of the Human Betterment League of North Carolina, an organization that was active in supporting eugenics after World War II. In 1944, Herndon wrote in the department's annual report of "a project aimed at eugenic improvement of the population of Forsyth County. . . . The project consists of a gradual, but systematic effort to eliminate certain genetically unfit strains from the local population. About thirty operations for sterilization have been performed." Making the local subjects for the operations available was the Forsyth County Health Officer, Dr. J. Roy Hege. The Forsyth County Commissioners funded the surgeries, all of which were performed at Forsyth County Hospital. Under Herndon's leadership in the 1950s, the Department of Medical Genetics acquired additional faculty members who, along with faculty from the Department of Obstetrics and Gynecology and the Department of Surgery, supported eugenics. Besides the leadership he provided at Bowman Gray, Herndon regularly taught a course on applied eugenics to medical students, nurses, and other healthcare professionals. The class, as he noted in November 1949, stressed sterilization (Begos et al. 2013, 35–39; Human Betterment League 2008, 41).

After World War II ended, two additional actors would enter the postwar story of eugenic sterilizations in North Carolina. The first was James G. Hanes, the president and chairman of the board of Hanes Hosiery Mills in Winston-Salem. One of the state's wealthiest citizens and a member of several boards of national corporations, Hanes was nevertheless active in the civic life of Winston-Salem. At various times between 1918 and 1950, he was elected to the Board of Aldermen of the city and to the Board of Commissioners of Forsyth County. Between 1921 and 1925, he served as mayor of Winston-Salem and for twenty-two years was the chair of the Commissioners. As a part of his public service, he championed public school construction and funding, and, after the Supreme Court's 1954 *Brown v. Board of Education* decision, he led local efforts for school desegregation and for the formation of the Winston-Salem County Relations Project that brought black and white leaders together to create ways for social change. In 1965, the North Carolina Conference for Social Service gave him its highest award for being an exemplary "leader, benefactor and servant of the people" (Green 1988).

In 1947, at the age of sixty-one, Hanes became one of the Founders of the Human Betterment League of North Carolina. The founding of the League introduced the second important actor in the postwar story of eugenics in North Carolina, Dr. Clarence J. Gamble.

Gamble, the grandson of one of the founders of the Proctor and Gamble Soap Company, was, like Hanes, wealthy. But, unlike Hanes, Gamble was never involved in the family's business. Instead, after graduating from Princeton University, he completed a medical degree at the Harvard Medical School in 1920. Around the time of his 1924 marriage to Sarah Merry Bradley, Gamble began work that would preoccupy him for the rest of his life. That preoccupation was birth control. Over the next two decades, from his home in Milton, Massachusetts, he carried out research on birth control devices, trying in the process to identify simple and inexpensive methods that ordinary women could use. He used his own funds to carry out the research and to establish a birth control clinic in several communities in the United States. He most often referred to his work as the "Great Cause" (Reed 2014, 225–226; Williams and Williams 1978, 3–197).

Gamble's involvement in North Carolina began in 1938 when he funded a one-year project to provide birth control clinics throughout the state. Unlike most of the states in the Northeast and upper Midwest, North Carolina did not have a large Roman Catholic population and thus, as Gamble perceived, efforts to provide birth control in North Carolina would not draw national attention. Likewise, among the

Southern states, North Carolina prided itself in having excellent universities and colleges, as well as wealthy families who, like Gamble, considered themselves to be progressive and enlightened. By the end of the decade, the state had sixty-two birth control clinics, each dispensing Gamble's favorite form of birth control—foaming powder and sponges. Working with local medical authorities, the project maintained its "enlightened" policies by providing birth control equally to both black and white women. What linked these women was their poverty (Carey 1998; Hansen and King 2013, 172–174, 240–241; Hubbard 1990; E. Schneider 1981; Schoen 2005, 33; Wharton 1939; Williams and Williams 1978, 128–148).

Thus, in 1947, when Gamble provided the funding to launch the Human Betterment League of North Carolina, he was already known to many of the state's academic and industrial elites. In addition to Hanes (who was listed in the League's charter not as the President of Hanes Hosiery Mills but as the Chairman of the Board of Commissioners of Forsyth County), the League's members from Winston-Salem included Nat S. Crews, the Forsyth County attorney; Nash Herndon, still an assistant professor at the Bowman Gray School of Medicine; and Jessie McMillan Stroup, a librarian at Salem College for Women, who served as the league's secretary. From Chapel Hill, the founding members of the League included four members who were associated with the University of North Carolina: Gordon W. Blackwell, the director of the Institute for Research in Social Science; A. M. Jordan and W. D. Perry, each a professor of educational psychology and both involved in intellectual testing; and Robert W. Madry, the director of the university's news bureau and chosen to lead the League's publicity committee. The three remaining charter members were Helen Hunter, the president of the North Carolina Mental Hygiene Society, from Charlotte; George H. Lawrence, a social worker and superintendent of the Buncombe County Welfare Department in Asheville; and Katharine R. H. Lyman, a social worker married to Dr. Richard S. Lyman, a neuropsychiatrist at Duke University in Durham. From its founding in 1947 until it disbanded in 1988, the League's selected membership included many prominent North Carolinians.[9] They were all white and always well-to-do.

At its first meeting, the ten inaugural members of League approved a statement of four objectives:

1. The study of the care of the insane and feebleminded of North Carolina
2. The encouragement of the best treatment and training of such patients; and the assurance of measures which will prevent such mental handicaps
3. Since no child can be brought up satisfactorily by an insane or feebleminded parent, the League will devote a part of its efforts to the solution of this important problem.
4. The League shall, in addition, educate the public in this field in order to assure the best possible care of the insane, the feebleminded and the children of these groups.

Although its objectives made no mention of eugenic sterilization, at its second meeting in November, Hanes moved that an "educational questionnaire" funded by

Gamble entitled "What Do You Know About Sterilization" be printed, thus making clear the central purpose of the organization. At its third meeting in May 1948, the League's Committee on Publicity and Publications reported that it had sent 110,000 questionnaires to a mailing list of 40,000 "upper class college students, faculty members, physicians, nurses, ministers, public officials, etc." At the same meeting, the minutes indicate that the mailing generated requests for additional information, especially from social workers in county welfare offices. In November, at its fourth meeting, Gamble persuaded the League to send a letter to every newspaper in the state that would give an estimate of the number of feebleminded people born in each newspaper's community "and suggesting sterilization" (Human Betterment League 2008, 21–25, 29).

In 1947, the same year that he funded the Human Betterment League, Gamble published a poem, "Lucky Morons," that focused on the good fortune of what Gamble characterized as the otherwise poor, uneducated, but ever fertile Tar Heel moron (Schaffer 2014, 95–96). The North Carolina moron, presumably unlike morons in some other states, was institutionalized in the state's institution for feeble minds, the Caswell Training School. In that setting, his intellectual deficiency became apparent from an intelligence test, and there the moron learned a trade. Soon he was able to return to his community to become self-supporting. But, Gamble wrote, with capitalized words for emphasis: "after a while he met a GIRL . . . and a surgeon had PROTECTED her from UNWANTED CHILDREN, without making her different in any other way from other women." The poem concludes, "And with just the two in the Family, they kept on being SELF SUPPORTING, and they were very thankful they lived in NORTH CAROLINA. And the WELFARE DEPARTMENT DIDN'T have to feed them and the SCHOOLS didn't have to waste their efforts on any of their children who weren't very bright. And because they had been STERILIZED, the taxpayers of North Carolina had saved THOUSANDS OF DOLLARS and the North Carolina MORONS LIVED HAPPILY EVER AFTER."[10] For Gamble and his fellow League members, as the poem unself-consciously shows, every North Carolinian would benefit from state-sponsored eugenic sterilizations of morons (see also Gamble 1946, 1949).

In the decades of the 1950s and 1960s, the state would fulfill the League's mission through its rejuvenation of the state's Eugenics Board. Like other states that authorized the sterilization of feeble minds earlier in the century, North Carolina had by the end of World War II nearly discontinued the practice. With the financial and managerial support of Gamble and Hanes after 1947, the League would reverse this trend and, in the process, turn the state into the nation's most active sterilizer. Sterilizations sanctioned by the Eugenics Board were almost always involuntary, and they were primarily of two kinds—the institutional sterilizations and the county sterilizations. In the state's three (and later four) residential institutions, adults, who through the 1950s continued to be labeled "morons," were regularly sterilized with the authority that the Eugenics Board gave to institutional authorities. Male morons, who received vasectomies, usually had the surgery performed at the institution. Female morons, who required the more complex tubal ligation, usually had the procedure done in a local public hospital, although some of these sterilizations were, like vasectomies, carried out at the institution. Institutional officials believed that sterilizations were especially important for morons who might be placed back into communities where, away from institutional control, they were likely to be sexually active.

The other type of sterilization in North Carolina—the one that received most of the attention after 2002—was sterilization performed in communities, usually with the approval of the Eugenics Board and carried out by local social welfare and public health agencies. Here, involuntary eugenic sterilization most often came under the purview of social workers, many of whom had received their education at what was then the state's only school of social work at the University of North Carolina. The Chapel Hill social work program through the decades of the 1950s and 1960s remained in close alliance with both the Eugenics Board and the Human Betterment League, especially through the efforts of Ellen B. Winston, the North Carolina Commissioner of Public Welfare between 1944 and 1963. Winston was an enthusiastic proponent of eugenics sterilization. She participated in League activities, and she influenced the faculty members at the School of Social Work to teach eugenics as a part of its curriculum on family planning. Going even further, she persuaded the Eugenics Board to allow social workers to petition the Board for approving sterilizations for their clients, most of whom were poor and uneducated and were threatened with losing their public assistance if they refused the procedure (Hansen and King 2013, 240–244; Schoen 2005, 105–109; see also Largent 2008).

Trained to appreciate eugenic sterilization and influenced by a respected authority like Winston, North Carolina social workers, more than their counterparts in other states, used sterilization as a means of what Frances Fox Piven and Richard Cloward (1971) called "regulating the poor." In virtually all of the state's 100 counties, social workers, along with public health nurses, used sterilization to control the breeding or potential breeding of clients who received cash assistance from the Aid for Dependent Children program, later known as Aid for Families with Dependent Children. The use was especially prevalent in so-called enlightened counties that contained the state's urban communities. Here, welfare recipients—and, by the late 1950s, especially black welfare recipients—were often given the choice of either sterilization and a monthly welfare check or no sterilization and no welfare assistance.

In Charlotte, the county seat of Mecklenburg County, for example, Wallace H. Kuralt was the Director of Public Welfare from 1945, when he finished his master of social work degree at the University of North Carolina, until his retirement in 1972. A New Deal progressive, Kuralt advocated for sterilization, along with birth control devices and abortion, as a major way to eliminate poverty. During his tenure as welfare director, Mecklenburg County sterilized 403 of its welfare recipients. One of the sterilized was a twelve-year-old girl. Most of the sterilized were poor black women with "too many children." In a 1993 interview, Kuralt stressed that the sterilizations were always voluntary, "except perhaps in case of some very seriously retarded children" (Schoen 1993, 6). This claim was disingenuous; he signed the sterilization papers for hundreds of petitions to the Eugenics Board. Many, perhaps most, of the clients were never tested. Today, the building that houses the Mecklenburg County Department of Social Services is named for Kuralt; after a gift from his son, television personality Charles Kuralt, the University of North Carolina's School of Social Work created a distinguished professorship in his name.[11]

None of the actors who created the widespread and publically sanctioned involuntary eugenics sterilization program in North Carolina between 1929 and 2003 were invidious people. Most were socially liberal, and most saw sterilizations as a form of birth control, which before the 1960s was one of the few effective forms of such control. None espoused overtly racist rhetoric or views; indeed, given the racist atmosphere in the state before the 1970s, their concern for racial harmony and racial political equality (but hardly racial integration) made them progressives. In fact, the Human Betterment League in the 1970s invited Durham's black business executive Asa T. Spaulding and his wife to be members. Nor were the proponents of eugenic sterilization likely to blame the poor for their poverty. Charles Kuralt remembered the persistent stinginess of the Mecklenburg County Commissioners when it came to welfare assistance. His father, according to Kuralt, was often branded a liberal and often criticized in the local newspaper (Academy of Achievement 1996). Yet, the practice of eugenic sterilizations operated by a state-mandated board and supported by an influential voluntary association continued to operate and even thrive long after it had waned in other parts of the nation.

It did so because, in a time before an effective birth control method that could be used by women, social welfare authorities saw eugenic sterilizations as a means to stop pregnancies of poor women in particular and poor families in general. From their social work education at the University of North Carolina, legitimated by academic and medical authorities at Wake Forest and Duke Universities, as well as by a well-funded voluntary association like the Human Betterment League and a state-sponsored Eugenics Board, North Carolina social workers maintained a system that they believed served their clients well.[12]

The program was never hidden from the public. Indeed, the Human Betterment League frequently place advertisements in several of the state's newspapers and magazine. One of these appeared in May 1953, in the popular weekly, *The State: Down Home in North Carolina*. The advertisement's title read, "Know About Eugenic Sterilization." It warned the reader that,

> Morons are now doubling their number with each generation. More than half the hospital beds in this country are occupied by mentally ill or mentally defective parents, and over-crowded institutions cannot begin to accommodate their increasing numbers. . . .
>
> Selective sterilization should be used when children must be shielded from being born to a heritage of insanity or feeblemindedness, when defenseless children must be saved the suffering and unhappiness of being brought up by an insane or feebleminded parent. (Human Betterment League of North Carolina 1953, 12)

Yet eugenic sterilization in North Carolina never received press scrutiny, in part because it received the active support of public influentials like Durham newspaper editor H. C. Bradshaw, a long-time League member. Like the Tuskegee syphilis experiments of nearly the same period, the cauldron of academic, governmental, and moneyed elite created, in the name of assistance and good will, an ordinary but still effective system that resulted in the involuntary sterilizations of more than 7,600 North Carolinians.

By 2011, a task force convened to recommend compensation for sterilized victims determined that less than 3,000 of the sterilized were living. The members of the task force recognized what, a generation earlier, would have been impossible to imagine, "We also acknowledge that no amount of money can replace or give value to what has been done to nearly 7,600 people—men, women, boys, girls, African Americans, Whites, American Indians, the poor, undereducated, and disabled— who[m] our state and its citizens judged, targeted, and labeled 'morons,' 'unfit,' and 'feebleminded.'" Several people gave testimony to the task force; some were victims and some were relatives of victims. One of the speakers was Melissa Hyatt, who spoke for Charles Holt, a man whom authorities had sterilized in 1966 while he lived at Murdoch Center, a large residential institution for mentally retarded people that the state opened after World War II (Task Force to Determine 2011; see also Castles 2002):

> Charles wasn't aware that he may never have a child of his own. I don't even think he knew what the surgery meant. He was just told he had to have [it].
>
> At the age of twenty he met a woman who he fell in love with and became ready to pursue a life with her only to find out at the time he was not able to have children. He went to the doctor and learned that the surgery he had in Murdoch wouldn't allow him to have children. This made him very disappointed and he became depressed. Now someone had finally explained the effects of the surgery. To make it worse, the woman that he had grown to love left him and made fun of him because he couldn't have children. With the love of his life leaving that too caused more grief. . .
>
> Afterwards he got a job with the City of High Point. . . . Still at the same job, he met another woman and she had three children. He remained working hard and spending time with his new children. . . Being one of those children that Charles raised, I picked him out to be my dad. My dad passed away when I was ten and Charles has always been very good to me. . . .
>
> And I just made a note from his court papers from back when he was in the institution. . . . [T]here was a psychological evaluation that looked like either the courts used or maybe even the Murdoch Center used to decide for this procedure. According to the evaluation, Charles was an attractive, neat appearing boy of average physical development. He bears no physical signs of retardation. His speech is of average complexity. There was nothing about his behavior which could be called unusual. The evaluation goes on to talk about his steady relationship with a girlfriend and basically how he is normal. Nothing wrong with him. And after reading the whole evaluation how can anyone [find] it is for your own good? You don't need to have a baby. You don't need to experience the wonders of being a parent. Who are they to say?

And number two, Charles has always offered his services to the public and at many places where he has worked has ultimate respect for him. For how well he's done these services whether he was working for the city for thirty years, doing street maintenance, helping the elderly at nursing homes, and manufacturing products in a factory, delivering your daily newspaper, or working in your nearest grocery store. . . . So why was it good for the public that he didn't have children?

There was nothing in his reports that stated Charles, at nineteen, was even told what the surgery meant for his life.

And in Charles' position that's all he's ever wanted was children. He's been so good us. He's been so good to any child that I've ever seen him. He loves a child. He's always wanted to have one of his own. He would have love to have one with my mother—I know that. . . .

DOWN SYNDROME, "SEVERE DISABILITY," AND THE END OF FEEBLE MINDS

In August 2007, the September issue of *Vanity Fair* arrived on stands across the United States. In it, Suzanna Andrews wrote a 5000-word "investigation" about Daniel Miller, a forty-one-year-old man born in 1966 to the playwright Arthur Miller and his third wife, the photojournalist Inge Morath. The article, "Arthur Miller's Missing Act," told the story of Daniel's birth with Down syndrome and his father's denial—publicly and privately—of a place for Daniel in the Miller family. Almost immediately after Daniel's birth, Arthur, over the objections of Inge, placed the baby in a private home for disabled infants. When he was four, the family moved him to Southbury Training School, Connecticut's second residential institution for intellectually disabled people. Although Inge visited him from time to time, Arthur never visited, and the family never mentioned him nor did they acknowledge his existence. When he entered the training school, it was a crowded facility with more than 2,300 inmates. Like other institutions of the early 1970s, Southbury was an appalling place. Yet, from all accounts, Danny Miller was a happy, friendly, and gregarious boy (Andrews 2007).

When he was about seventeen, Southbury, like most other state facilities under pressure to deinstitutionalize, placed Danny Miller in a community group home. His parents, to the surprise of the Southbury staff, did not object. In the group home, he received training in community living skills that he had never before received. By all accounts, he did well in the community. By the mid-1990s, Danny had moved to an apartment with a roommate. He held a job and had a bank account. Later, he joined the self-advocacy group, People First, and participated in a several athletic activities and events.

Father and son met publicly for the first time in September 1995 at a conference on false confessions in Hartford. Arthur gave a talk about Richard Lapointe, a man with intellectual disability who had been convicted of the murder of his wife's grandmother. Many people, like Miller, had come to believe that Lapointe's conviction had been based on a coerced confession. Danny attended the event with a group from People First. During the meeting, Danny, informed that Arthur was his father, ran to him to give the stunned speaker a hug. A photograph of the two was taken, and Danny "was thrilled." After this meeting, Arthur met Danny a few more times, but when Inge died in 2002, Danny did not attend the funeral, nor was there mention of him in her obituary. After Arthur's death in 2005, Danny received a portion of his father's estate, which served to make him ineligible for the Medicaid and SSI assistance he had been receiving (Andrews 2007).

Daniel Miller is by all accounts a delightful person who "leads a very active, happy life, surrounded by people who love him." The shame that caused Arthur Miller to deny his son resulted far more in his loss than his son's loss. Even in 1966, medical authorities (many of whom knew better) were still telling the parents of children with intellectual disabilities like the Millers that their disabled newborn was condemned to a life of endless medical problems, with no hope for academic or occupational success, and would be an ongoing psychological burden to their otherwise happy family. Fifty years later, this rhetoric of disaster with its promise of deliverance through institutionalization is rarely heard. Physicians, social workers, educators, psychologists, and occupational therapists have been socialized to provide parents with a rhetoric of hope through education and socialization. As noted earlier, intellectually disabled children and adults are more integrated into everyday social institutions that at any time since the founding of institutions in the 1840s (D. Wright 2011). Beginning in the 1990s, the parents of children with Down syndrome have written and spoken about the full, exciting, joyful, and even ordinary lives of their children (e.g., R. Adams 2013; Bérubé 1996, 2004; Estreich 2013; Riel-Smith 2014).

By the 2010s, people with Down syndrome, along with individuals with many other intellectual and developmental disabilities, have become more present by their absence. The advent of reliable and convenient prenatal testing has led 67 percent of the tested women in the United States who are carrying a fetus with Down syndrome to terminate the pregnancy (Burke et al. 2011; de Graaf, Buckley, and Skotko 2015; Sandel 2009; Schrad 2015). Pregnant women knowing that they will have child with Down syndrome, but who nevertheless bring the fetus to full term, are often criticized for doing so by healthcare providers, friends, and family. Some have argued that the 33 percent of the tested population who choose to have a Down syndrome child are the ones who can best care for such children. But others, like philosopher Peter Singer, argue that with prenatal testing, no parent who chooses to have a "severely" disabled child should receive any governmental healthcare support or coverage from private insurance companies. Repeatedly referring to a disabled child as "it," Singer argues that the killing of severely disabled infants is "quite reasonable." Besides, he added, "You know, I don't want my health insurance premiums to be higher so that infants who can experience zero quality of life can have expensive treatments" (Khuse and Singer 1985; Klein 2015).

Still others have supported the use of so-called growth attenuation therapy to stop the maturation of "severely disabled" children. By using large doses of estrogen and progesterone, Seattle physicians Gunther and Diekma announced in 2006 that they had successfully stopped the growth of a six-year-old girl with multiple disabilities including intellectual disability. The point of the therapy, according to Gunther and Diekma, was to render the disabled child smaller than she would naturally become so as to make the care she required easier for her family. That the family, much less the girl herself, would benefit from the procedure was a presupposition that interveners did not seem to have questioned (Gunther and Diekma 2006).[13]

In 2016, healthcare authorities are not likely to tell parents who have infants with Down syndrome or with other intellectual disability that their children are doomed to a "life not worth living." Nor are they likely to use the rhetoric of "zero quality of life." Disabled infants and children are hardly ever placed in institutions because there are few institutions and because parents have alternative options from an array of healthcare services to an assortment educational assistance. Likewise, two generations of North Americans have attended schools and been in voluntary association with intellectually disabled people. Disabilities are not the aberrations they once were, when so many disabled people were hidden away in institutions. Today, nondisabled people have disabled people as their classmates, friends, coworkers, and neighbors. Jason Kingsley, Mitchell Levitz (2007), Rosa Marcellino, Jamie Bérubé, Laura Estreich, Walker Smith, and Henry Connolly have in various ways articulated their place in ordinary day-to-day life, and, contra Singer, shown the high quality of their lives.

So, it is ironic that with the growth of greater openness to disability in the general population has also come the advent of designer human beings. The new eugenics of prenatal testing and of "growth attenuation" has replaced the old eugenics of segregation and sterilization. The new euthanasia of the "severely" disabled has replaced the old "menace of the feebleminded." Social demands for abortion and euthanasia may allow us to become a more perfect people. But what will we have gained, and, more importantly, what will we have lost? The loss may be imagined most poignantly in a June 2015 Facebook posting by the philosopher Eva Kittay (2015; see also Kittay 2000, 2001), who recounts the experience of Sesha, her disabled daughter:

Last night Sesha acquired a new favorite composer: Mahler (rollover Beethoven). I played her the Mahler 9th and she was spellbound from the first note. At times— the loud, dramatic, ones that feel like ocean waves, she could hardly contain her excitement. During the sweet soft times, a lovely smile would form on her face. I was holding her hand, and I could feel the pressure change as the mood of the piece changed. It was breathtaking—the Mahler and Sesha's response to it.

NOTES

1. Two other examples of a questionable institutionalization were Junius Wilson and John Doe No. 24. In 1916, officials placed Wilson in the North Carolina School for Colored Deaf and Blind in Raleigh. During his six year at the facility, he received almost no formal education. In 1922, he returned to Castle Hayne, his hometown

near Wilmington, where a few years later he was accused of rape. The circumstances of the rape accusations were unclear; nevertheless, in 1925, a local court declared him insane and feebleminded and ordered him sent to the Hospital for Colored Insane in Goldsboro where, in 1932, hospital officials surgically castrated him. He remained in the facility until 1992. His only disability was his deafness (Burch and Joyner 2007). John Doe No. 24 was also deaf. In 1945, police in Jacksonville, Illinois, found the nameless man wandering the streets. Shortly thereafter, officials sent the man to the Lincoln State School and Colony where institutional authorities labeled him John Doe. After his death in 1993, Mary Chapin Carpenter's song, "John Doe No. 24," made him famous in death (Bakke 2000).

2. On eugenics, assessment, and the Illinois commitment laws at the time of Darger's placement in the Illinois asylum, see Michael A. Rembis (2004).

3. The 2014 Minnesota study (S. Larson et al. 2014, 7) estimates that the total population—reported and not reported—was about 6,000 individuals larger, for a total of 28,146 residents.

4. There is limited evidence to suggest that private schools in the United States have not achieved this degree of integration because most private school simply refuse to accept intellectually disabled students or, for that matter, students with other disabilities.

5. I have changed the names of my friend and his sister to the fictitious names of Edward and Lois.

6. Even before Congress enacted the Fair Labor Standards Act in 1938, some residential institutions had developed workshops, usually in communities adjacent to the institution. The first opened in Massachusetts a century earlier. In the early 1840s, Samuel G. Howe founded a workshop for some of his blind students who had graduated from the Perkins Institution but had been unsuccessful in finding gainful community employee. After Howe opened the Massachusetts School for Idiotic Youth in 1848, he would add some intellectually disabled graduates of the school to the workshop. Howe reluctantly opened this workshop as an alternatives to community-based employment, wishing instead that his students would find gainful work in their own community (J. Trent 2012, 65–66).

7. Many citizens of the state knew that the Eugenics Board existed, and they may well have read the leaflets produced in the late 1940s and early 1950s by the North Carolina Human Betterment League. These leaflets were distributed to individual citizens throughout the state, and they were made available in the offices of physicians, hospitals, and public health facilities. However, the work and daily operations of the Eugenics Board were not usually reported on by leading newspapers in the state.

8. The North Carolina General Assembly created the Eugenics Board at the same time as Erskine Caldwell's novels *Tobacco Road* (1932) and *God's Little Acre* (1933) began drawing the interest of the nation's and the state's progressives. Although set in Georgia, the novels represented the plight and struggles of the South's desperate poor. Caldwell saw eugenics as a means of dealing with the apparently intractable problems that poverty spawned (Keely 2002; Lancaster 2007).

9. The names of the members of the North Carolina Human Betterment League are on lists (some dated and some not dated) that are in the records of the League in the Wilson Library at the University of North Carolina–Chapel Hill (Human Betterment League 2008) Most of these lists contain names from membership rolls of the 1960s and 1970s, but some are older. Most of the names of these North Carolinians appear on several lists, making them members for multiple years. Some

of the members, in addition to paying annual dues, contributed additional annual funds for the League's operations. Often their contributions to the League are noted in its membership lists. Although some of these names represented members whose positions on social and economic issues linked them to political conservatives, many members identified themselves as liberals. Human Betterment League members included Mary D. B. T. Semans, George Watts Hill, Ellen Winston, Gordon W. Blackwell, Alice S. Gray, H. C. Bradshaw, Eugene A. Hargrove, Charles H. Hendricks, Harold O. Goodman, Arthur M. Jordan, and John W. Davis III.

10. Gamble's 1947 poem, "The Lucky Morons," may be found in Schaffer (2014, 94–95) at http://digitalcommons.bard.edu/cgi/viewcontent.cgi?article=1082&context=sen proj_s2014.

11. Johanna Schoen, whose excellent book on the history of eugenic sterilization in North Carolina is the definitive work on the topic, is nevertheless far too enamored of Kuralt as a result of her 1993 interview with the welfare director. County and Eugenic Board records fail to back up Kuralt's claim that the 403 sterilizations under his directorship were mostly voluntary.

12. Most of these North Carolina social workers were women. On the role of women in the eugenics movement in the South, see Edward J. Larson (1995*b*).

13. For more information, pro and con, on the attenuated growth procedure, see the several articles on the topic in the first issue of the 2010 edition of *The American Journal of Bioethics* and Bersani (2007*a*).

Epilogue

On Suffering Fools Gladly

For ye suffer fools [*idios*] gladly, seeing ye yourselves are wise.
St. Paul, *2 Corinthians 11:19*

In the spring of 1991, now more than twenty years ago, I toured for the first time the Lincoln (Illinois) Development Center, the institution whose history I had already come to know intimately. Two parts of the tour have remained most prominent in my thinking, showing how complicated such a simple story of progress really is.

First, I spent well over an hour walking through the old administration building of the facility. The oldest structure on the grounds, "the Main," was built in 1877, and, for the next decade, this building constituted all there was of the Illinois School. Here, the superintendent, Charles Wilbur, his family, most of his staff, and the institution's inmates lived, worked, and were educated together. From Chicago and East St. Louis, from Moline and Decatur, intellectually disabled children came to learn and, if their relatives and communities would take them back, to renew the lives they had left. Unused by residents for nearly twenty years and by the administration for more than ten, the building in 1991 had been left in disrepair, awaiting legislative appropriations for its demolition. Stepping over chips of paint and fallen plaster, rotten floors, and vermin decaying on stairways, I made my way to the large dayrooms on each of the three stories (one was the room shown in Figure I.2 in the Introduction). Knowing Charles Wilbur's initial hopes and later frustrations, and his enduring affection for what he had built at Lincoln, I felt an unexpected sadness at the building's condition and fate.

My second vivid memory was of a drive out to what had been the institution's farm colonies. Created in the 1920s and modeled after those of Charles Bernstein in New York, the Lincoln farms had, by the 1930s, become concentrated in one location about two miles southeast of the institution's main "campus." There, the institution began to build "cottages" for the inmates who supplied most of its produce, dairy products, and meat. By the early 1950s, when Lincoln was the largest facility of its kind in the nation, the farm colonies had become "the colony," an institution within an institution. By then, only a minority of the nearly 2,000 colony inmates actually worked the 1,300 acres under cultivation; most were there to relieve crowding on the main campus. Soon, even the farm colony with its row after row of "cottages" had its own crowding problems.

Near the farm colony were the institution's graves. In these hundreds of graves lay the last vestige of the farm colony (see also Corcoran 1991). In the early 1980s, the state of Illinois converted the farm colony cottages into a medium-security prison and next to it built a minimum-security prison as well. My tour guides on the staff of the Development Center commented, only half-jokingly, that the closing of the state school had merely shifted the venue of incarceration: many of the prison's inmates would in earlier times have been inmates of the state school. Begun as a stepping stone "back to the community," the farm colony had become a containment site, first for feeble minds and now for wrongdoers. Through the 1990s and into the first decades of the twentieth-first century, this conversion has only increased (Parsons 2011).

Both the elimination of structures (like "the Main") and the changes in their function from one form of incarceration to another can serve as symbols for contemporary shifts in our treatment of people we label intellectually disabled. Put simply, we have been more successful in correcting the horrors of the state institutions than we have in developing humane alternatives in American cities and towns.

To be sure, over the past four decades the focus of intellectual disability has shifted to the community. In 1973, with the stroke of a pen, the American Association on Mental Deficiency changed the criterion for "mental retardation" from one to two standard deviations below the IQ norm (R. Cooper 2014; Grossman 1973; see also Mercer 1972*b*). In that year, too, civil libertarian interest in closing institutions converged with state interest in reducing expenses. As the change in definition accompanied changes in consciousness and funding, many people in the 1970s, 1980s, and 1990s who had been officially considered intellectually disabled were, by the end of the century, freed from the label and from the accompanying structures of state control. Even the label "mental retardation" by the first decade of the new century became unacceptable, soon replaced by the latest label, "intellectual disability."

At the same time, in state after state, these people often lost services they had enjoyed. For many, the loss of the label and the services was a good thing. The label and even the services had only stood in their way; freed from them, as Edgerton and Bercovici (1976) showed in the 1970 and many others have shown since (e.g., G. Dybwad and Bersani 1996, D. Ferguson, Ferguson, and Wehmeyer 2013), they could blend into the day-to-day life of communities. For others, however, things did not go so well. No better, that is, than for some individuals not burdened with the labels of mental retardation and intellectual disability. Many people, "normal" and "disabled" alike, live their lives more among "the lonely crowd" than in what we almost euphemistically call "community." Not surprisingly, some people once labeled mentally retarded have had trouble integrating into "normal" patterns of community life. Some have thrived in new and exciting living arrangements; others, as we saw in Chapters 7 and 8, have been reinstitutionalized in "community institutions" operated not by the state but by various nonprofit and for-profit organizations; still others have also been reinstitutionalized, this time in jails and prisons.

How can the history of intellectual disability in the United States help us better understand this dilemma, and what can it suggest for the future? Let me suggest three themes I have found woven through this history.

First, I have argued that superintendents, with the assistance of social welfare authorities, closely linked the care and control of people labeled intellectually disabled. Especially in institutions but also in special-education classes and schools, care and control, rather than being in tension, complemented each other. In the name of care, superintendents developed teaching facilities and then turned them into custodial institutions. Increasingly depending on the language, tools, and procedures of medicine, these officials absorbed growing numbers of clientele into their sphere of authority. As they did so, they devised ways to carry out efficiently the complex requirements of care. Never opposed to growth, they found in the control of "high-grade" moral imbeciles, fallen women, and defective delinquents a way of ensuring care for "low grades" at a reasonable cost to the state. As their populations grew beyond even their own expectations after World War I, they began to be attracted to "the community" where trained, well-behaved, and often sterilized high-functioning inmates could be paroled and eventually discharged, thus making space available for new clientele. To be sure, the Great Depression and World War II frustrated their experiment in community placement, and new demands and increased state control over the administration of their facilities led to the growth of their facilities in the 1950s and 1960s. By the 1970s, institutional control had become part of a rationalized set of administrative policies and procedures promulgated increasingly by federal resources and regulations.

It would be wrong to see in the care given to intellectually disabled people a conspiracy of control. Most superintendents believed they were helping people and families whose lives had been damaged. Often their efforts were vitiated by factors beyond their immediate control. Samuel Howe and Hervey Wilbur were sincere when they advocated against custodial institutions for their pupils. Charles Wilbur and W. H. C. Smith expressed honest emotions when they wrote each other remembering with affection the inmates they had known. When Wilbur wrote Smith in 1909, his private doubts hardly reflected conspiracy; there had been, he confessed, unintended consequences of a policy that he had earlier supported (Beverly Farm Records, 1909).

Yet it would also be naïve to see benign intent in their interest in caring for more and more intellectually disabled people in larger and larger facilities in more and more states, in their call for the total segregation of feeble minds and in their near hysterical warnings about the menace of the feebleminded. Likewise, it would be wrong to ignore their cultivation of elites like Mary Averell Harriman and Samuel Fels and later for elites like James G. Hanes and Clarence Gamble who cultivated them. For their efforts, they created professional legitimacy and personal privilege, in many cases winning authority over their institutions for many decades. What they could not control, of course, were changes in the fabric of the nation—economic hard times, wars, centralization of state authority. Nevertheless, many of them learned to manipulate their institutions in ways that would likely maintain and expand their professional and personal influence. Until the Great Depression (and in some cases, beyond), they were successful more often than not. The care that they gave people whom they labeled intellectually disabled, then, was never separated from, nor incompatible with, the personal and professional legitimacy that the control over these same people brought them.

My reading of the history of sterilization policy can serve as an example of this linkage. As I argued in Chapter 6, superintendents justified their support for and use of sterilization quite apart from any purely medical or technical purpose. At first, castration served as a way to control sexual behavior that deviated from the norms of the well-ordered institution and thus protected the institution from embarrassment occasioned by visitors' observation of that behavior. It maintained the internal integrity of the smoothly functioning institution and provided "damage control" for the institution's relationships with the world outside. Later, as these same professionals became involved in the eugenics movement, they promoted sterilization, especially vasectomies and tubal ligations, as part of their response to the menace of the feebleminded, a menace they created and sustained.

Behind their involvement, as we have seen, was their desire to enlarge existing institutions and create new ones. In 1927, after many superintendents had abandoned their earlier enthusiasm for sterilization, the Supreme Court provided the legal authority to sterilize intellectually disabled people. Ironically, much of the impetus for sterilization generated by the eugenics movement was on the wane, and superintendents had little involvement in the Court's decision. After 1927, however, taking up where they left off, superintendents formulated a new reason for sterilization. In growing institutions, whose populations began to increase rapidly after the advent of the Great Depression, superintendents saw in sterilization a linkage with parole. If sterilized inmates could be paroled, superintendents could safely integrate them into communities, making room in the process for new inmates. In the end, the Supreme Court provided the authority and the Great Depression the incentive for a new rationale for sterilization. The control of particular intellectually disabled people through the technological tool of sterilization, then, developed out of complex institutional and sociopolitical factors. Superintendents could not shape the parameters of either, but, in their individual institutions and professional associations, they constructed sterilization to fit their need for legitimacy and institutional stability in the context of what they saw as social and political demands and constraints.[1]

When he wrote about controlling feeblemindedness in 1924, the sociologist Stanley P. Davies used the idea of social control in a way quite different from the meaning applied to the idea beginning in the 1960s. For Davies and his contemporaries, drawing on a tradition begun by E. A. Ross, socially controlling intellectually disabled people meant providing a social context for their proper adaptation and adjustment to the social world of the institution or the special classroom and to the larger world of the community where, if their adjustment was successful, they might return. Implied in Davies's use of the expression, social control was the rational socialization of intellectually disabled people into the norms of smoothly functioning communities where they could become part of the well-ordered fabric of American life. The term thus seemed innocent of larger pertinent issues and ideologies, but this innocence was belied by the special interest taken in intellectual disability by American moneyed elites in the decades before and after World War I. Despite superficial differences (for example, between old-moneyed Republicans like Harriman and new-moneyed Democrats like Fels), these elites saw feeblemindedness as a threat to a vision of order and stability that they were interested in preserving. At the same time, among the professional class, self-proclaimed conservatives like Henry Goddard and Charles Davenport and progressives like Alexander Johnson were united both in linking feeblemindedness to eugenics and in using the elites' largess to enlarge their own professional territory. The history of the social control of people labeled intellectually disabled has thus had much larger professional and political implications than could be seen either in Davies's restricted usage or in the narrow political differences of other interested parties.

A second theme that has emerged in the history of intellectual disability is the reliance on particularistic and technical ways of understanding and dealing with the problem. By "particularistic" I mean the tendency to analyze the problem of intellectual disability into ever smaller pieces that can be more easily isolated and manipulated. Thus, a particular group of people like those labeled intellectually disabled are removed from the general social and economic context; categories of learning deficiency or social friction are differentiated and refined; particular techniques are then devised for intervening at particular physical, behavioral, or cognitive points. Certainly, particular people with intellectual limitations have particular needs that require careful study and, in many cases, involve technical problems of classroom practice, medical treatment, and living arrangements. In the history of intellectual disability, however, there has been an almost obsessive concern with the particularistic and the technical. If we can wake dormant senses from their lethargy, open the sutures of skulls to allow brains to expand, find the flawed chromosome, isolate and measure intelligence and social adaptation, refine educational technology, or condition people to behave acceptably, perhaps then we can better care and control the thing—which ironically enough we have labeled a no-thing—that is "mindlessness."

The problem with this focus in the history of intellectual disability is that it has kept our gaze on the person labeled intellectually disabled. In so doing, research questions and policy formulations have almost always placed the burden of change on the disabled person. It is her medical-pathological flaw that must be understood, his intelligence measured, her behavior modified, or his social maladjustment reshaped. None would argue that there are no needs particular to some people with intellectual disability. Yet most needs of people labeled intellectually disabled are the same as those of people not labeled intellectually disabled: meaningful work and economic security, fulfilling personal and community relations, dignity and a measure of control over one's own life. By restricting the gaze to the person with "it," issues of the maldistribution of resources, status, and power so prominent in the history of the lives of most intellectually disabled (and intellectually abled) people remain muted.

Thus, what is striking today in reviewing Edward Seguin's system of physiological education is how little fundamental educational innovation has occurred since his time. Although educators have refined his procedures and developed new techniques, much of what he devised remains current, even if the language he used has changed. Even the well-intended principle of normalization formulated by Wolfensberger (1972) to train intellectually disabled people "to live in normal community settings," despite its revolutionary importance in alerting the public to the repressive nature of institutions, suffers from its narrow focus on intellectually disabled people and their immediate environments. The weight of normalization has remained on fine-tuning the deviant person to make her or him more "normal" in his or her "normal" immediate environment; the good health of the "community" has uncritically been taken as a given.[2]

The use of operant conditioning, which behaviorists first employed on pigeons and then perfected on institutionalized disabled people, is an example of this particularistic and technical way of dealing with "problems" of intellectual disability. Beginning in the 1960s, behavioral psychologists began to compete with cognitive, IQ-testing psychologists for an alternative way of inventing the feeble mind. From token economies set up to reward "appropriate" behaviors, to aversive electric shock "therapy" devised to suppress "inappropriate" behaviors—all often in the settings of the institutions' back wards—these psychologists experimented with operant conditioning while also focusing "the problem" of intellectual disability on the person with the condition. With the advent of deinstitutionalization, this focus transferred to the community, where community living was often grounded in the behaviorists' paradigm of proper behavior.

Third, this focus on technical and particularistic approaches to intellectual disability has blinded us to another dimension of the larger context. In a nation where economic vulnerability is a consistent if unacknowledged part of everyday life, Americans with intellectual disability are especially vulnerable. This vulnerability has persisted through the American history of the disability. It was the economic and social change brought on by a depression and civil war that frustrated the expectations and efforts of Hervey Wilbur, Samuel G. Howe, Henry Knight, and James Richards. In the 1840s and 1850s, the remarkable success they claimed even among their most disabled clientele was confirmed by parents, neighbors, and public officials. They began to modify these claims only after their pupils, especially pupils from working-class parents, could not find community employment. With the next generation of superintendents, a mythology of the uneducability of intellectually disabled people for community life began to grow and be believed. For nearly a century, people who were quite capable of working for a living were sequestered in public facilities where their work and their lives were controlled by the state. During the history of this incarceration, their vulnerability was constructed first as a *burden* for their parents and community and second as a *menace* to the fundamental social fabric. In publicly financed institutions, intellectually disabled workers would neither burden their family nor pollute the national gene pool; they could stay out of trouble and their work could help in the care of minds believed to be even weaker than their own. For a hundred years, this construction of meaning about intellectual disability, despite various modifications, seemed to virtually all actors to work.

In social and economic good times, the contours of control could afford to appear progressive and enlightened. During the 1920s, when employment opportunities were for a time plentiful, superintendents who only a few years earlier had warned of the menacing moron were ready for nearly a decade to send sterilized morons back into the community. The Great Depression and subsequent world war put an end to the progress. In bad times, the meaning of intellectual disability entailed incarceration.

In the late 1960s, the principal locus of incarceration appeared to be a "Christmas in Purgatory." The rapid and continuous growth of state schools over the previous twenty years began to strain the budgets of several "flagship" states like New York, Pennsylvania, Illinois, and California. In response, the 1970s saw a period of de-institutionalization similar to that of the 1920s, except that institutions in the 1970s could not add new residents to make up for discharged clientele. The principal scheme for making the large institution economically self-supporting was no longer feasible because federal courts had declared unpaid or underpaid inmate labor to be involuntary servitude. Unable to work the institutional farm or care for lower functioning residents, many institutionalized intellectually disabled people, like many other Americans before them, joined in the exodus of rural America to new urban centers. Many left for private profit-making or private nonprofit urban group homes, intermediate care facilities/mental retardation (ICF/MRs), nursing homes, family-care facilities, and foster homes; others found ways of blending into the wash of urban America.

Across the nation, professionals stressed "normalization" in living arrangements, work, and personal relations, and many people previously labeled "mentally retarded" met these new challenges successfully (e.g., Gollay et al. 1978, 127–135; Janicki, Krauss, and Seltzer 1988). Once institutionalized residents have married, had children, and joined local neighborhoods and voluntary associations. Some have found work,[3] many others receive financial and emotional support from family and friends. Since the early 1980s, many have become involved in the self-advocacy movement (Biklen 1988; G. Dybwad 1989; G. Dybwad and Bersani 1996; Ferguson et al. 2008). On television, in local restaurants, in neighborhood groceries, it has become a familiar sight to see people working who most of us once labeled mentally retarded. Many of us have gotten to know them and have developed close friendships with them.

Their work, however, as it has been since the late 1850s, is quite vulnerable to economic change. As Gunnar Dybwad (1990), a national authority on intellectual disability, remarked, rooted even in the most successful examples of deinstitutionalization is the problem of employment and work. Supporting Dybwad's observation, Gollay et al. (1978, 149–153; see also Hoffman 2013; Rusch and Dattilo 2012) found that intellectually disabled people's dissatisfaction with work (or, in some cases, lack of work) was a major factor in their dissatisfaction with community living. In a society whose economic arrangements leave many Americans vulnerable, intellectually disabled people are especially susceptible to economic fluctuation. And with that vulnerability, there lurk social constructions of reality that manipulate and even hide the association of meaning and vulnerability. In the 1980s, when the Philip Becker case drew headlines around the country, few recognized that most commentators, even as they quite rightly stressed the moral implications of the case, failed to acknowledge that it was Philip Becker's worth that was being debated. Was Philip Becker worth keeping alive? Nearly two decades later, on an April 2012 television episode of the *Dr. Phil* show, psychologist Phil McGraw portrayed the story of a mother with two adult children with Sanfilippo syndrome, a rare genetic condition that includes physical and intellectual limitations along with behavioral disturbances. The clear message of the show was that "merciful killing" was a valid outcome for such conditions. In a society where economic worth and productive capability shape the meaning given to human beings, there will continue to be some who remain vulnerable, even when the contours of vulnerability change over history (G. Dybwad 1983; see also Herr 1984; Shearer 1984).

Only a few decades ago, authorities in intellectual disability studies tended to debate deinstitutionalization as an issue of institution versus community. In this framework, criticism of one, more often than not, indicated support for the other. Appeals to science tended to come from champions of the institution and appeals to morality from champions of the community. The former accused the latter of being too ideological, and the latter suggested the former lacked common sense (see, e.g., Bruinicks 1990; Krauss 1990; Landesman and Butterfield 1987; Zigler, Hodapp, and Edison 1990).

What was usually missing from these otherwise thoughtful and informative debates was a recognition that, in a society that defines and confines all meaning and worth in terms of production, profit, and pervasive greed, intellectually disabled people will likely be exploited. In this macrosociological context, even the most vigilant advocates, whether in institutions or communities, cannot stop the exploitation. The debate, if it is to free itself from "either . . . or," must look beyond the locus of services to the content of production and to the place of disabled people in that content. Thus reframed, the issue of place becomes not just a matter of location, but also a matter of production. Thus, one can imagine that, in a world where the definition and value of human beings are not based on their productive capabilities, intellectually disabled people would be participating members of, for example, a boarding school or a kibbutz-like settlement, either of which would resemble an institution. At the same time, one could imagine in such a world intellectually disabled people who live alone in apartments but who have close circles of friends, all of whom also live alone but share with each other common time and experiences. Likewise, we know (we do not have to imagine) that both institutions and communities can be inhumane and exploitive; each mirrors the world around us. A return to Christmas-in-Purgatory institutions is in the interest of no disabled citizen; nor is it in the interest of any citizen to return to the modern equivalent of county poorhouses, local jails, and outdoor relief.

History cannot predict the future. What it can provide are touchstones—memories and visions of what was and what might have been. The future of intellectual disability must move beyond its focus on the intellectually disabled person and begin to look at intellectual ability, at the constructors of intellectual disability and their relationship to "screens of ideology" that link their constructions to the world of resources, status, and power and that hide intellectually disabled persons themselves. In this future, the problem of intellectual disability will be seen as the problem of intellectual ability or what I once called "mental acceleration," with all the threat and the magnificent promise that this implies.

NOTES

1. Most interest in intellectual disability from a social constructionist outlook (an interest I also share) has remained focused on the interaction of the constructors and the constructed (Bogdan and Taylor 1982, 1989, 1994; Dexter 1960*a*, 1960*b*, 1964; Edgerton 1967; Edgerton and Bercovici 1976; Ferguson 1987; Mercer 1973; Perry 1966). This focus is appropriate but limited.

   In his subtle and sophisticated study of juvenile delinquency in the United States, Sutton (1988, 3–5) "explores both systemic and entrepreneurial influences on American strategies of child control." But he also stresses that this dual-focused content of reform remained in a historically limited framework. He writes, "The logic of reform is historical: reformers in each generation worked from a set of assumptions inherited from the generation before and sought to achieve their own local interests within those assumptions." Thus, for Sutton, systemic and entrepreneurial influences by themselves cannot explain the content of reform.

   By emphasizing this point, Sutton suggests (perhaps a bit unfairly) that theories of social control that emphasize "system imperatives" or "reform entrepreneurs" are necessarily incompatible or that both are unappreciative of the historical impact of local interests on the one hand or competing institutional and political tensions on the other. I should also add that this distinction is related to the debate between "strict constructionists" and "contextual constructionists" (see note 2 in the Introduction). Also see the provocative take on intellectual disability and social constructionism in Rapley (2004).

2. For another reinterpretation of normalization from one of its American originators, see G. Dybwad 1982.

3. Craig and Boyd (1990) have shown that most intellectually disabled people who have jobs work in private and public services and in transportation.

REFERENCES

Abeson, Alan. 1977. "Legal Change for the Handicapped through Litigation." Pp. 351–389 in *An Alternative Textbook in Special Education: People, Schools, and Other Institutions*, edited by B. Blatt, D. Biklin, and R. Bogdan. Denver, CO: Love Publishing.

Academy of Achievement. 1996. "Interview: Charles Kuralt, Life on the Road." Retrieved September 29, 2015 (http://www.achievement.org/autodoc/print-member/kur0int-1).

Adams, Rachel. 2001. *Sideshow USA.: Freaks and the American Cultural Imagination*. Chicago: University Chicago Press.

Adams, Rachel. 2013. *Raising Henry: A Memoir of Motherhood, Disability, and Discovery*. New Haven, CT: Yale University Press.

Adams, Susan. 2013. "Does Goodwill Industries Exploit Disabled Workers?" *Forbes* July 30. Retrieved August 3, 2015 (http://www.forbes.com/sites/susanadams/2013/07/30/does-goodwill-industries-exploit-disabled-workers/).

Addams, Jane. 1910. "The President's Address: Charity and Social Justice." *Proceedings of the National Conference of Charities and Correction*, 1–18.

Allen, Garland E. 1975. "Genetics, Eugenics, and Class Struggle." *Genetics* 79:29–45.

Allen, Garland E. 1986. "The Eugenics Record Office at Cold Spring Harbor, 1910–1940: An Essay in Institutional History." *Osiris* 2(2d ser.):225–264.

American Association for the Study of the Feeble-Minded. 1905. "Discussion." *Journal of Psycho-Asthenics* 9:108–110.

American Association for the Study of the Feeble-Minded. 1910. "Minutes." *Journal of Psycho-Asthenics* 14:131–149.

American Association for the Study of the Feeble-Minded. 1913. "Minutes of the Association." *Journal of Psycho-Asthenics* 18:46–62.

American Association for the Study of the Feeble-Minded. 1917. "Minutes." *Journal of Psycho-Asthenics* 22:39.

American Association for the Study of the Feeble-Minded. 1918. "Discussion" [of A. W. Wilmarth's "The Practical Working Out of Sterilization"]. *Journal of Psycho-Asthenics* 23:28.

American Association for the Study of the Feeble-Minded. 1924. "Incomplete List of State and Private Institutions." *Proceedings and Minutes of the Association*, 365–373.

American Association for the Study of the Feeble-Minded. 1930. "Minutes of the Association." *Journal of Psycho-Asthenics* 35:260.

American Association on Mental Deficiency. 1933. "Business Sessions." *Proceedings and Addresses of the Association*, 381–421.

American Association on Mental Deficiency. 1934a. "Discussion" [of Mabel Ann Matthews's 'Some Effects of the Depression on Social Work with the Feebleminded']. *Proceedings and Addresses of the Association*, 52.

American Association on Mental Deficiency. 1934*b*. "Discussion" [of Lloyd Yepsen's 'Newer Trends in the Rehabilitation of the Mentally Deficient']. *Proceedings and Addresses of the Association*, 112–113.

American Association on Mental Deficiency. 1934*c*. "Discussion" [of L. Potter Harshman's 'Medical and Legal Aspects of Sterilization in Indiana']. *Proceedings and Addresses of the Association*, 203.

American Association on Mental Deficiency. 1965. *Directory of Residential Facilities for the Mentally Retarded*. Washington, DC: American Association on Mental Deficiency.

American Psychiatric Association. 1952. *Diagnostic and Statistical Manual: Mental Disorders*. Washington, DC: American Psychiatric Association.

American Sunday School Union. ca. 1840. "The Idiot." In *Children's Books*, vol. 14, n.p. Philadelphia: American Sunday School Union.

Amesbury Villager. 1851. "Letters." From Jacob Rowells and John Greenleaf Whittier to Samuel G. Howe, 6 March.

Amoros y Ondeano, Francisco. 1834. *Manuel de l'éducation physique, gymnastique et morale*. Paris: Roret.

Amoros y Ondeano, Francisco. 1848. *De l'éducation physique, gymnastique et morale*. Paris: Roret.

Andrews, Suzanna. 2007. "Arthur Miller's Missing Act." *Vanity Fair*. Retrieved February 9, 2016 (http://www.vanityfair.com/culture/2007/09/miller200709).

Angell, Stephen L., Jr. 1944. "Training Schools – And CPS." *Reporter* 3(July 15):3–5.

ARC. 2012. "Employment Issues of People with Disabilities." Retrieved May 23, 2015 (http://www.thearc.org/FINDS).

Arnold, G. B. 1938. "A Brief Review of the First Thousand Patients Eugenically Sterilized at the State Colony for Epileptics and Feebleminded." *Proceedings of the American Association on Mental Deficiency* 43:56–63.

Association of Medical Officers of American Institutions for Idiotic and Feeble-Minded Persons. 1877. *Proceedings, 1876*.

Association of Medical Officers of American Institutions for Idiotic and Feeble-Minded Persons. 1892. *Proceedings, 1892*.

Association of Medical Officers of American Institutions for Idiotic and Feeble-Minded Persons. 1897. *Proceedings, 1895*.

Atkinson, William B. 1880. "Edouard Seguin." Pp. 252–253 in *A Biographical Dictionary of Contemporary American Physicians and Surgeons*, 2d ed. Philadelphia: Brinton.

Axinn, June, and Herman Levin. 1982. *Social Welfare: A History of the American Response to Need*. New York: Longman.

Bagatell, Nancy. 2010. "From Cure to Community: Transforming Notions of Autism." *Ethos* 38:33–55.

Bagley, William. 1924. "The Army Tests and the Proto-Nordic Propaganda." *Educational Review* 67:179–186.

Baker, Benjamin W. 1927. "Address of the President of the Association." *Proceedings and Addresses of the American Association for the Study of the Feeble-Minded*, 169–178.

Bakke, Dave. 2000. *God Knows His Name: The True Story of John Doe No. 24*. Carbondale and Edwardsville: Southern Illinois University Press.

Bank-Mikkelsen, Niels Erik. 1969. "A Metropolitan Area in Denmark: Copenhagen." Pp. 227–254 in *Changing Patterns of Residential Services for the Mentally Retarded*, edited by R. Kugel and W. Wolfensberger. Washington, DC: President's Committee on Mental Retardation.

Barbetta, Pietro, Andree Bella, and Enrico Valtellina. 2014. "The Complete Idiot's Guide to Idiocy. Or, What 'Oligophrenia' Tells Us." *Trauma and Memory* 2(2):57–66.

Barker, David. 1983. "How to Curb the Fertility of the Unfit: The Feebleminded in Edwardian Britain." *Oxford Review of Education* 9:197–211.

Barker, David. 1989. "The Biology of Stupidity: Genetics, Eugenics, and Mental Deficiency in the Inter-War Years." *British Journal of the History of Science* 22:347–375.

Barr, Martin W. 1892. *Cerebral Meningitis: Its History, Diagnosis, Prognosis, and Treatment.* Detroit, MI: George S. Davis.

Barr, Martin W. 1897. "President's Annual Address." *Journal of Psycho-Asthenics* 2:1–13.

Barr, Martin W. 1898. "Defective Children: Their Needs and Their Rights." *International Journal of Ethics* 8(July):481–490.

Barr, Martin W. 1899. "The How, the Why, and the Wherefore of the Training of Feeble-Minded Children." *Journal of Psycho-Asthenics* 4:204–212.

Barr, Martin W. 1902a. "The Imbecile and Epileptic versus the Tax-Payer and the Community." *Proceedings of the National Conference of Charities and Correction,* 161–165.

Barr, Martin W. 1902b. "The Imperative Call of Our Present to Our Future." *Journal of Psycho-Asthenics* 7:5–8.

Barr, Martin W. 1904a. *Mental Defectives: Their History, Treatment, and Training.* Philadelphia: Blakiston Press.

Barr, Martin W. 1904b. "What Can Teachers of Normal Children Learn from the Teachers of Defectives." *Journal of Psycho-Asthenics* 8:55–59.

Barr, Martin W. 1934. "A Brief Review of the Life of Isaac Newton Kerlin." *Proceedings and Addresses of the American Association on Mental Deficiency,* 144–150.

Barrick, Mac E. 1980. "The Helen Keller Joke Cycle." *Journal of American Folklore* 93:441–449.

Bass, Jack. 1993. *Taming the Storm: The Life and Times of Judge Frank M. Johnson, Jr. and the South's Fight over Civil Rights.* New York: Doubleday.

Bateman, Newton, Paul Selby, and J. Seymour Currey. 1920. *Historical Encyclopedia of Illinois,* vol. 1. Chicago: Munsell.

Baughman, Ernest W. 1943. "'Little Moron' Studies." Pp. 17–18 in *Hoosier Folklore Bulletin,* edited by H. Halpert, vol. 2. Bloomington, IN: Hoosier Folklore Society.

Beeghley, Leonard, and Edgar W. Butler. 1974. "The Consequences of Intelligence Testing in Public Schools before and after Desegregation." *Social Problems* 21(June):740–754.

Beers, Clifford W. 1908. *A Mind That Found Itself.* New York: Longmans, Green.

Begos, Kevin, Danielle Deaver, Jon Railey, and Scott Sexton. 2013. *Against Their Will: North Carolina's Sterilization Program and the Campaign for Reparations.* Apalachicola, FL: Gray Oak Books.

Bellingham, Bruce. 1986. "Institution and Family: An Alternative View of Nineteenth-Century Child Saving." *Social Problems* 33:S33–S57.

Ben-Moshe, Liat. 2013. "Disabling Incarceration: Connecting Disability to Divergent Confinements in the USA." *Critical Sociology* 39(3):385–403.

Berkowitz, Edward D. 1980. "The Politics of Mental Retardation during the Kennedy Administration." *Social Science Quarterly* 61:128–143.

Berkson, Gershon, and Sharon Landesman-Dwyer. 1977. "Behavioral Research on Severe and Profound Mental Retardation (1955–1974)." *American Journal of Mental Deficiency* 81:428–454.

Bernstein, Charles. 1907. "Training School for Attendants for the Feeble-Minded." *Journal of Psycho-Asthenics* 12:31–43, 88–92.

Bernstein, Charles. 1913. "Discussion." *Journal of Psycho-Asthenics* 18:39.

Bernstein, Charles. 1921. "Colony Care for Isolation Defective and Dependent Cases." *Journal of Psycho-Asthenics* 26:43–54.

"Bernstein Dies; Hospital Official." 1942. *New York Times,* 16 June, 46.

Bersani, Hank. 2007a. "Growth Attenuation: Unjustifiable Non-therapy." *Archives of Pediatrics and Adolescent Medicine,* 161(May):521–522.

Bersani, Hank. 2007b. "The Past is Prologue: 'MR,' Go Gentle Into That Good Night." *Intellectual and Developmental Disabilities* 45(December):399–404.

Bérubé, Michael. 1996. *Life as We Know It: A Father, a Family, and an Exceptional Child.* New York: Pantheon Books.

Bérubé, Michael. 2004. "Family Values." Pp. 494–500 in *Mental Retardation in America: A Historical Reader,* edited by S. Noll and J. W. Trent Jr. New York: New York University Press.

Best, Joel. 1989. "Extending the Constructionist Perspective: A Conclusion and an Introduction." Pp. 243–253 in *Typifying Contemporary Social Problems,* edited by J. Best. New York: Aldine de Gruyter.

Beverly Farm Records. 1885–1976. *Beverly Farm Papers* [unsorted letters, papers, documents, and photographs]. Lovejoy Library, Southern Illinois University at Edwardsville.

Beyer, Henry A. 2000. "Bulkeley: The Other Emerson." *Journal of Religion, Disability & Health* 4(1):81–85.

"The Bicêtre Asylum." 1848. *Westminster Review and Foreign Quarterly* 49:70–84.

Biesenbach, Klaus, ed. 2014. *Henry Darger.* Munich: Prestel.

Biklen, Douglas. 1977. "The Politics of Institutions." Pp. 29–84 in *An Alternative Textbook in Special Education: People, Schools, and Other Institutions,* edited by B. Blatt, D. Biklen, and R. Bogdan. Denver, CO: Love Publishing.

Biklen, Douglas. 1988. "Empowerment: Choices and Change." *TASH Newsletter* 14:6.

Binet, Alfred, and Theodore Simon. 1905a. "Application des méthodes nouvelles au diagnostic du niveau intellectuel chez des enfants normaux et anormaux d'hospice et d'école primaire." *L'année psychologique* 11:245–336.

Binet, Alfred, and Theodore Simon. 1905b. "Méthodes nouvelles pour le diagnostic du niveau intellectuel des anormaux." *L'année psychologique* 11:191–244.

Binet, Alfred, and Theodore Simon. 1905c. "Sur la nécessité d'un diagnostic scientifique des états inférieurs de l'intelligence." *L'année psychologique* 11:161–190.

Bining, Arthur C., and Thomas C. Cochran. 1964. *The Rise of American Economic Life.* 4th ed. New York: Charles Scribner's Sons.

Birnbrauer, J. S. 1968. "Generalization of Punishment Effects – A Case Study." *Journal of Applied Behavioral Analysis* 1(Fall):201–211.

Bix, Amy Sue. 1997. "Experiences and Voices of Eugenics Field-Workers: 'Women's Work' in Biology." *Social Studies of Science* 27(August):625–668.

Black, Edwin. 2003. *The War against the Weak: Eugenics and America's Campaign to Create a Master Race.* Expanded Edition. Westport, CTCT: Dialog Press.

Blatt, Burton. 1973. *Souls in Extremis: An Anthology on Victims and Victimizers.* Boston: Allyn and Bacon.

Blatt, Burton, and C. Mangel. 1967. "Tragedy and Hope of Retarded Children." *Look* 31(October 31):96–99.

Blatt, Burton, and Fred Kaplan. 1966. *Christmas in Purgatory: A Photographic Essay on Mental Retardation.* Boston: Allyn and Bacon.

Bledstein, Burton. 1976. *The Culture of Professionalism: The Middle Class and the Development of Higher Education in America.* New York: Norton.

Block, Pamela. 2000. "Sexuality, Fertility, and Danger: Twentieth-Century Images of Women with Cognitive Disabilities." *Sexuality and Disability* 18(4):239–254.

Bogdan, Robert. 1988. *Freak Show: Presenting Human Oddities for Amusement and Profit.* Chicago: University of Chicago Press.

Bogdan, Robert. 2014. "Race, Showmen, Disability and the Freak Show." Pp. 195–208 in *The Invention of Race: Scientific and Popular Representations of Race,* edited by N. Bancel, T. David and D. Thomas. New York: Routledge.

Bogdan, Robert, Elks, Martin, and Knoll, James A. 2012. *Picturing Disability: Beggar, Freak, Citizen, and Other Photographic Rhetoric.* Syracuse, NY: Syracuse University Press.

Bogdan, Robert, and Steven Taylor. 1982. *Inside Out: The Social Meaning of Mental Retardation.* Toronto: University of Toronto Press.

Bogdan, Robert, and Steven Taylor. 1989. "Relationships with Severely Disabled People: The Social Construction of Humanness." *Social Problems* 36:135–148.

Bogdan, Robert, and Steven Taylor. 1994. *The Social Meaning of Mental Retardation: Two Life Stories.* New York: Teachers College Press.

Bogdan, Robert, Steven Taylor, Bernard de Grandpre, and Sondra Haynes. 1974. "Attendants' Perspectives and Programming on Wards in State Schools." *Journal of Health and Social Behavior* 15:141–151.

Bogenschutz, Matthew D., Amy Hewitt, Derek Nord, and Renee Hepperlen. 2014. "Direct Support Workforce Supporting Individuals with IDD: Current Wages, Benefits, and Stability." *Intellectual & Developmental Disabilities* 52(October):317–329.

Boggs, Elizabeth. 1975. "Legal, Legislative, and Bureaucratic Factors Affecting Planned and Unplanned Change in the Delivery of Services to the Mentally Retarded." Pp. 441–458 in *The Mentally Retarded and Society,* edited by M. Begab and S. A. Richardson. Baltimore, MD: University Park Press.

Bosco, Ronald A., and Joel Myerson. 2005. *The Emerson Brothers: A Fraternal Biography in Letters.* New York: Oxford University Press.

Botkin, B. A. 1944. *A Treasury of American Folklore, Stories, Ballads, and Traditions of the People.* New York: Crown.

Bourneville, Desire Magloire. 1880. "Nécrologie: E. Séguin." *Archives de neurologie* 1:636–640.

Bourneville, Desire Magloire. 1895. *Assistance traitement et éducation des enfants idiots et dégénerés.* Paris: Bureaux du Progrès Médical.

Bowles, Samuel, and Herbert Gintis. 1976. *Schooling in Capitalist America: Educational Reform and the Contradiction of Economic Life.* New York: Basic Books.

Boyd, William. 1914. *From Locke to Montessori.* London: George G. Harrap.

Brace, Charles L. 1872. *The Dangerous Classes of New York and Twenty Years Work among Them.* New York: Wynkoop and Hallenbeck.

Brace, Charles L. 1880. "The Best Methods of Founding Children's Charities in Towns and Villages." *Proceedings of the National Conference of Charities and Correction,* 227–241.

Braddock, David L. 1987. *Federal Policy toward Mental Retardation and Developmental Disabilities.* Baltimore: Brookes.

Braddock, David L. 2007. "Washington Rises: Public Financial Support for Intellectual Disability in the United States, 1955–2004." *Mental Retardation and Developmental Disabilities Research Reviews* 13:169–177.

Braddock, David L, Richard Hemp, Glenn Fujiura, Lynn Bachelder, and Dale Mitchell. 1990. *The State of the States in Developmental Disabilities.* Baltimore: Brookes.

Braddock, David L., Richard E. Hemp, Mary C. Rizzolo, Emily Shea Tanis, Laura Haffer, and Jiang Wu. 2015. *The State of the States in Intellectual and Developmental Disabilities.* Washington, DC: American Association on Intellectual and Developmental Disabilities.

Bragar, Madeline C. 1977. *The Feeble-Minded Female: An Historical Analysis of Mental Retardation as a Social Definition, 1890-1920.* Ph.D. diss., Syracuse University, New York.

Braginsky, Dorothea, and Benjamin Braginsky. 1971. *Hansels and Gretels: Studies of Children in Institutions for the Mentally Retarded.* New York: Holt, Rinehart and Winston.

Brands, H.W. 2010. *American Colossus: The Triumph of Capitalism, 1865–1900.* New York: Doubleday.

Brigham, Carl C. 1923. *A Study of American Intelligence.* Princeton, NJ: Princeton University Press.

Brockett, Linus P. 1855. "Idiots and Institutions for Their Training." *American Journal of Education* 1:593–608.

Brockett, Linus P. 1856a. "Idiots and the Efforts for Their Improvement." In *Report of the Commissioners on Idiocy to the Legislature of the State of Connecticut, May, 1856.* New Haven, CT: Carrington and Hotchkiss.

Brockett, Linus P. 1856b. "Visit to the New York Asylum." In *Report of the Commissioners on Idiocy to the Legislature of the State of Connecticut, May, 1856,* Connecticut General Assembly. New Haven: Carrington and Hotchkiss.

Brockett, Linus P. 1858. "Cretins and Idiots: What Has Been and What Can Be Done for Them." *Atlantic Monthly* 1:410–419.

Brockett, Linus P. 1881. "Remarks by Dr. L. R. Brockett." *In Memory of Edouard Seguin, M.D.* Supplement to *Proceedings of the Association of Medical Officers of American Institutions for Idiotic and Feeble-Minded Persons,* 7–23.

Brockett, Linus P. 1882. "The Seguin Physiological School." *New York Times,* October 29, 5.

Brockley, Janice. 2004. "Rearing the Child Who Never Grew: Ideologies of Parenting and Intellectual Disability in American History." Pp. 130–164 in *Mental Retardation in America: A Historical Reader,* edited by S. Noll and J. W. Trent Jr. New York: New York University Press.

Brown, Catherine W. 1887. "The Future of the Educated Imbecile." *Proceedings of the Association of Medical Officers of American Institutions for Idiotic and Feeble-Minded Persons, 1886,* 401–406.

Brown, Catherine W. 1892. "In Memoriam, George Brown, M.D." *Proceedings of the Association of Medical Officers of American Institutions for Idiotic and Feeble-Minded Persons,* 267–273.

Brown, Catherine W. 1897. "Reminiscences." *Journal of Psycho-Asthenics* 1:134–140.

Brown, Elizabeth, and Sarah S. Genheimer. 1969. *Haven on the Neuse, A History of Caswell Center, Kinston, North Carolina, 1911–1964.* New York: Vantage Press.

Brown, George. 1884. "In Memory – Hervey B. Wilbur." *Proceedings of the Association of Medical Officers of American Institutions for Idiotic and Feeble-Minded Persons, 1884,* 291–295.

"Brown, George." 1929. Pp. 117–118 in *Dictionary of American Biography,* edited by Dumas Malone. New York: Charles Scribner's Sons.

Brown, JoAnne. 1992. *The Definition of a Profession: The Authority of Metaphor in the History of Intelligence Testing, 1890–1930.* Princeton, NJ: Princeton University Press.

Bruckner, Leona S. 1954. *Triumph of Love: An Unforgettable Story of the Power of Goodness.* New York: Simon and Schuster.

Bruininks, Robert H. 1990. "There Is More Than a Zip Code to Changes in Services." *American Journal of Mental Retardation* 96:13–15.

Bruinius, Harry. 2007. *Better for All the World: The Secret History of Forced Sterilization and America's Quest for Racial Purity.* New York: Vintage Books.

Bruno, Frank J. 1957. *Trends in Social Work, 1874–1956: A History Based on the Proceedings of the National Conference of Social Work*. New York: Columbia University Press.

Buck, Pearl S. 1950. *The Child Who Never Grew*. New York: John Day.

Bunyan, John. 1856. *The Pilgrim's Progress*. Hartford, CT: S. Andrus.

Burch, Susan and Hannah Joyner. 2007. *Unspeakable: The Story of Junius Wilson*. Chapel Hill: University of North Carolina Press.

Burke, Wylie, Beth Tarini, Nancy A. Press, and James P. Evans. 2011. "Genetic Screening." *Epidemiologic Reviews* 33(June):148–164.

"Burned Asylum." 1881. *Cleveland Herald*, 6 December, 1–2.

Burnham, John C. 1968. "The New Psychology: From Narcissism to Social Control." Pp. 351–398 in *Change and Continuity in Twentieth-Century America: The 1920s*, edited by J. Braemon, Robert H. B. and D. Brody. Columbus: Ohio State University Press.

Burrage, Walter L. 1923. *A History of the Massachusetts Medical Society, 1781–1922*. Norwood, MA: Plimpton Press.

Butler, Amos W. 1907. "The Burden of Feeble-Mindedness [President's Address]." *Proceedings of the National Conference of Charities and Correction*, 1–10.

Butler, Amos W. 1915. *The "C" Family*. Indianapolis: Indiana Academy of Science.

Butler, Amos W. 1923. "Some Families as Factors in Anti-Social Conditions." Pp. 387–390 in *The Second International Congress of Eugenics: Eugenics, Genetics, and the Family*, edited by H. H. Laughlin. Baltimore: Williams and Wilkins.

Butterfield, Earl C. 1976. "Some Basic Changes in Residential Facilities." Pp. 15–34 in *Changing Patterns in Residential Services for the Mentally Retarded*, edited by R. B. Kugel and A. Shearer. Washington, DC: President's Committee on Mental Retardation.

Byers, Joseph P. 1934. *The Village of Happiness: The Story of the Training School*. Vineland, NJ: Vineland Training School.

Caldwell, Erskine. 1932. *Tobacco Road*. New York: Grosset and Dunlap.

Caldwell, Erskine. 1933. God's Little Acre. New York: Grosset and Dunlap.

Caldwell, Joe, Katie K. Arnold, and Mary Kay Rizzolo. 2012. *Envisioning the Future: Allies in Self-Advocacy Final Report*. Chicago: University of Illinois at Chicago, Institute on Disability and Human Development.

Campbell, Persia. 1971. "Mary Williamson Averell Harriman." Pp. 140–142 in *Notable American Women, 1607–1950*, edited by E. T. James, vol. 2. Cambridge, MA: Belknap and Harvard Presses.

Cahn, Susan. 1998. "Spirited Youth or Fiends Incarnate: The Samarcand Arson Case and Female Adolescence in the American South." *Journal of Women's History* 9(Winter):152–180.

Caplan, Gerald. 1961. *An Approach to Community Mental Health*. New York: Grune and Stratton.

Carey, Allison C. 1998. "Gender and Compulsory Sterilization Programs in America, 1907–1950." *Journal of Historical Sociology* 11(March):74–105.

Carlson, Elof A. 1980. "R. L. Dugdale and the Jukes Family: A Historical Injustice Corrected." *Bioscience* 30:535–539.

Carlson, Licia. 2001. "Cognitive Ableism and Disability Studies: Feminist Reflections on the History of Mental Retardation." *Hypatia* 16(Fall):124–146.

Carlson, Licia. 2010. *The Faces of Intellectual Disability: Philosophical Reflections*. Bloomington and Indianapolis: Indiana University Press.

Carson, J. C. 1891a. "Presidential Address, 1889." *Proceedings of the Association of Medical Officers of American Institutions for Idiotic and Feeble-Minded Persons, 1889*, 12–17.

Carson, J. C. 1891b. "Report on New York, 1890." *Proceedings of the Association of Medical Officers of American Institutions for Idiotic and Feeble-Minded Persons, 1890*, 77–79.

Castel, Robert. 1988. *The Regulation of Madness: The Origins of Incarceration in France*. Translated by W. D. Hall. Berkeley and Los Angeles: University of California Press.

Castellani, Paul J. 2005. *From Snake Pit to Cash Cow: Politics and Public Institutions in New York*. Albany: State University of New York Press.

Castles, Katherine. 2002. "Quiet Eugenics: Sterilization in North Carolina's Institutions for the Mentally Retarded, 1945–1965." *Journal of Southern History*, 68(November):849–878.

Castles, Katherine. 2004. "'Nice, Average Americans': Postwar Parents' Groups and the Defense of the Normal Family." Pp. 351–370 in *Mental Retardation in America: A Historical Reader*, edited by S. Noll and J. W. Trent, Jr. New York: New York University Press.

Caswell Training School. 1926. *Report of the Committee on Caswell Training School in Its Relation to the Problem of Feebleminded of the State of North Carolina*. Raleigh: Capital Printing.

Cavalier, Albert R., and Ronald B. McCarver. 1981. "Wyatt v. Stickney and Mentally Retarded Individuals." *Mental Retardation* 19:209–214.

Cave, F. C. 1911. "Report of Sterilization in Kansas State Home for Feeble Minded." *Proceedings of the American Association for the Study of the Feeble-Minded*, 123–125.

Chace, Lydia G. 1904. "Public School Classes for Mentally Deficient Children." *Proceedings of the National Conference of Charities and Correction*, 390–401.

"Chamber of Commerce on Defective Immigrants." 1912. *Survey* 27:1824–1825.

Chamberlain, Houston S. 1911. *Foundations of the Nineteenth Century*. New York: John Lane.

"A Chapter on Idiots." 1854. *Harper's Magazine* 9:101–104.

Chase, Allan. 1977. *The Legacy of Malthus: The Social Costs of the New Scientific Racism*. New York: Knopf.

Childs, Donald J. 2001. *Modernism and Eugenics: Woolf, Eliot, Yeats and the Culture of Degeneration*. New York: Cambridge University Press.

Chomsky, Noam. 1972. "Psychology and Ideology." *Cognition* 1(1): 11–46.

"City Takes Ownership of Fernald Property." 2014. *Boston Globe* (December 28). Retrieved September 15, 2015 (http://www.bostonglobe.com/metro/regionals/west/2014/12/28/city-takes-ownership-fernald-property/5QYCwdqRg1FeDZWJ55AKxH/story.html).

Clark, Martha Louise. 1894. "The Relation of Imbecility to Pauperism and Crime." *The Arena* 10:55(November):788–794.

Clausen, Johannes. 1967. "Mental Deficiency – Development of a Concept." *American Journal of Mental Deficiency* 71:727–745.

Cocke, Elton C. 1948. "A Brief History of the Department of Biology of Wake Forest College." *Bios* 19:3(October): 179–184.

Collier, Peter, and David Horowitz. 1984. *The Kennedys: An American Drama*. New York: Summit Books.

"Commission in Insanity." 1894. *Lincoln Daily News-Herald*, 12 December, p. 3, Lincoln, Illinois.

Committee on Education of the AAMD [American Association on Mental Deficiency]. 1951. "Report on Characteristic Population Trends in Institutions for Mental Defectives." *American Journal of Mental Deficiency* 56:229–231.

Committee on Protection of the Feeble-Minded, Massachusetts Society for the Prevention of Cruelty to Children. 1913. *The Menace of the Feeble-Minded*. Boston: Griffth-Stillings.

"A Committee to Eradicate Feeblemindedness." 1915. *Survey* 34:369.

"Conditions in Mental Hospitals." 1946. Letter to the editor [name withheld]. *Christian Century* 63(April 10): A65–66.

Connecticut General Assembly. 1856. *Report of the Commissioners on Idiocy to the Legislature of Connecticut.* New Haven: Carrington and Hotchkiss.

Connolly, Margaret. 1925. *Life Story of Orison Swett Marden: A Man Who Benefited Men.* New York: Thomas Y. Crowell.

Conolly, John. 1845. "Notice of the Lunatic Asylums of Paris." *British and Foreign Medical Review* (January):281–298.

Conolly, John. 1847. "Analytical and Critical Reviews." *British and Foreign Medical Review* (July):1–22.

Coolidge, Calvin. 1921. "Whose Country Is This?" *Good House-keeping* 72(February):14.

Cooper, Rachel. 2014. "Shifting Boundaries between the Normal and the Pathological: The Case of Mild Intellectual Disability." *History of Psychiatry* 25(June):171–186.

Cooper, Sarah B. 1896. "Reports from the States: California." *Proceedings of the National Conference of Charities and Correction,* 22–23.

Corcoran, David. 1991. "Nameless Headstones for the Forgotten Mentally Retarded." *New York Times,* 9 December, p. B12.

"CPS Camps and Units." 1944. *Reporter* 3(15 July):2, 7.

Craig, Delores E., and William F. Boyd. 1990. "Characteristics of Employers of Handicapped Individuals." *American Journal of Mental Retardation* 96:40–43.

Craig, Oscar, W. F. Slocum Jr., Herbert A. Forrest, Samuel G. Smith, and M. D. Follett. 1893. "History of State Boards." *Proceedings of the National Council of Charities and Correction,* 33–51.

Cravens, Hamilton. 1978. *The Triumph of Evolution: American Scientists and the Heredity-Environment Controversy, 1900–1941.* Philadelphia: University of Pennsylvania Press.

Creadick, Anna G. 2010. *Perfectly Average: The Pursuit of Normality in Postwar America.* Amherst: University of Massachusetts Press.

Cremin, Lawrence. 1961. *The Transformation of the School.* New York: Alfred A. Knopf.

Crissey Marie S. 1975. "Mental Retardation: Past, Present, and Future." *American Psychologist* 30:800–808.

Crist, Judith. 1950. "Not Quite Bright!" *Better Homes and Gardens* 28:148–149, 151–152, 154–156.

Curti, Merle. 1951. *The Growth of American Thought.* New York: Harper and Brothers.

Dana, Charles L. 1924. "The Seguins of New York, Their Careers and Contributions to Science and Education." *Annals of Medical History* 6:475–479.

Danforth, Scot. 2008. "John Dewey's Contributions to an Educational Philosophy of Intellectual Disability." *Educational Theory* 58(February):45–62.

Danforth, Scot. 2009. *The Incomplete Child: An Intellectual History of Learning Disabilities.* New York: Peter Lang.

Daniels, Jonathan. 1966. *The Time between the Wars: Armistice to Pearl Harbor.* Garden City, NY: Doubleday.

D'Antonio, Michael. 2005. *The State Boys Rebellion.* New York: Simon and Schuster.Darger, Henry Joseph. ca. 1960 [2014]. *The History of My Life.* Pp. 281–313 in *Henry Darger,* edited by Klaus Biesenbach. Munich: Prestel.

Darrow, Clarence. 1926. "The Eugenic Cult." *American Mercury* 8:129–137.

Davenport, Charles B. 1910. "News and Notes." *American Breeders' Magazine* 1:306.

Davenport, Charles B. 1911. *Heredity in Relation to Eugenics.* New York: Henry Holt.

Davenport, Charles B. 1912. "The Nams: The Feeble-Minded as Country Dwellers." *Survey* 27:1844–1845.

Davenport, Charles B. 1913. *State Laws Limiting Marriage Selection.* Cold Spring Harbor, N.Y: Eugenics Record Office.

Davenport, Charles B., and Florence H. Danielson. 1912. *The Hill Folk: Report on a Rural Community of Hereditary Defectives.* Cold Spring Harbor, N.Y: Press of the New Era Printing Co.

Davenport, Charles B., Harry H. Laughlin, David Weeks, E. R. Johnstone, and Henry H. Goddard. 1911. *The Study of Human Heredity: Methods of Collecting, Charting, and Analyzing Data* [Eugenics Record Office Bulletin No. 2]. Cold Spring Harbor, NY: Eugenics Record Office.

Davenport, Charles B., and Morris Steggerda. 1929. *Race Crossing in Jamaica. Publication no. 395.* Washington, DC: Carnegie Institution.

Davidson, Levette Jay. 1943. "Moron Stories." *Southern Folklore Quarterly* 7:101–104.

Davies, Stanley P. 1923. *Social Control of the Feebleminded: A Study of Social Programs and Attitudes in Relation to the Problem of Mental Deficiency.* New York: National Committee for Mental Hygiene.

Dayton, Neil A. 1931. "Mortality in Mental Deficiency over a Fourteen Year Period: Analysis of 8,976 Cases, and 878 Deaths in Massachusetts." *Proceedings of the American Association for the Study of the Feeble-Minded,* 127–212.

"Death of Elsie Seguin." 1930. *Journal of Psycho-Asthenics* 35:260.

Decroly, Ovide, and J. Degand. 1906. "Les Tests de Binet et Simon pour la mésure de l'intelligence: Contribution critique." *Archive de psychologie* 6:17–130.

Degler, Carl N. 1991. *In Search of Human Nature: The Decline and Revival of Darwinism in American Social Thought.* New York: Oxford University Press.

de Graaf, Gert, Frank F. Buckley, and Brian G. Skotko. 2015. "Estimates of the Live Births, Natural Losses, and Elective Terminations with Down Syndrome in the United States." *American Journal of Medical Genetics* Part A 167A:756–767.

deLone, Richard H. 1979. *Small Futures: Children, Inequality, and the Limits of Liberal Reform.* New York: Harcourt Brace Jovanovich.

D'Emilio, John, and Estelle B. Freedman. 1988. *Intimate Matters: A History of Sexuality in America.* New York: Harper and Row.

DeSelincourt, Ernest, ed. 1935. *The Early Letters of William and Dorothy Wordsworth (1787–1805).* Oxford, UK: Oxford University Press.

Deutsch, Albert. 1937. *The Mentally Ill in America: A History of Their Care and Treatment from Colonial Times.* New York: Doubleday.

Deutsch, Albert. 1948. *The Shame of the States.* New York: Harcourt, Brace.

Deutsch, Albert. 1949. *The Mentally Ill in America: A History of Their Care and Treatment from Colonial Times.* 2d ed. New York: Columbia University Press.

Deutsch, Albert. 1950. *Our Rejected Children.* Boston: Little, Brown.

Deutsch, Nathaniel. 2009. *Inventing America's "Worst" Family: Eugenics, Islam, and the Fall and Rise of the Tribe of Ishmael.* Berkeley: University of California Press.

Dexter, Lewis A. 1960a. "Research on Problems of Mental Subnormality." *American Journal of Mental Deficiency* 64:835–838.

Dexter, Lewis A. 1960b. "The Sociology of Adjustment: Who Defines Mental Deficiency?" *American Behavioral Scientist* 4:13–15.

Dexter, Lewis A. 1964. *The Tyranny of Schooling: An Inquiry into the Problem of "Stupidity."* New York: Basic Books.

Diament, Michelle. 2012. "Protests to Target Low Pay at Goodwill." *Disability Scoop* August 21. Retrieved August 25, 2015 (http://www.disabilityscoop.com/2012/08/21/protests-target-goodwill/16285/).

Dickens, Charles. 1871. *Barnaby Rudge.* London: Chapman and Hall.

"Discussions: Accidents in Institutions for Feeble-Minded and Epileptics." 1909. *Journal of Psycho-Asthenics* 13:100–107.

Dixon, Thomas. 1902. *The Leopard's Spots: A Romance of the White Man's Burden, 1865–1900.* New York: Doubleday, Page.

Dixon, Thomas. 1905. *The Clansman: An Historical Romance of the Ku Klux Klan.* New York: Doubleday, Page.

Doll, Eugene E. [ca. 1976]. "Before the Big Time: The Early History of the Training School at Vineland and Its Influence." Typescript. In the collection of Gunnar Dybwad, Goldfarb Library, Brandeis University, Waltham, MA.

Dolmage, Jay. 2011. "Disabled upon Arrival: The Rhetorical Construction of Disability and Race at Ellis Island." *Cultural Critique* 77(Winter):24–69.

Donald, David H. 1960. *Charles Sumner and the Coming of the Civil War.* Chicago: University of Chicago Press.

Doren, Gustavus A. 1854–1905. Manuscripts [thirteen boxes, approximately 4,000 items]. Ohio Historical Society, Archives and History Division, Columbus.

Doren, Gustavus A. 1887. "Report on Ohio." *Proceedings of the Association of Medical Officers of American Institutions for Idiotic and Feeble-Minded Persons, 1886,* 461–462.

Doren, Gustavus A. 1902 [1891]. "Costodial [sic] Care of Idiots." Pp. 21–37 in *Our Defective Classes,* edited by G. A. Doren. Columbus, Ohio: Fred. J. Heer.

Dorey, Annette K. Vance. 1999. *Better Baby Contests: The Scientific Quest for Perfect Childhood Health in the Early Twentieth Century.* Jefferson, NC: McFarland & Co.

Douglass, Mary I. 1914. "Special Lines of Work and Results Sought." *Journal of Psycho-Asthenics* 19:135–149.

Dowbiggn, Ian Robert. 1997. *Keeping America Sane: Psychiatry and Eugenics in the United States and Canada 1880-1940.* Ithaca, NY: Cornell University Press.

Dowling, P. J., and W. K. Towlinson. 1974. "The Role of Cultural Minorities in the Decline of Moral Treatment – A Recurring Pattern in American Psychiatry." Pp. 438–444 in *Proceedings of the Twenty-third International Congress of the History of Medicine.* London: Wellcome Institute of the History of Medicine.

Down, J. Langdon. 1866. "Observations on an Ethnic Classification of Idiots." *Clinical Lecture Reports of the London Hospital* 3:259–262.

Down, J. Langdon. 1867. "Observations on an Ethnic Classification of Idiots." *Journal of Mental Science* 13:121–123.

"Dr. Charles Eliot Norton, Who Favors Death for Hopelessly Incurable Persons." [ca. 1896]. Undated newspaper clipping in the Beverly Farm Collection.

"Dr. Smith Protests." 1908. *Lincoln Daily News-Herald,* 7 March, p. 2, Lincoln, Illinois.

DuBois, Philip. 1970. *A History of Psychological Testing.* Boston: Allyn and Bacon.

Dugdale, Richard L. 1877a. "Hereditary Pauperism." *Proceedings of the National Conference of Charities and Correction,* 81–95.

Dugdale, Richard L. 1877b. *The Jukes: A Study in Crime, Pauperism, Disease, and Heredity.* New York: Putnam.

Dulberger, Judith A. 1996. *"Mother Donit fore the Best": Correspondence of a Nineteenth-Century Orphan Asylum.* Syracuse, NY: Syracuse University Press.

Dummer, Ethel S. 1948. "Life in Relation to Time." In *Orthopsychiatry, 1923–1948: Retrospect and Prospect,* edited by Lawson G. Lowrey and Victoria Sloane. Menasha, WI: George Bantam.

Dunphy, Mary C. 1908. "Modern Ideals of Education Applied to the Training of Mental Defectives." *Proceedings of the National Conference of Charities and Correction,* 325–336.

Dwyer, Ellen. 1987. *Homes for the Mad: Life inside Two Nineteenth-Century Asylums*. New Brunswick, NJ: Rutgers University Press.

Dybwad, Gunnar. 1964. "Are We Retarding the Retarded?" Pp. 19–25 in *Challenges in Mental Retardation*, edited by Gunnar Dybwad. New York: Columbia University Press.

Dybwad, Gunnar. 1969. "Action Implications, USA. Today." Pp. 383–428 in *Changing Patterns in Residential Services for the Mentally Retarded*, edited by R. Kugel and W. Wolfensberger. Washington, DC: President's Committee on Mental Retardation.

Dybwad, Gunnar. 1973. "New Patterns of Living Demand New Patterns of Service: Is Normalization a Feasible Principle of Rehabilitation?" Address to the International Conference on Models of Service for the Multi-Handicapped Adult, New York. Photocopy.

Dybwad, Gunnar. 1982. "Normalization and Its Impact on Social and Public Policy." In *Advancing Your Citizenship: Normalization Re-Examined*. Proceedings of a National Conference on Normalization and Contemporary Practice in Mental Retardation. Eugene, OR: Rehabilitation and Training Center on Mental Retardation.

Dybwad, Gunnar. 1983. "Infants with Birth Defects: Who May Live? Who must Die?" Address to the King's Fund Centre, King Edward's Hospital Fund for London, 11 May 1983. Photocopy.

Dybwad, Gunnar. 1989. "Self-Determination: Influencing Public Policy." Paper given at the National Self-Determination Conference, Arlington, VA. Photocopy.

Dybwad, Gunnar. 1990. Interview with author. Transcribed June 12–14.

Dybwad, Gunnar, and Hank Bersani Jr., eds. 1996. *New Voices: Self-advocacy by People with Disabilities*. Cambridge, MA: Brookline.

Dybwad, Rosemary F. 1990*a*. Interview with author. Transcribed June 12–14.

Dybwad, Rosemary F. 1990*b*. *Perspectives on a Parent Movement: The Revolt of Parents of Children with Intellectual Limitations*. Brookline, MA: Brookline Books.

Dyck, Ericka. 2013. *Facing Eugenics: Reproduction, Sterilization, and the Politics of Choice*. Toronto: University of Toronto Press.

Eadline, James D. 1963. *A Brief History: The Training School at Vineland, New Jersey*. Vineland: Training School.

Edgerton, Robert B. 1967. *The Cloak of Competence: Stigma in the Lives of the Mentally Retarded*. Berkeley and Los Angeles: University of California Press.

Edgerton, Robert B., and S. Bercovici. 1976. "The Cloak of Competence – Years Later." *American Journal of Mental Deficiency* 80:485–497.

Edgerton, Robert B., and Cecile R. Edgerton. 1973. "Becoming Mentally Retarded in a Hawaiian School." Pp. 211–233 in *Sociobehavioral Studies in Mental Retardation: Papers in Honor of Harvey F. Dingman*, edited by G. Tarjan, R. K. Eyman, and C. E. Meyers. Los Angeles: American Association on Mental Deficiency.

Edgerton, Robert B., and Georges Sabagh. 1962. "From Mortification to Aggrandizement: Changing Self-Concepts in the Careers of the Mentally Retarded." *Psychiatry* 25:263–272.

"Education of Idiots." 1847. *Living Age* 15:423–425.

"Education of Idiots." 1849. *Southern Literary Messenger* 15:65–68.

"Education of Idiots at the Bicêtre." 1847. *Living Age* 13:369–371.

Edwards, R.A.R. 2012. *Words Made Flesh: Nineteenth-Century Deaf Education and the Growth of Deaf Culture*. New York: New York University Press.

Eggers, Barbara. 1986. "Jesse Donaldson Hodder." Pp. 376–379 in *Biographical Dictionary of Social Welfare in America*, edited by W. I. Trattner. New York: Greenwood Press.

Elks, Martin A. 2004. "Believing is Seeing: Visual Conventions in Barr's Classification of the 'Feeble-Minded'." *Mental Retardation* 42(5):371–382.

Elks, Martin A. 2005. "Visual Indictment: A Contextual Analysis of the Kallikak Family Photographs." *Mental Retardation* 43(4):268–280.

Elledge, Jim. 2013. *Henry Darger, Throwaway Boy: The Tragic Life of an Outsider Artist.* New York: Overlook Books.

Emerick, E. J. 1917. "Progress in the Care of the Feeble-Minded in Ohio." *Journal of Psycho-Asthenics* 22:73–79.

English, Horace B. 1922. "Is America Feeble-minded?" *Survey* 49:79–81.

Esquirol, Jean-Etienne. 1818. "Idiotisme" Pp. 507–524 in *Dictionnaire des sciences médicales*, vol. 23. Paris: Panckoucke.

Esquirol, Jean-Etienne. 1838. *Des maladies mentales, considerées sous les rapports médical, hygienique, et médico-legal.* Paris: Baillière. English translation: *Mental Maladies.* New York: Hafner, 1965.

Esquirol, Jean-Etienne, and Edouard Séguin. 1839. *Résumé de ce que nous avons fait pendant quatorze mois.* Paris: Porthmann.

Estabrook, Arthur H. 1916. *The Jukes in 1915.* Washington, DC: Carnegie Institution.

Estabrook, Arthur H. 1923. "The Tribe of Ishmael." Pp. 398–404 in *The Second International Congress of Eugenics: Eugenics, Genetics, and the Family*, edited by H. H. Laughlin. Baltimore: Williams and Wilkins.

Estabrook, Arthur H., and Charles B. Davenport. 1912. *The Nam Family: A Study in Cacogenics.* Cold Spring Harbor, NY: New Era Printing.

Estabrook, Arthur H., and Ivan E. McDougle. 1926. *Mongrel Virginians: The Win Tribe.* Baltimore: Williams and Wilkins.

Estreich, George. 2013. *The Shape of the Eye: A Memoir.* New York: Tarcher.

Experimental School for the Instruction and Training of Idiots and Feeble-Minded Children in the State of Illinois. 1865–70. *Minutes of the Board.* Illinois State Archives, record no. 254.1, Springfield.

Eyal, Gil. 2013. "For a Sociology of Expertise: The Social Origins of the Autism Epidemic." *American Journal of Sociology* 118(January):863–907.

Fairchild, Amy. L. 2003. *Science at the Borders: Immigrant Medical Inspection and the Shaping of the Modern Industrial Labor Force.* Baltimore, MD: Johns Hopkins University Press.

Felicetti, Daniel A. 1975. *Mental Health and Retardation Politics: The Mind Lobbies in Congress.* New York: Praeger.

Ferguson, Dianne L., Philip M. Ferguson, and Michael L. Wehmeyer. 2013. "The Self-Advocacy Movement: Late Modern Times (1980 CE to Present)." Pp. 233–277 in *The Story of Intellectual Disability: An Evolution of Meaning, Understanding, and Public Perception*, edited by M. L. Wehmeyer. Baltimore: Brookes.

Ferguson, Philip M. 1987. "The Social Construction of Mental Retardation." *Social Policy* 18:51–56.

Ferguson, Philip M. 1994. *Abandoned to Their Fate: Social Policy and Practice toward Severely Retarded People in America, 1820–1920.* Philadelphia, PA: Temple University Press.

Ferguson, Philip M. 2013. "The Development of Systems of Supports: Intellectual Disability in Middle Modern Times (1800 CE to 1899 CE)." Pp. 79–115 in *The Story of Intellectual Disability: An Evolution of Meaning, Understanding, and Public Perception*, edited by M. L. Wehmeyer. Baltimore: Brookes.

Fernald, Walter E. 1893. "History of the Treatment of the Feebleminded." *Proceedings of the National Association of Charities and Correction*, 203–221.

Fernald, Walter E. 1894. "Some of the Methods Employed in the Care and Training of Feeble-Minded Children of the Lower Grades." *Proceedings of the Association of Medical Officers of American Institutions for Idiotic and Feeble-Minded Persons,* 450–457.

Fernald, Walter E. 1902. "The Massachusetts Farm Colony for the Feeble-Minded." *Proceedings of the National Conference of Charities and Correction,* 487–490.

Fernald, Walter E. 1904a. "Discussion on Defectives and the Public Schools." *Proceedings of the National Conference of Charities and Correction,* 486–489.

Fernald, Walter E. 1904b. "Mentally Defective Children in the Public Schools." *Journal of Psycho-Asthenics* 8:25–35.

Fernald, Walter E. 1907. "Possibilities of the Colony." *Proceedings of the National Conference of Charities and Correction,* 411–418.

Fernald, Walter E. 1909. "The Imbecile with Criminal Instincts." *Journal of Psycho-Asthenics* 14:16–36.

Fernald, Walter E. 1919. "After-Care Study of the Patients Discharged from Waverly for a Period of Twenty-five Years." *Ungraded* 5:25–31.

Fernald, Walter E. 1920. "An Out-Patient Clinic in Connection with a State Institution for the Feeble-Minded." *American Journal of Insanity* 77:227–235 and *Journal of Psycho-Asthenics* 25:81–89.

Fernald, Walter E. 1922. "The Inauguration of a State-Wide Public School Mental Clinic in Massachusetts." *Mental Hygiene* 6:471–486.

Fernald, Walter E. 1924. "Thirty Years Progress in the Care of the Feeble-Minded." *Journal of Psycho-Asthenics* 29:206–219.

Fernald, Walter E., E.E. Southard, and Annie E. Taft. 1918 and 1921. *Waverley Researches in the Pathology of the Feeble-Minded. Memoirs of the American Academy of Arts and Sciences* 14:2(May 1918), 1–128; and 14:3(December 1921), 129–207.

Fink, Arthur. 1938. *Causes of Crime: Biological Theories in the United States, 1800–1915.* Philadelphia: University of Pennsylvania Press.

Finlayson, Anna. 1916. *The Dack Family: A Study in Hereditary Lack of Emotional Control.* Eugenics Record Office, bulletin no. 15. Cold Spring Harbor, NY: Eugenics Record Office.

Fish, William B. 1879. *A Thesis on Idiocy.* M.D. thesis, Albany Medical College, Albany, New York.

Fish, William B. 1889. "Institutional Discipline." *Proceedings of the Association of Medical Officers of American Institutions for Idiotic and Feeble-Minded Persons, 1887,* 45–48.

Fish, William B. 1892. "The Colony Plan." *Proceedings of the National Conference of Charities and Correction,* 161–165.

Foley, Henry A., and Steven S. Sharfstein. 1983. *Madness and Government: Who Cares for the Mentally Ill?* Washington, DC: American Psychiatric Press.

"The Folly of Freedom for Fools." 1918. *Survey* 39:657.

Folsom, Franklin. 1991. *Impatient Armies of the Poor: The Story of Collective Action of the Unemployed, 1808–1942.* Niwot: University Press of Colorado.

Foucault, Michel. 1973. *The Birth of the Clinic: An Archaeology of Medical Perception.* New York: Pantheon Books.

Foucault, Michel. 1979. *Discipline and Punish: The Birth of the Prison.* New York: Random House.

Fox, Richard W. 1978. *So Far Disordered in Mind: Insanity in California 1870–1930.* Berkeley and Los Angeles: University of California Press.

Frank, John P. 1952. *My Son's Story.* New York: Alfred A. Knopf.

Fredrickson, George M. 1965. *The Inner Civil War: Northern Intellectuals and the Crisis of the Union*. New York: Harper and Row.

Freeman, Joshua B. 2012. *American Empire:The Rise of a Global Power, the Democratic Revolution at Home, 1945–2000*. New York: Viking.

Fynne, Robert J. 1924. *Montessori and Her Inspirers*. London: Longman, Green.

Gallagher, Nancy L. 1999. *Breeding Better Vermonters: The Eugenics Project in the Green Mountain State*. Hanover, NH: University Press of New England.

Galt. John M.II. 1859. *A Lecture on Idiocy*. Richmond, VA: Enquirer Book and Job Office.

Galton, Francis. 1883. *Inquiries into Human Faculty and Its Development*. London: Macmillan.

Gamble, Clarence J. 1946. "Sterilization of the Mentally Deficient under State Laws." *American Journal of Mental Deficiency* 51(2):164–169.

Gamble, Clarence J. 1948. "Sterilizations of the Mentally Deficient in 1946." *American Journal of Mental Deficiency* 52:375–378.

Gamble, Clarence J. 1949. "Preventive Sterilization in 1948." *Journal of the American Medical Association* 141(11):773.

Garraty, John A. 1987. *The Great Depression: An Inquiry into the Causes, Course, and Consequences of the Worldwide Depression of the Nineteen-Thirties as Seen by Contemporaries and in the Light of History*. New York: Anchor Books.

Garrison, Maxine. 1956. *The Angel Spreads Her Wings*. Westwood, NJ: Revell.

Gelb, Steven A. 1995. "The Beast in Man: Degeneration and Mental Retardation, 1900–1920." *Mental Retardation* 33(February): 1–9.

Gelb, Steven A. 1999. "Spilled Religion: The Tragedy of Henry H. Goddard." *Mental Retardation*, 37(3):240–243.

Genthe, Arnold. 1944. "Letchworth Village: Arnold Genthe Photographs a Famed Village for Mental Deficients." *US Camera* (November):27–33.

Giddings, Franklin H. 1910. "Introduction." Pp. iii–v in *The Jukes: A Study in Crime, Pauperism, Disease, and Heredity*, by Robert Dugdale. 4th ed. New York: G. P. Putnam's Sons.

Gillham, Nicholas Wright. 2001. *Sir Francis Galton: From African Exploration to the Birth of Eugenics*. New York: Oxford University Press.

Gilman, Sander L., ed. 1976. *The Face of Madness: Hugh Diamond and the Origin of Psychiatric Photography*. New York: Brunner/Mazel.

Gish, Lowell. 1972. *Reform at Osawatome State Hospital*. Lawrence: University of Kansas Press.

Gittens, Joan. 1994. *Poor Relations: The Children of the State in Illinois, 1818–1990*. Urbana and Chicago: University of Illinois Press.

Givens, Larry D. 1986. "Frederick Howard Wines." Pp. 777–779 in *Biographical Dictionary of Social Welfare in America*, edited by W. I. Trattner. New York: Greenwood Press.

"Gladys Burr, 82." 1989. Obituary. *St Louis Post-Dispatch*. 19 December.

Glenna, Leland, Margaret A. Gollnick and Stephen S. Jones. 2007. "Eugenic Opportunity Structures: Teaching Genetic Engineering at US Land-Grant Universities since 1911." *Social Studies of Science* 37(April):281–296.

Gobineau, Comte Joseph-Arthur de. 1915. *The Inequality of Human Races*. New York: G. P. Putnam's Sons.

Goddard, Henry. 1907a. "Psychological Work among the Feeble-Minded." *Journal of Psycho-Asthenics* 12:18–30.

Goddard, Henry. 1907b. "The Research Work." Supplement to the *Training School Bulletin* 1:1–13.

Goddard, Henry. 1908*a*. "The Binet and Simon Tests of Intellectual Capacity." *Training School Bulletin* 5:3–9.

Goddard, Henry. 1908*b*. "The Grading of Backward Children." *Training School Bulletin* 5:12–14.

Goddard, Henry. 1908*c*. "Two Months among the European Institutions for the Mentally Defective." *Training School Bulletin* 5:11–16.

Goddard, Henry. 1909*a*. "A Growth Curve for Feeble-Minded Children, Height and Weight." *Journal of Psycho-Asthenics* 14:9–13.

Goddard, Henry. 1909*b*. "Suggestions for a Prognostical Classification of Mental Defectives." *Journal of Psycho-Asthenics* 14:48–52.

Goddard, Henry. 1909*c*. "Will the Backward Child Outgrow Its Backwardness?" *Training School Bulletin* 5:1–3.

Goddard, Henry. 1910*a*. "The Application of Educational Psychology to the Problems of the Special Class." *Journal of Educational Psychology* 1:521–531.

Goddard, Henry. 1910*b*. *Feeble-Minded Children with Dangerous Tendencies*. Washington, DC: Bulletin de la Committée Pénitentiaire Internationale.

Goddard, Henry. 1910*c*. "Four Hundred Feeble-Minded Children Classified by the Binet Method." *Journal of Psycho-Asthenics* 15:17–30.

Goddard, Henry. 1910*d*. "Heredity of Feeble-Mindedness." *American Breeders' Magazine* 1:165–178.

Goddard, Henry. 1910*e*. "What Can the Public School Do for Normal Children?" *Training School Bulletin* 7:242–247.

Goddard, Henry. 1911*a*. "The Menace of the Feeble-Minded." *Pediatrics* 23:1–8.

Goddard, Henry. 1911*b*. "Measuring Scale of Intelligence." *Pediatric Seminar* 18:232–259.

Goddard, Henry. 1911*c*. "Two Thousand Normal Children Tested by the Binet Scale." *Training School Bulletin* 7:310–312.

Goddard, Henry. 1912*a*. "The Feeble-Minded Immigrant." *Training School Bulletin* 9(November-December):109–113.

Goddard, Henry. 1912*b*. "Feeble-Mindedness and Immigration." *Training School Bulletin* 9(October):91–94.

Goddard, Henry. 1912*c*. *The Kallikak Family: A Study in the Heredity of Feeble-Mindedness*. New York: Macmillan.

Goddard, Henry. 1912*d*. "Sterilization and Surgery." *Bulletin of the American Academy of Medicine* 13:1–7.

Goddard, Henry. 1913*a*. "The Binet Tests in Relation to Immigration." *Journal of Psycho-Asthenics* 18(December):105–107.

Goddard, Henry. 1913*b*. "The Hereditary Factor in Feeblemindedness." *Institutional Quarterly* 4(June):9–11.

Goddard, Henry. 1914. *Feeble-Mindedness: Its Causes and Consequences*. New York: Macmillan.

Goddard, Henry. 1917*a*. "Mental Levels of a Group of Immigrants." *Psychological Bulletin* 14(February):68–69.

Goddard, Henry. 1917*b*. "Mental Tests and the Immigrant." *Journal of Delinquency* 2(September):243–279.

Goddard, Henry. 1928. "Feeblemindedness: A Question of Definition." *Journal of Psycho-Asthenics* 33:219–227.

Goddard, Henry. 1942. "In Defense of the Kallikak Study." *Science* 95:574–576.

Goddard, Henry. 1943. "In the Beginning." *Training School Bulletin* 40:154–161.

Goddard, Henry H., and Helen F. Hill. 1911. "Feebleminded and Criminality." *Training School Bulletin* 8:3–6.

Godding, W. W. 1883. "Memorial to H. B. Wilbur." *American Psychological Journal* 1:27–29.

Goffman, Erving. 1961. *Asylums: Essays on the Social Situation of Mental Patients and Other Inmates.* New York: Doubleday.

Goldstein, H. 1959. "Population Trends in US Public Institutions for the Mentally Deficient." *American Journal of Mental Deficiency* 63:599–604.

Goldstein, Jan. 1987. *Console and Classify: The French Psychiatric Profession in the Nineteenth Century.* Cambridge, UK: Cambridge University Press.

Gollay, Elinor, Ruth Freedman, Marty Wyngaarten, and Norman R. Kurtz. 1978. *Coming Back: The Community Experiences of Deinstitutionalized Mentally Retarded People.* Cambridge, MA: Abt Books.

Good, Harry G. 1962. *A History of American Education.* New York: Macmillan.

Goode, David, Darryl B. Hill, Jean Reiss, and William Bronston. 2013. *History and Sociology of the Willowbrook State School.* Washington, DC: AAIDD.

Goodey, C.F. 2011. *A History of Intelligence and "Intellectual Disability": The Shaping of Psychology in Early Modern Europe.* Surrey, UK: Ashgate.

Goodheart, Lawrence B. 2004. "Rethinking Mental Retardation: Education and Eugenics in Connecticut, 1818–1917." *Journal of the History of Medicine and the Allied Sciences* 59(1):90–111.

Goodwin, Doris Kearnes. 1987. *The Fitzgeralds and the Kennedys: An American Saga.* New York: Simon and Schuster.

Gorwitz, Kurt. 1974. "Census Enumeration of the Mentally Ill and the Mentally Retarded in the Nineteenth Century." *Health Services Reports* 89:180–187.

Gossett, Thomas F. 1965. *Race: The History of an Idea.* New York: Schocken Press.

Gould, Stephen Jay. 1981. *The Mismeasure of Man.* New York: W. W. Norton.

Gould, Stephen Jay. 1984. "Carrie Buck's Daughter" *Natural History* 93, 7(July):14–18.

Gould, Stephen Jay. 2002. *The Structure of Evolutionary Theory.* Cambridge, MA: The Belknap Press of Harvard University Press.

Gramm, Eugene. 1951. "New Hope for the Different Child." *Parents' Magazine* 26(9):48, 152–156.

Graney, Bernard J. 1980. *Hervey Backus Wilbur and the Evolution of Policies and Practices toward Mentally Retarded People.* Ph.D. diss., Syracuse University, New York.

Grant, Madison. 1916. *The Passing of the Great Race.* New York: Charles Scribner's Sons.

Grant, Madison, ed. 1930. *The Alien in Our Midst, or Selling Our Birthright for a Mess of Pottage.* New York: Galton.

Grant, Madison. 1933. *The Conquest of a Continent, or, Expansion of Races in America.* New York: Charles Scribner's Sons.

Green, C. Sylvester. 1988. "Hanes, James Gordon, Sr." *NCpedia.* Retrieved September 1, 2015 (http://ncpedia.org/biography/hanes-james-gordon-sr).

Greenspan, Steven. 1995. "Selling DSM: The Rhetoric of Science in Psychiatry." *American Journal on Mental Retardation* 99:683–685.

Grinspoon, Reid. 2013. "The Burden of Feeble-mindedness: The History of Eugenics and Sterilization in Massachusetts." *New England Journal of History* 70 (Fall):1–20.

Grob, Gerald N. 1973. *Mental Institutions in America: Social Policy to 1875.* New York: Free Press.

Grob, Gerald N. 1977. "Rediscovering Asylums: The Unhistorical History of the Mental Hospital." *Hastings Center Report* 7:33–41.

Grob, Gerald N. 1980. "Institutional Origins and Early Transformation, 1830–1855." Pp. 19–44 in *The Enduring Asylum: Cycles of Institutional Reform at Worcester State Hospital,* edited by J. P. Morrissey, H. H. Goldman, and L. V. Klerman. New York: Grune and Stratton.

Grob, Gerald N. 1983. *Mental Illness and American Society, 1875–1940*. Princeton, NJ: Princeton University Press.

Grob, Gerald N. 1985. *The Inner World of American Psychiatry, 1890–1940: Selected Correspondence*. New Brunswick, NJ: Rutgers University Press.

Grob, Gerald N. 1990. "Marxian Analysis and Mental Illness." *History of Psychiatry* 1:223–232.

Grob, Gerald N. 1991. *From Asylum to Community: Mental Health Policy in Modern America*. Princeton, NJ: Princeton University Press.

Groce, Nora. 1992. "'The Town Fool': An Oral History of a Mentally Retarded Individual in Small Town Society." Pp. 175–196 in *Interpreting Disability: A Qualitative Reader*, edited by P. M. Ferguson, D. L. Ferguson, and S. J. Taylor. New York: Teachers College Press.

Grossman, H. J., ed. 1973. *Manual on Terminology and Classification in Mental Retardation*. Washington, DC: American Association on Mental Deficiency.

Grossman, H. J., ed. 1983. *Manual on Terminology and Classification in Mental Retardation*. Washington, DC: American Association on Mental Deficiency.

Gugliotta, Angela. 1998. "'Dr. Sharp with His Little Knife': Therapeutic and Punitive Origins of Eugenic Vasectomy in Indiana, 1892–1921." *Journal of the History of Medicine* 3(October):371–406.

Gunther, Daniel F., and Douglas Diekema. 2006. "Attenuating Growth in Children with Profound Developmental Disability: A New Approach to an Old Dilemma." *Archives of Pediatrics and Adolescent Medicine* 160:1013–1017.

Gusfield, Joseph R. 1989. "Constructing the Ownership of Social Problems: Fun and Profit in the Welfare State." *Social Problems* 36:431–441.

Hacking, Ian. 1999. *The Social Construction of What?* Cambridge, MA: Harvard University Press.

Hahn, Nicholas F. [Nicole H. Rafter]. 1980. "Too Dumb to Know Better: Cacogenic Family Studies and the Criminology of Women." *Criminology* 18:3–25.

"A Half-Million Dollars for Randall's Island." 1915. *Survey* 34:369.

Hall, Randal L. 2000. *William Louis Poteat: A Leader of the Progressive-Era South*. Lexington: University Press of Kentucky.

Haller, John S., Jr. 1971. *Outcasts from Evolution: Scientific Attitudes of Racial Inferiority, 1859–1900*. Urbana: University of Illinois Press.

Haller, Mark. 1963. *Hereditarian Attitudes in American Thought*. New Brunswick, NJ: Rutgers University Press.

Hansen, Betty. 1961. "Let Them Be Normal." *News and Notes* (October). Saginaw County Association for Retarded Children, Michigan.

Hansen, Randall, and Desmond King. 2013. *Sterilized by the State: Eugenics, Race, and the Population Scare in Twentieth-Century North America*. New York: Cambridge University Press.

Hardt, Harry G. 1909. "Accidents in Institutions for Feeble-Minded and Epileptics." *Journal of Psycho-Asthenics* 13:37–42.

Haring, Helen Garnsey. 1930. "Deficient." *Atlantic Monthly* 146:78–82.

Harkins, Anthony. 2004. *Hill Billy: A Cultural History of an American Icon*. New York: Oxford University Press.

"Harriman, Mary Williamson Averell." 1933. In *National Cyclopedia of American Biography*, vol. 23, 187. New York: James T. White.

Harris, Theodore F. 1969. *Pearl S. Buck: A Biography*. Vol. 1. New York: John Day.

Harris, Theodore F. 1971. *Pearl S. Buck: A Biography*. Vol. 2. New York: John Day.

Harshman, L. Potter. 1934. "Medical and Legal Aspects of Sterilization in Indiana." *Proceedings and Addresses of the American Association on Mental Deficiency*, 183–199.

Hasain, Marouf Arif. 1996. *The Rhetoric of Eugenics in Anglo-American Thought*. Athens: University of Georgia Press.

Hash, Phillip M. 2010. "Music at the Illinois Asylum for Feeble-Minded Children, 1865–1920." *Journal of Historical Research in Music Education* 32(October):37–56.

Hassencahl, Frances J. 1969. *Harry H. Laughlin: "Expert Eugenics Agent" for the House Committee on Immigration and Naturalization, 1921 to 1931*. Ph.D. diss., Case Western Reserve University, Cleveland, OH.

Hawke, C. C. 1950. "Castration and Sex Crimes." *American Journal of Mental Deficiency* 55:220–226.

Hays, W. M. 1910. "Editorials." *American Breeders' Magazine* 1:223.

Health Law Library Bulletin. 1979. Report on 43 *Federal Register* 52146(8 November 1978). Vol. 4.

Healy William. 1915. *The Individual Delinquent: A Textbook of Diagnosis and Prognosis for All Concerned in Understanding Offenders*. Boston: Little, Brown.

Healy William. 1918. "Normalities of the Feeble-Minded." *Proceedings and Addresses of the American Association for the Study of the Feeble- Minded*, 175–184.

Heber, Rick. 1961. *A Manual on Classification and Terminology in Mental Retardation* (2nd ed.). Washington, DC: American Association on Mental Deficiency.

Herald. 1913–1946. A monthly newspaper also known as the *Rome Custodial Herald* and the *Custodial Herald*. Rome, NY: Rome State School.

Herr, Stanley. 1983. *Rights and Advocacy for Retarded People*. Lexington, MA: D. C. Heath.

Herr, Stanley. 1984. "The Philip Becker Case Resolved: A Chance for Habilitation." *Mental Retardation* 22:30–35.

Herrick, Helen. 1959. "The Parent: Passive Recipient, Angry Lobbyist, or Responsible Team Member." Address to the Annual Conference of the National Association for Retarded Children. Collection of Gunnar Dybwad.

Herrnstein, Richard C. 1971. "IQ." *Atlantic Monthly* 228(September):43–58, 63–64.

Herrnstein, Richard C. 1973. *IQ. and the Meritocracy*. Boston: Little, Brown.

Hexter, Maurice B., and Abraham Myerson. 1924. "13.77 versus 12.05; A Study in Probable Error: A Critical Review of Brigham's *American Intelligence*." *Mental Hygiene* 8:69–82.

Higham, John. 1963. *Strangers in the Land: Patterns of American Nativism, 1860–1925*. New York: Atheneum.

Hill, Helen F. 1945. "Vineland Summer School for Teachers." *Journal of Exceptional Children* 11:203–209.

Hitchens, Christopher. 1992. "Voting in the Passive Voice." *Harper's Magazine* 28 4(April):45–52.

Hoffman, Laura C. 2013. "An Employment Opportunity or a Discrimination Dilemma? Sheltered Workshops and the Employment of the Disabled." *University of Pennsylvania Journal of Law and Social Change* 16:151–179.

Hollander, Russell. 1986. "Mental Retardation and American Society: The Era of Hope." *Social Service Review* 60:395–420.

Holman, Henry. 1914. *Seguin and His Physiological Method of Education*. London: Sir I. Pitman and Sons.

Holman, Joseph G. 1966. "Provision for the Mentally Retarded, Being an Historical Survey of the Changing Concepts of State Care for the Mentally Deficient in Kansas." *Journal of the Kansas Medical Society* 67:501–512.

Holmes, Samuel J. 1921. *The Trends of the Race: A Study of Present Tendencies in the Biological Development of Civilized Mankind*. New York: Harcourt, Brace.

Holt, L. Emmett, Jr. 1955. "The Children's Center: The Retarded Child." *Good Housekeeping* 141(10):158, 160.

Hornick, Robert. 2012. *The Girls and Boys of Belchertown: A Social History of the Belchertown State School for the Feeble-Minded*. Amherst: University of Massachusetts Press.

Howard, Robert P. 1988. *Mostly Good and Competent Men: Illinois Governors, 1818–1988*. Springfield: Illinois State Historical Society.

Howe, Daniel Walker. 2007. *What Hath God Wrought: The Transformation of America, 1815–1848*. New York: Oxford University Press.

Howe, Samuel G. 1848*a*. "Apologetical and Explanatory." *Massachusetts Quarterly Review* 1:509–512.

Howe, Samuel G. 1848*b*. *Report Made to the Legislature of Massachusetts upon Idiocy*. Boston: Coolidge and Wiley.

Howe, Samuel G. 1848*c*. "Review" [of *De la misère des classes laborieuses en Angleterre et en France, 1840* and *Report of the Massachusetts Commissioners Appointed to Inquire into the Conditions of Idiots in the Commonwealth, 1848*]. *Massachusetts Quarterly Review* 1:308–331.

Howe, Samuel G. 1874. *The Causes and Prevention of Idiocy*. Boston: Wright and Potter.

Hubbard, Ruth. 1990. *The Politics of Women's Biology*. New Brunswick, NJ: Rutgers University Press.

Human Betterment League of North Carolina, Inc. 1953. "Know About Eugenic Sterilization." *The State: Down Home in North Carolina* 20 (May 2):12.

Human Betterment League of North Carolina, Inc. 2008. *Records, 1947–1988*. Southern Historical Collection, University of North Carolina, Chapel Hill. Retrieved August 2, 2015 (http://www2.lib.unc.edu/mss/inv/h/Human_Betterment_League_of_North_Carolina.htmlfolder_501).

Hutchinson, Charles X., Jr. 1946. "It's Different in Connecticut." *Christian Century* 63:241–242.

"Idiocy in Massachusetts." 1847. *Living Age* 13:259–260.

"Idiocy in Massachusetts." 1849. *Southern Literary Messenger* 15:367–370.

"Idiots." 1851. *Household Works: A Weekly Journal* 7:313–317.

Illinois Asylum for Feeble-Minded Children. 1865–1906. *Admissions Applications*. 53 vols. Illinois State Archives, record no. 254.4, Springfield.

Illinois Board of Administration. 1914. *Biennial Reports of the Board of Administration*. Springfield: Illinois State Journal.

Illinois Board of State Commissioners of Public Charities. 1879. *Fifth Biennial Report*. Springfield: Weber, Magie.

Illinois Board of State Commissioners of Public Charities. 1885. *Eighth Biennial Report*. Springfield: H. W. Rokker.

Illinois Department of Public Welfare. 1930. *Ninth Report of Statistician, Year Ending June 30, 1930*. Pontiac: Illinois State Reformatory.

Illinois General Assembly. 1908. *Investigation of Illinois State Institutions: Testimony, Findings, and Debate*. Chicago: Regan Printing House.

Illinois Institution for the Education of Feebleminded Children. 1873. *Annual Report*. Lincoln: n.p.

Illinois State Charities Commission. 1912. *Second Annual Report*. Springfield: Illinois State Journal.

"Influence of Music on Idiots." 1857. *Living Age* 52:310–312.

The Institutional Bulletin: Quarterly Announcement of the California Home for the Care and Training of Feeble-Minded Children 1891. 3(September):8–9.

Ireland, William W. 1877. *On Idiocy and Imbecility*. London: J. and A. Churchill.

Jackson, Mark. 2000. *The Borderland of Imbecility: Medicine, Society and the Fabrication of the Feeble Mind in Late Victorian and Edwardian England*. Mancester, UK: Mancester University Press.

Janicki, Matthew P., Marty W. Krauss, and Marsha M. Seltzer. 1988. *Community Residences for Persons with Developmental Disabilities: Here to Stay*. Baltimore: Brookes.

Jencks, Christopher. 1969. "A Reappraisal of the Most Controversial Educational Document of Our Time." *New York Times Magazine* (10 August):12–13.

Jencks, Christopher, and Mary Jo Bane. 1973. "Five Myths about Your I.Q." *Harper's Magazine* 246(February):28, 32–34, 38–40.

Jensen, Arthur R. 1969. "How Much Can We Boost I.Q. and Scholastic Achievement?" *Harvard Educational Review* 39(Winter):1–123.

Jensen, Arthur R. 1972. "The Heritability of Intelligence." *Saturday Evening Post* 244(2):9, 12, 149.

Jezer, Marty. 1982. *The Dark Ages: Life in the United States, 1945–1960*. Boston: South End Press.

Johnson, Alexander. 1903. "Report of Committee on Colonies for Segregation of Defectives." *Proceedings of the National Conference of Charities and Correction*, 245–254.

Johnson, Alexander. 1908. "Custodial Care." *Proceedings of the National Conference of Charities and Correction*, 333–336.

Johnson, Alexander. 1914. "Discussion" [of E. R. Johnstone's "The Extension of the Care of the Feeble-Minded"]. *Journal of Psycho-Asthenics* 19:15–18.

Johnson, Alexander. 1923. *Adventures in Social Welfare: Being Reminiscences of Things, Thoughts, and Folks during Forty Years of Social Work*. Fort Wayne, IN: Fort Wayne Printing.

Johnstone, Edward R. 1904. "President's Address." *Journal of Psycho-Asthenics* 8:63–68.

Johnstone, Edward R. 1906. "Defectives: Report of the Committee." *Proceedings of the National Conference of Charities and Correction*, 235–243.

Johnstone, Edward R. 1908. "Practical Provision for the Mentally Deficient." *Proceedings of the National Conference of Charities and Correction*, 316–325.

Johnstone, Edward R. 1909. "The Summer School for Teachers of Backward Children." *Journal of Psycho-Asthenics* 13:122–128.

Johnstone, Edward R. 1911. "The Feeble-Minded of Pennsylvania Are an Expense to the Taxpayer." Pp. 6–7 in *Public Provision for the Feeble-Minded: A Symposium*. Philadelphia, PA: Department of Public Health and Charities of Philadelphia.

Johnstone, Edward R. 1914. "The Extension of the Care of the Feeble-Minded." *Journal of Psycho-Asthenics* 19:3–15.

Johnstone, Edward R. 1923. *Dear Robinson: Some Letters on Getting Along*. Vineland, NJ: Smith Printing House.

Jones, Jacqueline. 1992. *Dispossessed: America's Underclasses From the Civil War to the Present*. New York: Basic Books.

Jones, Kathleen W. 1999. *Taming the Troublesome Child: American Families, Child Guidance, and the Limits of Psychiatric Authority*. Cambridge, MA: Harvard University Press.

Jones, Kathleen W. 2004. "Education for Children with Mental Retardation: Parent Activism. Public Policy, and Family Ideology in the 1950s." Pp. 322–350 in *Mental Retardation in America: A Historical Reader*, edited by S. Noll and J. W. Trent, Jr. New York: New York University Press.

Juvenile Protective Association of Cincinnati. 1915. *The Feeble-Minded; or, The Hub to Our Wheel of Vice, Crime, and Pauperism: Cincinnati's Problem*. Cincinnati, OH: Juvenile Protective Association.

Kamin, Leon J. 1974. *The Science and Politics of IQ.* New York: Halstead Press.

Kanner, Leo. 1938. "Habeas Corpus Releases of Feebleminded Persons and Their Consequences." *American Journal of Psychiatry* 94(5):1013–1033.

Kanner, Leo. 1943. "Autistic Disturbances of Affective Contact." Pp. 1–43 in *Childhood Psychosis: Initial Studies and New Insights.* Washington, DC: Winston & Sons.

Kanner, Leo. 1964. *A History of the Care and Study of the Mentally Retarded.* Springfield, IL: Charles C. Thomas.

Katz, Michael B. 1968. *The Irony of Early School Reform: Educational Innovations in Mid-Nineteenth Century Massachusetts.* Boston: Beacon Press.

Keely, Karen A. 2002. "Poverty, Sterilization, and Eugenics in Erskine Caldwell's Tobacco Road." *Journal of American Studies* 36:23–42.

Keen, William W. 1892. "Linear Craniotomy for the Relief of Idiotic Conditions." *Proceedings of the Association of Medical Officers of American Institutions for Idiotic and Feeble-Minded Persons,* 344–350.

Keller, Helen A. 1903. *Optimism.* New York: Thomas Y. Crowell.

Keller, Helen A. 1905. *The Story of My Life.* New York: Doran.

Kerby, Phil. 1967. "The Reagan Backlash: Revolt against the Poor." *Nation* 205(25 November):262–267.

Kerlin, Isaac N. 1858. *The Mind Unveiled; or, A Brief History of Twenty-two Imbecile Children.* Philadelphia, PA: U. Hunt and Son.

Kerlin, Isaac N. 1877. "The Organization of Establishments for Idiotic and Imbecile Classes." *Proceedings of the Association of Medical Officers of American Institutions for Idiotic and Feeble-Minded Persons,* 19–28.

Kerlin, Isaac N. 1879. "Juvenile Insanity." *Proceedings of the Association of Medical Officers of American Institutions for Idiotic and Feeble-Minded Persons,* 86–94.

Kerlin, Isaac N. 1887a. "Idiotic and Feeble-Minded Children: Report of Standing Committee to the Eleventh National Conference of Charities and Correction, St. Louis, 1884." *Proceedings of the Association of Medical Officers of American Institutions for Idiotic and Feeble-Minded Persons, 1886,* 465–507.

Kerlin, Isaac N. 1887b. "James B. Richards in Pennsylvania." *Proceedings of the Association of Medical Officers of American Institutions for Idiotic and Feeble-Minded Persons, 1886,* 417–418.

Kerlin, Isaac N. 1888. "Report on Pennsylvania, 1888." *Proceedings of the Association of Medical Officers of American Institutions for Idiotic and Feeble-Minded Persons,* 81–82.

Kerlin, Isaac N. 1889. "Moral Imbecility." *Proceedings of the Association of Medical Officers of American Institutions for Idiotic and Feeble-Minded Persons, 1887,* 32–37.

Kerlin, Isaac N. 1890. "The Moral Imbecile." *Proceedings of the National Conference of Charities and Correction,* 244–250.

Kerlin, Isaac N. 1891a. *The Manual of Elwyn, 1864–1891.* Philadelphia, PA: J. B. Lippincott.

Kerlin, Isaac N. 1891b. "Status of the Work – Pennsylvania." *Proceedings of the Association of Medical Officers of American Institutions for Idiotic and Feeble-Minded Persons, 1890,* 69–70.

Kerlin, Isaac N. 1892a. "'Discussion' of J. C. Carson's paper, A Case of Moral Imbecility." *Proceedings of the Association of Medical Superintendents of American Institutions for Idiotic and Feeble-Minded Persons, 1891,* 190–198.

Kerlin, Isaac N. 1892b. "Dr. Joseph Parrish." *Proceedings of the Association of Medical Officers of American Institutions for Idiotic and Feeble-Minded Persons, 1891,* 247–249.

Kerlin, Isaac N. 1892c. "President's Annual Address." *Proceedings of the Association of Medical Officers of American Institutions for Idiotic and Feeble-Minded Persons,* 274–285.

Kerlin, Isaac N. 1892*d*. "Status of the Work – Pennsylvania." *Proceedings of the Association of Medical Superintendents of American Institutions for Idiotic and Feeble-Minded Persons,* 381–382.

Kesey, Ken. 1962. *One Flew over the Cuckoo's Nest.* New York: Viking.

Kevles, Daniel J. 1985. *In the Name of Eugenics: Genetics and the Use of Human Heredity.* New York: Alfred Knopf.

Key, Wilhelmine E. 1920. *Heredity and Social Fitness: A Study of Differential Mating in a Pennsylvania Family.* Publication no. 296. Washington, DC: Carnegie Institute.

Key, Wilhelmine E. 1923. "Heritable Factors in Human Fitness and Their Social Control." Pp. 405–412 in *The Second International Congress of Eugenics: Eugenics, Genetics, and the Family,* edited by H. H. Laughlin. Baltimore, MD: Williams and Wilkins.

Khuse, Helga, and Peter Singer. 1985. *Should the Baby Live? The Problem of Handicapped Infants.* Oxford, UK: Oxford University Press.

Kingsley, Jason, and Mitchell Levitz. 2007. *Count Us In: Growing Up with Down Syndrome.* New York: Harcourt Books.

Kirkbride, Franklin B. 1909. "Letchworth Village, New York State's New Institution for Defectives." *Proceedings of the National Conference of Charities and Correction,* 85–91.

Kirkbride, Thomas S. 1854. *On the Construction, Organization, and General Arrangements of Hospitals for the Insane.* Philadelphia, PA: Lindsay and Balkiston.

Kite, Elizabeth H. 1912*a*. "Two Brothers." *Survey* 27:1861–1864.

Kite, Elizabeth H. 1912*b*. "Unto the Third Generation." *Survey* 28:789–791.

Kite, Elizabeth H. 1913. "The Pineys." *Survey* 31:7–13.

Kittay, Eva. 1998. *Love's Labor: Essays on Women, Equality, and Dependency.* New York: Routledge.

Kittay, Eva. 2000. "Relationality, Impairment and Peter Singer on the Fate of Severely Impaired Infants." *APA Newsletter on Philosophy and Medicine* 99:253–256.

Kittay, Eva. 2001. "When Caring Is Just and Justice Is Caring: Justice and Mental Retardation." *Public Culture* 13(3):557–579.

Kittay, Eva. 2015. Facebook entry 22 June. Retrieved June 23, 2015 (https://www.facebook.com/eva.f.kittay?fref=ts).

Klein, Aaron. 2015. "Interview with Peter Singer." Retrieved September 30, 2015 (https://soundcloud.com/atfyfe/interview-with-peter-singer).

Kline, Wendy. 2001. *Building a Better Race: Gender, Sexuality, and Eugenics from the Turn of the Century to the Baby Boom.* Berkeley and Los Angeles: University of California Press.

Knight, George H. 1889. "Report on Connecticut." *Proceedings of the Association of Medical Officers of American Institutions for Idiotic and Feeble-Minded Persons, 1888,* 67–68.

Knight, George H. 1892. "The Colony Plan for All Grades of Feeble-Minded." *Proceedings of the National Conference of Charities and Correction,* 155–160.

Knight, Henry M. 1850–1890. "Henry Martyn Knight Manuscripts" [three folders of approximately 100 pages of handwritten speeches and notes]. Frank Knight Sanders Papers. Yale Divinity School Library, Yale University, New Haven, CT.

Knox, Howard A. 1914. "Tests for Mental Defects: How the Public Health Service Prevents Contamination of Our Racial Stock by Turning Back Feeble-Minded Immigrants." *Journal of Heredity* 5:122–130.

Kollings, P. F. 1962. "Story of a Father and Mother Who Have Solved the Most Perplexing Problem Parents Can Face." *Better Homes and Gardens* 40:56–57.

Koren, John. 1906. "Feeble-Minded in Institutions." Pp. 205–230 in Department of Commerce and Labor, Bureau of Census, *Insane and Feeble-Minded in Hospitals and Institutions, 1904.* Washington, DC: Government Printing Office.

Kostir, Mary S. 1916. *Family of Sam Sixty*. Mansfield, OH: Press of the Ohio State Reformatory.

Kraft, Ivor. 1961. "Edouard Seguin and the Nineteenth Century Moral Treatment of Idiots." *Bulletin of the History of Medicine* 35:393–418.

Krause, Arnold, and Grant M. Stolzfus. 1948. *Forgotten Children: The Story of Mental Deficiency*. Philadelphia, PA: National Mental Health Foundation.

Krauss, Marty W. 1990. "In Defense of Common Sense." *American Journal of Mental Retardation* 96:19–21.

Krentz, Christopher. 2005. "'Vacant Receptacle'? Blind Tom, Cognitive Difference, and Pedagogy." *PMLA* 120(2):552–557.

Kugel, Robert B., and Wolf Wolfensberger. 1969. *Changing Patterns in Residential Services for the Mentally Retarded*. Washington, DC: Government Printing Office.

Kuhl, Stefan. 1994. *The Nazi Connection: Eugenics, American Racism, and German National Socialism*. New York: Oxford University Press.

Kunzel, Regina. 1995. *Fallen Women, Problem Girls: Unmarried Mothers and the Professionalization of Social Work, 1890–1945*. New Haven, CT: Yale University Press.

Kurtz, Richard A. 1967. "Sex and Age Trends in Admissions to an Institution for the Mentally Retarded, 1910–1959." *Nebraska State Medical Journal* 4:134–143.

Ladd-Taylor, Molly. 1997. "Saving Babies and Sterilizing Mothers: Eugenics and Welfare Politics in the Interwar United States." *Social Politics* 4(Spring):136–153.

Ladd-Taylor, Molly. 2014. "Contraception or Eugenics? Sterilization and 'Mental Retardation' in the 1970s and 1980s." *Canadian Bulletin of Medical History/Bulletin canadien d'histoire de la médecine* 31(1):189–211.

Lakin, K. Charlie, Sheryl A. Larson, Patrick Salmi, and A. Webster. 2010. *Residential Services for Persons with Developmental Disabilities: Status and Trends through 2009*. Research and Training Center on Community Living, Institute on Community Integration/UCEDD, College of Education and Human Development, University of Minnesota. Retrieved August 24, 2015 (http://rtc.umn.edu/docs/risp2009.pdf).

Lancaster, Ashley Craig. 2007. "Weeding Out the Recessive Gene: Representations of the Evolving Eugenics Movement in Erskine Caldwell's *God's Little Acre*." *Southern Literary Journal* 39(Spring):78–99.

Landesman, Sharon, and Earl Butterfield. 1987. "Normalization and Deinstitutionalization of Mentally Retarded Individuals: Controversy and Facts." *American Psychologist* 42:809–816.

Lane, Harlan. 1976. *The Wild Boy of Aveyron*. Cambridge, MA: Harvard University Press.

Largent, Mark A. 2008. *Breeding Contempt: The History of Coerced Sterilization in the United States*. New Brunswick, NJ: Rutgers University Press.

Larson, Edward J. 1995a. *Sex, Race, and Science: Eugenics in the Deep South*. Baltimore, MD: Johns Hopkins University Press.

Larson, Edward J. 1995b. "'In the Finest, Most Womanly Way': Women in the Southern Eugenics Movement," *American Journal of Legal Studies* 39(2):119–47.

Larson, Kate Clifford. 2015. *Rosemary: The Hidden Kennedy Daughter*. New York: Houghton, Mifflin, Harcourt.

Larson, Sheryl A., L. Hallas-Muchow, F. Aiken, A. Hewitt, S. Pettingell, L. L. Anderson, C. Moseley, M. Sowers, M.L. Fay, D. Smith, and Y. Kardell. 2014. *In-Home and Residential Long-Term Supports and Services for Persons with Intellectual or Developmental Disabilities: Status and Trends through 2012*. Minneapolis: University of Minnesota, Research and Training Center on Community Living, Institute on Community Integration.

Larson, Sheryl A. and K. Charlie Lakin. 2010. "Changes to the Primary Diagnosis of Students with Intellectual or Developmental Disabilities Ages 6 to 21 Receiving Special Education Services 1999 to 2008." *Intellectual and Developmental Disabilities* 48(June):233–238.

Laughlin, Harry H. 1923. *The Second International Exhibition of Eugenics, Held September 22 to October 22, 1921, in Connection with the Second International Congress of Eugenics*. Baltimore, MD: Williams and Wilkins.

Laughlin, Harry H. 1926. "The Eugenical Sterilization of the Feeble-Minded." *Journal of Psycho-Asthenics* 31:210–218.

Lavi, Shai. 2005. *The Modern Art of Dying: A History of Euthanasia in the United States* Princeton, NJ: Princeton University Press.

Leekley, Sheryle, and John Leekley. 1982. *Moments: The Pulitzer Prize Photographs*. Updated ed. New York: Crown.

Leiby, James. 1967. *Charity and Correction in New Jersey: A History of State Welfare Institutions*. New Brunswick, NJ: Rutgers University Press.

Leonard, Thomas C. 2003. "'More Merciful and Not Less Effective': Eugenics and American Economics in the Progressive Era." *History of Political Economy* 35(4):687–712.

Leonard, Thomas C. 2005. "Retrospectives Eugenics and Economics in the Progressive Era." *Journal of Economic Perspectives* 19(Fall):207–224.

Lerman, Paul. 1982. *Deinstitutionalization and the Welfare State*. New Brunswick, NJ: Rutgers University Press.

Letchworth, William P. 1894. "Provisions for Epileptics." *Proceedings of the National Conference of Charities and Correction*, 188–200.

Letchworth, William P. 1900. *Care and Treatment of Epileptics*. New York: G. P. Putnam's Sons.

Levinson, Abraham. 1952. *The Mentally Retarded Child*. New York: John Day.

Lewontin, Richard C. 1970. "Race and Intelligence." *Bulletin of the Atomic Scientists* 26(3):2–8.

"Life Subscribers and Donors to the Pennsylvania Training School for Feeble-Minded Children." 1859. Philadelphia, PA: privately printed pamphlet.

Lincoln, Abraham.1852. "Petition and Letter for the Pardon of John A. L. Crockett." Illinois Digital Archives. Retrieved July 23, 2015 (http://www.idaillinois.org/cdm/ref/collection/isa/id/1443).

Lincoln State School and Colony. 1880–1941. *Photographic Pile*. Illinois State Archives, record no. 254.123, Springfield.

Lincoln State School and Colony. 1935–36. *Sample Book*. Illinois State Archives, record no. 254.41, Springfield.

"The Lincoln State School and Colony." 1913. *Institution Quarterly* 4:80–81, 127–129.

Lippmann, Walter. 1922a. "The Mental Age of Americans." *New Republic* 32:213–215.

Lippmann, Walter. 1922b. "Tests of Hereditary Intelligence." *New Republic* 32:328–330.

Lippmann, Walter. 1923. "A Defense of Education." *Century* 106:96–106.

Little, Charles S. 1912. "Letchworth Village: The Newest State Institution for the Feeble-Minded and Epileptic." *Survey* 27:1869–1872.

Lively, Carrie E. 1983. "Reminiscences of a Mental Hospital Attendant." *Indiana Medical History Quarterly* 9:13–22.

Lombardo, Paul A. 2003. "Taking Eugenics Seriously: The Generations of ??? Are Enough?" *Florida State University Law Review* 30 (Winter):191–218.

Lombardo, Paul A. 2008. *Three Generations No Imbeciles: Eugenics, the Supreme Court, and Buck v. Bell*. Baltimore, MD: Johns Hopkins University Press.

Lombroso, Cesare. 1876. *L'Uomo Delinquente*. Milano: Ulrico Hoepli.Lombroso, Cesare. 1911. *Crime, Its Causes and Remedies*. Translated by Henry P. Horton. Boston: Little, Brown.

Lowell, Josephine Shaw. 1879. "One Means of Preventing Pauperism." *Proceedings of the National Conference of Charities and Correction*, 189–200.

Luckasson, Ruth, Coulter, David L., Polloway, E. A., Reiss, S., Schalock, Robert L., Snell, M. E., Spitalnick, D. M., Stark, J. A. 1992. *Mental Retardation: Definition, Classification and Systems of Supports* (9th ed.). Washington, DC: American Association on Mental Retardation.

Luckasson, Ruth, . Borthwick-Duffy, Sharon A., Buntinx, W. H. E., Coulter, David L., Craig, E. M., Reeve, A., Schalock, Robert L., Snell, M. E., Spitalnick, D. M., Spreat, S., & Tasse, M. J. 2002. *Mental Retardation: Definition, Classification and Systems of Supports* (10th ed.). Washington, DC: American Association on Mental Retardation.

Ludmerer, Kenneth M. 1972. *Genetics and American Society: A Historical Appraisal*. Baltimore, MD: Johns Hopkins University Press.

Lund, Alton F. 1959. "The Role of Parents in Helping Each Other." Pp. 62–70 in Woods Schools Conference, *Proceedings: Counseling Parents of Children with Mental Handicap*. Langhorne, PA: Woods Schools.

MacAndrew, C., and Robert Edgerton. 1964. "The Everyday Life of the Institutionalized 'Idiots'" *Human Organization* 23:312–318.

MacDonald, Carlos F. 1914. "President's Address." *American Journal of Insanity* 71:1–12.

MacGregor, John M. 2002. *Henry Darger: In the Realms of the Unreal*. New York: Delano Greenridge Editions.

Mackie, Romaine. 1969. *Special Education in the U.S: Statistics, 1948–1966*. New York: Teachers College (Columbia University) Press.

Macklin, Ruth, and Willard Macklin, eds. 1981. *Mental Retardation and Sterilization: A Problem of Competency and Paternalism*. New York: Plenum.

Malacrida, Claudia. 2015. *A Special Hell: Institutional Life in Alberta's Eugenic Years*. Toronto: University of Toronto Press.

Mann, Horace. 1891 [1844]. "Seventh Annual Report of the Honorable Horace Mann, Secretary of the Massachusetts Board of Education, 1843." Pp. 230–418 in *Life and Work of Horace Mann*, vol. 3, edited by Mary P. Mann. Boston: Lee and Shepard.

"Mann, Horace." 1893. In *National Cyclopedia of American Biography*, vol. 3, 78–79. New York: James T. White.

Mann, Mary Peabody. 1937. *Life of Horace Mann*. Centennial ed. Washington, DC: National Education Association.

Manne, Jack. 1936. "Mental Deficiency in a Closely Inbred Mountain Clan." *Mental Hygiene* 20:269–279.

Marden, Orison Sweet. 1894. *Pushing the Front, or Success under Difficulties: A Book of Inspiration and Encouragement to All Who Are Struggling for Self-Elevation along the Paths of Knowledge and of Duty*. New York: Thomas Y. Crowell.

Margolin, Leslie. 1994. *Goodness Personified: The Emergence of Gifted Children*. New York: Aldine de Gruyter.

May, Elaine Tyler. 1988. *Homeward Bound: Americans in the Cold War Era*. New York: Basic Books.

McCullagh, James G. 1988. "Challenging the Proposed Deregulation of P.L. 94–142: A Case Study of Citizens Advocacy." *Journal of Sociology and Social Welfare* 15:65–81.

McCulloch, Oscar C. 1888. "The Tribe of Ishmael: A Study in Social Degradation." In *Proceedings of the National Conference of Charities and Correction*, 154–159.

McDonagh, Patrick. 2001. "'Only an Almost': Helen MacMurchy, Feeble Minds, and the Evidence of Literature." *Journal on Developmental Disabilities* 8(2):61–74.

McDonagh, Patrick. 2008. *Idiocy: A Cultural History*. Liverpool, UK: Liverpool University Press.

McDonald, Margaret. 1956. "Because a Father Cared." *Rotarian* 89:12–14, 51–52.

McGovern, Constance M. 1985. *Masters of Madness: Social Origins of the American Psychiatric Profession*. Hanover, NH: University Press of New England.

McGrew, Roderick E. 1985. "Epilepsy." Pp. 111–114 in *Encyclopedia of Medical History*, edited by R. E. McGrew. New York: McGraw-Hill.

McLaren, Angus. 1986. "The Creation of a Haven for 'Human Thoroughbreds': The Sterilization of the Feeble-Minded and the Mentally Ill in British Columbia." *Canadian Historical Review* 67:127–150.

McPhee, John A. 1968. *The Pine Barrens*. New York: Farrar, Straus, and Giroux.

McPherson, George E. 1929. "Address of the President." *Proceedings and Addresses of the American Association for the Study of the Feeble-Minded*, 176–179.

Mercer, Jane R. 1972a. "I.Q.: The Lethal Label." *Psychology Today* 6(September):44–47, 95–97.

Mercer, Jane R. 1972b. "Who Is Normal? Two Perspectives on Mild Mental Retardation." Pp. 56–75 in *Patients, Physicians, and Illness: A Sourcebook in Behavioral Science and Health*, 2nd ed., edited by E. G. Jaco. New York: Free Press.

Mercer, Jane R. 1973. *Labeling the Mentally Retarded: Clinical and Social System Perspectives on Mental Retardation*. Berkeley and Los Angeles: University of California Press.

Mercer, Jane R. 1974. "A Policy Statement on Assessment Procedures and Rights of Children." *Harvard Educational Review* 44:328–344.

Meyer, Adolf. 1917. "Organization of Eugenics Investigation." *Eugenical News* 2:66–69. Reprinted in Pp. 511–516 in *The Commonsense Psychiatry of Dr. Adolf Meyer*, edited by A. Lief. New York, McGraw-Hill, 1948.

Meyer, Carrie A. 2007. *Days on the Family Farm: From the Golden Age to the Great Depression*. Minneapolis: University of Minnesota Press.

Michels-Peterson, Peg. 1978. "Biographical Sketch." Inventory of the Arthur Curtis Rogers Papers, 1885–1917 [six boxes]. Minnesota Historical Society, St. Paul.

Millias, Ward Winthrop. 1942. "Thirty Years of Colonies." *American Journal of Mental Deficiency* 46:414–423.

Milligan, Glenn E. 1961. "History of the American Association on Mental Deficiency." *American Journal of Mental Deficiency* 66:357–369.

Mills v. Board of Education of the District of Columbia. 1972. F. Supp. 866 (District of the District of Columbia).

Minton, Henry L. 1988. *Lewis M. Terman: Pioneer in Psychological Testing*. New York: New York University Press.

Miron, Janet. 2011. *Prisons, Asylums, and the Public: Institutional Visiting in the Nineteenth Century*. Toronto: University of Toronto Press.

Monroe, Will S. 1894. "Feeble-Minded Children in the Public Schools." *Proceedings of the National Conference of Charities and Correction*, 430–433.

Moore, Coyle Ellis. 1928. *The Cost and Administration of Public Welfare in Illinois, 1904–1925*. Ph.D. diss., University of Chicago.

Morris, Catherine, and Matthew Higgs, eds. 2014. *Judith Scott: Bound and Unbound*. New York: Prestel.

Morrison, J. L. 1965. "Illegitimacy, Sterilization, and Racism: A North Carolina Case History." *Social Science Review* 39:1–10.

Morrissey, Joseph P., and Howard H. Goldman. 1980. "The Paradox of Institutional Reform: Administrative Transition with Functional Stability." Pp. 247–280 in *The Enduring Asylum: Cycles of Institutional Reform at Worcester State Hospital,* edited by J. R. Morrissey, H. H. Goldman, and L. V. Klerman. New York: Grune and Stratton.

Mott, Alice J. 1894. "The Education and Custody of the Imbecile." *Proceedings of the National Conference of Charities and Correction,* 168–179.

"A Mountain Moves." 1954. *Newsweek* 44(December 12):39.

Mullins, J. B. 1971. "Integrated Classrooms." *Journal of Rehabilitation* 37(2):14–16.

Murdoch, J. M. 1909. "Report of Committee on Defectives – Quarantine Mental Defectives." *Proceedings of the National Conference of Charities and Correction,* 64–67.

Murdoch Center Resident. 1976. Interview with author. Transcribed at Butner, North Carolina, January 23, 1976.

Myerson, Abraham. 1917a. "Psychiatric Family Studies I." *Journal of Insanity* 73:355–486.

Myerson, Abraham. 1917b. "Psychiatric Family Studies II." *Journal of Insanity* 74:497–554.

National Conference of Charities and Correction. 1881. "Busines of the Conference." *Proceedings of the National Conference of Charities and Coreection, 1881,* xxxvi–xxxvii.

National Conference of Charities and Correction. 1884. "Business of the Conference (Resolution on the Death of Harvey [sic] B. Wilbur)." *Proceedings of the National Conference of Charities and Correction, 1883,* xxx–xxxii.

National Conference of Charities and Correction. 1889. "Discussion on the Care of the Feeble-Minded." *Proceedings of the National Conference of Charities and Correction, 1889,* 318–329.

National Core Indicators. 2012. *NCI Data Brief* Special Issue (October). Retrieved August 31, 2015 (http://www.thearc.org/what-we-do/public-policy/policy-issues/employment).

National Council on Disability. 2009. *Large State Institutions:Unfinished Business.* Retrieved July 2, 2015 (www.ncd.gov/rawmedia_repository/8cccd177_dd9e_4181_ade5_ce182376b347?document.docx).

National Council on Disability. 2012. *Deinstitutionalization: Unfinished Business Companion Paper to Unfinished Business Toolkit.* Washington, DC: National Council on Disability.

Nehring, Wendy M. 2004. "Formal Health Care at the Community Level: The Child Development Clinics of the 1950s and 1960s." Pp. 371–383 in *Mental Retardation in American a Historical Reader,* edited by S. Noll and J. W. Trent, Jr. New York: New York University Press.

Netchine, Gaby. 1970–71. "La répresentation psychologique de la déficience mentale, de Descartes à Binet." *Bulletin de psychologie* 24:403–414.

Netchine-Grynberg, Gaby. 1979. "De l'idiotie à la débilité mentale ou les étapes de abstraction nécessaire." Pp. 53–86 in *Les débilités mentales,* edited by R. Zazzo. 3d ed. Paris: A. Colin.

New Jersey. *Report of the Commissioners, Deaf and Dumb, Blind, and Feeble-Minded in the State of New Jersey for the Year 1873.* 1873. Trenton: State Gazette.

New York Asylum for Idiots. 1852. *First Annual Report of the Trustees.* Senate Document no. 30 (9 February), Albany.

New York Asylum for Idiots. 1854. *The Laying of the Corner-Stone, September 8, 1854.* Albany: J. Munsell.

New York Asylum for Idiots. 1861. *Tenth Annual Report.* Albany: Charles VanBenthuysen.

New York Asylum for Idiots. 1864. *Thirteenth Annual Report.* Albany: Charles VanBenthuysen.

New York Asylum for Idiots. 1874. *Twenty-third Annual Report.* Albany: Weed, Parsons.

New York Asylum for Idiots. 1875. *Twenty-fourth Annual Report*. Albany: Weed, Parsons.

New York State. Department of Mental Hygiene. 1937. *A Survey of Methods of Care, Treatment, and Training of the Feeble-Minded Together with a Program for the Future*. Thiells, NY: Letchworth Village.

New York State. Department of Mental Hygiene. 1948. *Life at Letchworth Village: The Fortieth Annual Report of the Board of Visitors for the Fiscal Year Ended March 3, 1948*. Albany: Department of Mental Hygiene.

New York State. Rome Custodial Asylum. 1915. *Annual Report of the Rome Custodial Asylum*. Rome: Custodial Press.

New York State. State Senate. 1846. *Report of the Committee on Medical Societies and Medical Colleagues, on that Portion of the Census Relating to Idiots*. Document no. 23(23 January).

New York State. State Senate. 1915. *Report of Advisory Committee on the Plan of Development of Letchworth Village*. Albany: J. B. Lyon.

New York Times. 1878. "Our Beauty Spots: Prof. Seguin before the Academy of Sciences," October 29, p. 5.

New York Times. 1880a. "Death of Dr. Edward Seguin, Sketch of the Life of the Celebrated Specialist." 39 October, p. 3.

New York Times. 1880b. "New Publications, A Suggestive Experiment: 'On the Psycho-Physiological Training of an Idiotic Hand' by Edward Seguin, M.D." April 4, p. 4.

New York Times. 1883. "Richard Dugdale Dies." Obituary. July 24, p. 5.

"Newberry, John Strong." 1899. In *National Cyclopedia of American Biography*, vol. 9, 235–236. New York: James T. White.

"Newberry, John Strong." 1934. Pp. 445–446 in *Dictionary of American Biography*, vol. 13, edited by Dumas Malone. New York: Charles Scribner's Sons.

Nirje, Bengt. 1970. "The Normalization Principle: Implications and Comments." *Journal of Mental Subnormality* 16:1662–1670.

Nisonger, Herschel W. 1963. "Changing Concepts in Mental Retardation." *American Journal of Mental Deficiency* 67:4–8.

Noll, Steven. 1991. "Southern Strategies for Handling the Black Feeble-minded: From Social Control to Profound Indifference." *Journal of Policy History* 3(2):130–151.

Noll, Steven. 1995. *Feeble-Minded in Our Midst: Institutions for the Mentally Retarded in the South, 1900–1940*. Chapel Hill: University of North Carolina Press.

Noll, Steven. 2005. "The Public Face of Southern Institutions for the 'Feeble-Minded' *The Public Historian* 27(Spring):25–41.

Noll, Steven, J. David Smith, and Michael L. Wehmeyer, 2013. "In Search of a Science: Intellectual Disability in Late Modern Times (1900 to 1930)." Pp. 117–156 in *The Story of Intellectual Disability: An Evolution of Meaning, Understanding, and Public Perception*, edited by M. L. Wehmeyer. Baltimore, MD: Brookes.

Norbury, Frank P. 1892. "Surgical versus Educational Methods for the Improvement of the Mental Condition of the Feeble-Minded." *Proceedings of the Association of Medical Officers of American Institutions for Idiotic and Feeble-Minded Persons*, 336–341.

Norbury, Frank P. 1894. "Operative Interference in Microcephalus: A Failure." *Proceedings of the Association of Medical Officers of American Institutions for Idiotic and Feeble-Minded Persons*, 421–425.

North Carolina General Assembly. 1977. "An Act to Repeal G.S. 143B-151 and G.S. 143B-152 so as to Abolish the Eugenics Commission." Retrieved August 30, 2015 (http://digital.ncdcr.gov/u?/p249901coll22,373414).

North Carolina General Assembly. 2003. "Sterilization of Persons Mentally Ill and Mentally Retarded." Retrieved August 30, 2015 (http://www.ncleg.net/ EnactedLegislation/Statutes/HTML/ByChapter/Chapter_35.html).

North Carolina State Archives. Department of Public Instruction. Office of the Superintendent. 1912–1917. Correspondence.

North Carolina State Archives. State Board of Public Welfare. *Schools and Hospitals, 1912–1956.* Caswell Training School Papers.

Norton, Charles Eliot. 1896. "Some Aspects of Civilization in America." *Forum* 20:641–651.

Nourse, Victoria F. 2008. *In Reckless Hands: Skinner v. Oklahoma and the Near Triumph of American Eugenics.* New York: W.W. Norton.

O'Brien, Gerald. 2004. "Rosemary Kennedy: the Importance of a Historical Footnote." *Journal of Family History* 29:225–236.

O'Brien, Gerald. 2013. *Framing the Moron: The Social Construction of Feeble-Mindedness in the American Eugenic Era.* Manchester, UK: Manchester University Press.

Odem, Mary. 1995. *Delinquent Daughters: Protecting and Policing Adolescent Female Sexuality in the United States, 1889–1920.* Chapel Hill: University of North Carolina Press.

Oettinger, K. B. 1963. "Opening Doors for the Retarded Child." *New York Times Magazine* (12 May):68–69.

Ohio Asylum for the Education of Idiotic and Imbecile Youth. 1858. *First Annual Report.* Columbus: Richard Nevine.

Ohio Asylum for the Education of Idiotic and Imbecile Youth. 1861. *Fourth Annual Report.* Columbus: Richard Nevine.

Ohio Asylum for the Education of Idiotic and Imbecile Youth. 1868. *Twelfth Annual Report.* Columbus: Richard Nevine.

Ohio Asylum for the Education of Idiotic and Imbecile Youth. 1878. *Twenty-second Annual Report.* Columbus: G. J. Brand.

Ohio Asylum for the Education of Idiotic and Imbecile Youth. 1881. *Twenty-fifth Annual Report.* Columbus: G. J. Brand.

Ohio Asylum for the Education of Idiotic and Imbecile Youth. 1889. *Thirty-third Annual Report.* Columbus: Wesbote Printers.

Ohio Department of Public Welfare. 1929. *Annual Report of the Department.* Columbus: Department of Public Welfare.

Ohio Department of Public Welfare. 1934. *Annual Report of the Department.* Columbus: Department of Public Welfare.

Ohio Institution for Feeble-Minded Youth. 1899. *Forty-third Annual Report.* Columbus: State Printers.

Ohio State Medical Society. 1856. *Transactions, 1846–1856.* Dayton: B. P. Dubois and Co.

Olmstead v. L.C. and E.W. 1999. Retrieved July 2, 2015 (https://supreme.justia.com/ cases/federal/us/527/581/case.html).

Olmsted, Frederick Law. 1937. "General Physical Plan." Pp. 45–65 in *A Survey of Methods of Care, Treatment, and Training of the Feebleminded Together with a Program for the Future.* Thiells, NY Letchworth Village.

Opie, Iona, and Peter Opie, eds. 1951. *The Oxford Dictionary of Nursery Rhymes.* Oxford, UK: Oxford University Press.

Ordover, Nancy. 2003. *American Eugenics: Race, Queer Anatomy, and the Science of Nationalism.* Minneapolis: University of Minnesota Press.

Osborne, A. E. 1892. "Report on California." *Proceedings of the Association of Medical Officers of American Institutions for Idiotic and Feeble-Minded Persons,* 367–369.

Osgood, Robert L. 2000. *For "Children Who Vary from the Normal Type": Special Education in Boston 1838–1930*. Washington, DC: Gallaudet University Press.

Osgood, Robert L. 2001. "The Menace of the Feebleminded: George Bliss, Amos Butler, and the Indiana Committee on Mental Defectives." *Indiana Magazine of History*, 47(December):253–277.

"Parrish, Joseph." 1904. In *National Cyclopedia of American Biography*, vol. 12, 486–487. New York: James T. White.

Parsons, Anne E. 2011. "From Asylum to Prison: The Story of the Lincoln State School." *Journal of Illinois History* 14(Winter):242–260.

"The Passing of the Dunce's Stool." 1918. *Survey* 39:423–424.

Pastore, Nicholas. 1949. *The Nature-Nurture Controversy*. New York: Columbia University Press.

Patterson, James T. 1986. *America's Struggle against Poverty, 1900–1985*. Cambridge, MA: Harvard University Press.

Paul, Diane B. 1995. *Controlling Human Heredity:1865 to the Present*. New York: Humanity Books.

Pauly, Philip J. 2000. *Biologists and the Promise of American Life: From Meriwether Lewis to Alfred Kinsey*. Princeton, NJ: Princeton University Press.

Pelicier, Yves, and Guy Thuillier. 1980. *Edouard Séguin (1812–1880), "l'instituteur des idiots."* Paris: Economica.

Pelicier, Yves, and Guy Thuillier. 1996. *Un pionnier de la psychiatrie de l'enfant: Edouard Séguin (1812–1880)*. Paris: Comité d'histoire de la Sécurité sociale.

Penley, Gary. 2002. *Della Raye: A Girl Who Grew Up in Hell and Emerged Whole*. Gretna, LA: Pelican.

Pennsylvania Association for Retarded Children v. Commonwealth of Pennsylvania. 1971. CA. 71–41, 334 F. Supp. 1257(Eastern District of Pennsylvania). 1972. 343 Supp. 279(Eastern District of Pennsylvania).

Pennsylvania Association for Retarded Children v. Commonwealth of Pennsylvania. 1972. 343 Supp. 279(Eastern District of Pennsylvania).

Pennsylvania Institution for Feeble-Minded Children [ca. 1885]. *Pennsylvania Institution for Feeble-Minded Children, located at Elwyn, Pennsylvania, USA*. [undated bound collection of photographs, no page numbers; photo of classroom blackboard dated 1884]. Elwyn Institutes, Elwyn, Penn.

Pennsylvania Training School for Feeble-Minded Children. 1853–1858. *Minutes of the Board of Directors*. Vol. 1. Unpublished manuscript. Archives of Elwyn Institutes, Elwyn, Penn.

Pennsylvania Training School for Feeble-Minded Children. 1858. *Fifth Annual Report*. Philadelphia: Henry B. Ashmead.

Pennsylvania Training School for Feeble-Minded Children. 1869. *Sixteenth Annual Report*. Philadelphia: Henry B. Ashmead.

Pennsylvania Training School for Feeble-Minded Children. 1871. *Eighteenth Annual Report*. Philadelphia: Vernon and Cooper.

Pennsylvania Training School for Feeble-Minded Children. 1873. *Twentieth Annual Report*. Philadelphia: Henry B. Ashmead.

Pennsylvania Training School for Feeble-Minded Children. 1894. *The Act of Incorporation with Amendments and By-Laws of the Pennsylvania Training School for Feeble-Minded Children, at Elwyn, PA*. Philadelphia: Avil Printing.

Pennsylvania Training School for Idiotic and Feeble-Minded Children. 1854. *First Annual Report*. Philadelphia: King and Baird.

Pernick, Martin S. 1996. *The Black Stork: Eugenics and the Death of "Defective" Babies in American Medicine and Motion Picture since 1915.* New York: Oxford University Press.

Perry, Stewart E. 1966. "Notes for a Sociology of Prevention in Mental Retardation." Pp. 145–182 in *Prevention and Treatment of Mental Retardation,* edited by I. Philips. New York: Basic Books.

Perske, Robert. 1972. "The Dignity of Risk and the Mentally Retarded." *Mental Retardation* 10 (l):24–26.

Perske, Robert. 1980. *New Life in the Neighborhood: How Persons with Retardation and Other Disabilities Can Help Make a Good Community Better.* Nashville, TN: Abington.

Perske, Robert. 1991. *Unequal Justice?* Nashville, TN: Abington.

Piccola, Frank. 1955. "We Kept Our Retarded Child at Home." *Coronet* 39 (November):48–52.

Pickens, Donald K. 1968. *Eugenics and the Progressives.* Nashville, TN: Vanderbilt University Press.

Piven, Frances Fox, and Richard A. Cloward. 1971. *Regulating the Poor: The Function of Public Welfare.* New York: Random House.

Platt, Anthony M. 1977. *The Child Savers: The Invention of Delinquency.* Chicago: University of Chicago Press.

Popplestone, John A., and Marion White McPherson. 1984. "Pioneer Psychology Laboratories in Clinical Settings." Pp. 196–272 in *Explorations in the History of Psychology in the United States,* edited by J. Brozek. Lewisburg, PA: Bucknell University Press.

Porteus, Stanley D. 1969. *A Psychologist of Sorts: The Autobiography and Publications of the Inventor of the Porteus Maze Tests.* Palo Alto, CA: Pacific Books.

Poteat, William Louis. 1925. "Can a Man Be a Christian To-Day?" *Social Forces* 3:4(May):691–698.

Potter, Alonzo, John K. Kane, James Martin, G. B. Wood, and Charles D. Cleaveland. 1853. *Education of Idiots: An Appeal to the Citizens of Philadelphia.* Philadelphia, PA: H. Evans.

Potter, Howard. 1965. "Mental Retardation: The Cinderella of Psychiatry." *Psychiatric Quarterly* 39:241–252.

Powell, F. M. 1887. "The Care and Training of Feeble-Minded Children." *Proceedings of the National Conference of Charities and Correction,* 250–260.

Powell, F. M. 1900. "Report of the Standing Committee on the Feeble-Minded and Epileptic." *Proceedings of the National Conference of Charities and Correction,* 70–82.

Proctor, Robert. 1988. *Racial Hygiene: Medicine under the Nazis.* Cambridge, MA: Harvard University Press.

Providence (Rhode Island) School Committee. 1896–97. *Report of the School Committee, 1896–1897.* Providence, RI: School Committee.

Pumphrey, Muriel. 1990. Interview with author. Transcribed August 17, 1990.

"Question of Priorities." 1967. *Nation* 205(20 November):516.

Quincy, Josiah. 1821. *Report of the Committee to Whom Was Referred the Consideration of the Pauper Laws of the Commonwealth.* Boston: Shaw and Shoemaker. Reprinted in *Poverty USA.: The Almshouse Experience,* compiled by the Children's Aid Society of New York City. New York: Arno Press, 1971.

Radford, John P. 1991. "Sterilization versus Segregation: Control of the 'Feebleminded' 1900–1938." *Social Science and Medicine* 33:449–458.

"Radiation Used on Retarded: Postwar Experiments Done at Fernald School" 1993. *Boston Globe* (December 26), pp. 1, 23.

Rafter, Nicole H. [Nicholas F. Hahn]. 1992a. "Claims-Making and Socio-Cultural Context in the First US Eugenics Campaign." *Social Problems* 39:17–34.

Rafter, Nicole H. [Nicholas F. Hahn]. 1992*b*. "Some Consequences of Strict Constructionism." *Social Problems* 39:38–39.

Rafter, Nicole H. [Nicholas F. Hahn], ed. 1988. *White Trash: The Eugenic Family Studies, 1877–1919.* Boston: Northeastern University Press.

Rafter, Nicole H. [Nicholas F. Hahn]. 1997. *Creating Born Criminals.* Urbana: University of Illinois Press.

Rafter, Nicole H. [Nicholas F. Hahn] 2010. "Lombroso's Reception in the United States. Pp. 1–16 in *The Eternal Recurrence of Crime and Control: Essays in Honour of Paul Rock,* edited by D. Downes, D. Hobbs, and T. Newburn. Oxford, UK: Oxford University Press.

Ramsay, H. H. [ca. 1920]. *Mississippi's Burden of Mental Defect* [a pamphlet]. Jackson, MS: Hederman Bros.

Ramsay, H. H. 1931. "President's Address." *Proceedings of the American Association for the Study of the Feeble-Minded,* 294–299.

Rapley, Mark. 2004. *The Social Construction of Intellectual Disability.* Cambridge, UK: Cambridge University Press.

Ray, Isaac. 1838. *A Treatise on the Medical Jurisprudence of Insanity.* Boston: Little and Brown.

Reaume, Geoffrey. 2009. *Remembrance of Patients Past: Patient Life at the Toronto Hospital for the Insane, 1870–1940.* Toronto: University of Toronto Press.

Reed, James. 2014. *The Birth Control Movement and American Society: From Private Vice to Public Virtue.* Princeton, NJ: Princeton University Press.

Reeves, Helen T. 1938. "The Later Years of a Noted Mental Defective." *Proceedings of the American Association for the Study of the Feebleminded,* 43:194–200.

Reilly, Philip R. 1991. *The Surgical Solution: A History of Involuntary Sterilization in the United States.* Baltimore, MD: Johns Hopkins University Press.

Rembis, Michael A. 2004. "'I ain't been reading while on parole': Experts, Mental Tests, and Eugenic Commitment Law in Illinois, 1890–1940," *History of Psychology* 7(3):225–247.

Rembis, Michael A. 2011. *Defining Deviance: Sex, Science, and Delinquent Girls, 1890–1960.* Urbana: University of Illinois Press.

"Report of Committee on Classification of Feeble-Minded." 1910. *Journal of Psycho-Asthenics* 15:61–62.

"Review of Edouard Seguin's *Traitement Moral Hygiene et Education des Idiots.*" 1847. *British and Foreign Medical Review* (July):1–22.

"Reviving an Old Scandal." 1895. *Kansas City Times,* August 25, p. 4.

Reynolds, David S. 2008. *Waking Giant: America in the Age of Jackson.* New York: Harper.

Rhode Island School for the Feeble-Minded. 1910. *Annual Report of the Superintendent, 1910.* Providence: State of Rhode Island.

Richards, James B. 1854. "Principal's Report." Pp. 14–18 in *First Annual Report of the Pennsylvania Training School for Idiotic and Feeble-Minded Youth.* Philadelphia, PA: King and Baird.

Richards, James B. 1856. "Causes and Treatment of Idiocy." *New York Journal of Medicine* (ser. 3) 1:378–387.

Richards, Laura E. 1935. *Samuel Gridley Howe.* New York: D. Appleton-Century.

Richards, Laura E, ed. 1906–09. *Letters and Journals of Samuel Gridley Howe.* 2 vols. Boston: D. Estes.

Richards, Penny. 2004. "'Beside Her Sat Her Idiot Child': Families and Developmental Disability in Mid-Nineteenth-Century America." Pp. 65–84 in *Mental Retardation in*

America: A Historical Reader, edited by S. Noll and J. W. Trent, Jr. New York: New York University Press.

Richards, Penny. 2014. "Thomas Cameron's 'Pure and Guileless' Life 1806–1870: Affection and Developmental Disability." Pp. 35–57 in *Disability Histories*, edited by Susan Burch and Michael Rembis. Urbana: University of Illinois Press.

Richards, Penny L., and George H. S. Singer. 1998. "'To Draw Out the Effort of His Mind': Educating a Child with Mental Retardation in Early Nineteenth Century America." *Journal of Special Education* 31(4):443–466.

Richardson, Channing B. 1946. "A Hundred Thousand Defectives." *Christian Century* 63(23 January):110–111.

Richardson, John T. E. 2011. *Howard Andrew Knox Pioneer of Intelligence Testing at Ellis Island*. New York: Columbia University Press.

Riel-Smith, Vici. 2014. Interview with author. Transcribed December 15.

Riggs, James C. 1936. *Hello Doctor: A Brief Biography of Charles Bernstein*. East Aurora, NY: Roycroft.

The Riot! 2015. (http://www.theriotrocks.org).

Rivera, Geraldo. 1972. *Willowbrook: A Report on How It Is and Why It Doesn't Have to Be That Way*. New York: Random House.

Robinson, Robert. 1953. "Don't Talk to Us about 'Living Death'." *Coronet Magazine* (July): 74-78.

Rochefort, David A. 1981. "Three Centuries of Care of the Mentally Disabled in Rhode Island and the Nation, 1650–1950." *Rhode Island History* 40:110–132.

Rogers, A. C. 1888. "Functions of a School for Feeble-Minded." *Proceedings of the National Conference of Charities and Correction*, 101–106.

Rogers, A. C. 1891*a*. "President's Address, Faribault Meeting, 1890." *Proceedings of the Association of Medical Officers of American Institutions for Idiotic and Feeble-Minded Persons*, 28–34.

Rogers, A. C. 1891*b*. "Report on Minnesota." *Proceedings of the Association of Medical Officers of American Institutions for Idiotic and Feeble-Minded Persons, 1890*, 68–69.

Rogers, A. C. 1892. "Report of Five Cases of Mental and Moral Aberration among the Feeble-Minded at the Minnesota School for Feeble-Minded." *Proceedings of the Association of Medical Officers of American Institutions for Idiotic and Feeble-Minded Persons*, 318–325.

Rogers, A. C. 1897. "Desexualization." *Journal of Psycho-Asthenics* 2:50.

Rogers, A. C. 1903. "Colonizing the Feeble-Minded." *Proceedings of the National Conference of Charities and Correction*, 254–258.

Rogers, A. C. 1907. "The Relation of the Institutions for Defectives to the Public School System." *Proceedings of the National Conference of Charities and Correction*, 469–477.

Rogers, A. C. 1911. "Dr. Charles T. Wilbur." *Journal of Psycho-Asthenics* 15:126–130.

Rogers, A. C. 1913. "The Desirability of Early Diagnosis of Mental Defect in Children, and Mental Tests as an Aid." *Journal of the American Medical Association* 61:2294–2297.

Rogers, A. C., and Maud A. Merrill. 1919. *Dwellers in the Vale of Siddem*. Boston: Richard G. Badger.

Rogers, Dale Evans. 1953. *Angel Unaware*. Westwood, NJ: Revell.

Rome Custodial Herald. 1913–1946. A monthly newspaper also known as the *Herald* and the *Custodial Herald*. Rome, NY: Rome State School.

Roos, Philip. 1970. "Normalization, De-Humanization, and Conditioning: Conflict or Harmony?" *Mental Retardation* 8(4):12–14.

Roosevelt, Theodore R. 1904. "Twisted Eugenics." *Outlook* 106:30–34.

Rorty, Richard. 1989. *Contingency, Irony, and Solidarity*. Cambridge, UK: Cambridge University Press.

Rosanoff, Aaron J. 1915. "Some Neglected Phases of Immigration in Relation to Heredity." *American Journal of Insanity* 72:45–58.

Rosanoff, Aaron J., and Gertrude L. Cannon. 1911. "Preliminary Report of a Study of Heredity in Insanity in the Light of the Mendelian Laws." *Journal of Nervous and Mental Diseases* 38:272–279.

Rosanoff, Aaron J., and Florence I. Orr. 1911. "A Study of Heredity of Insanity in the Light of Mendelian Theory." *American Journal of Insanity* 73:221–261.

Rose, Sarah Frances. 2008. *No Right To Be Idle: The Invention of Disability, 1850–1930*. Ph.D. diss., University of Illinois, Chicago.

Roselle, Ernest N. 1942. "Increased Cost of Institution Operation under Present Economic Conditions and Some Suggestions for Meeting It." *American Journal of Mental Deficiency* 46:424–429.

Rosen, Christine. 2004. *Preaching Eugenics: Religious Leaders and the American Eugenics Movement*. New York: Oxford University Press.

Rosenberg, Charles E. 1961. "Charles Benedict Davenport and the Beginnings of Human Genetics." *Bulletin of the History of Medicine* 35:266–276.

Rosenberg, Charles E. 1987. *The Care of Strangers: The Rise of America's Hospital System*. New York: Basic Books.

Ross, Dorothy. 1972. *G. Stanley Hall: The Psychologist as Prophet*. Chicago: University of Chicago Press.

Ross, Dorothy. 1991. *The Origins of American Social Science*. Cambridge, UK: Cambridge University Press.

Ross, E. A. 1914. *The Old World in the New: The Significance of Past and Present Immigration to the American People*. New York: Century.

Rothman, David J. 1971. *The Discovery of the Asylum: Social Order and Disorder in the New Republic*. Boston: Little, Brown.

Rothman, David J. 1980. *Conscience and Convenience: The Asylum and Its Alternatives in Progressive America*. Boston: Little, Brown.

Rothman, David J. 1981. "Social Control: The Uses and Abuses of the Concept in the History of Incarceration." *Rice University Studies* 67:9–20.

Rothman, David J., and Sheila M. Rothman. 1984. *The Willowbrook Wars*. New York: Harper and Row.

Rothman, Sheila M. 1978. *Women's Proper Place: A History of Changing Ideals and Practices*. New York: Basic Books.

Rusch, Frank R., and John Dattilo. 2012. "Employment and Self-Management: A Meta-Evaluation of Seven Literature Reviews." *Intellectual and Developmental Disabilities* 50 (1):69–75.

Rush, Benjamin. 1812. *Medical Inquiries and Observations upon the Diseases of the Mind*. Philadelphia, PA: Kimber and Richardson.

Ryan, Mary P. 2006. *Mysteries of Sex: Tracing Women and Men through American History*. Chapel Hill: University of North Carolina Press.

Ryan, Patrick J. 1997. "Unnatural Selection: Intelligence Testing, Eugenics, and American Political Cultures." *Journal of Social History* 30:669–685.

Ryan, Patrick J. 2007. "'Six Blacks from Home': Childhood, Motherhood, and Eugenics in America." *Journal of Policy History* 19(3):253–281.

Saint-Simon, Henri. 1825. *Nouveau Christianisme*. Paris: Bassange.

Sample Book. 1935–36. Lincoln State School and Colony. Illinois State Archives, record no. 254.41, Springfield.

Sanborn, Franklin B. 1881. "Opening Address by the President." *Proceedings of the National Conference of Charities and Correction*, 4–19.

Sanborn, Franklin B. 1892. "Minutes and Discussions." *Proceedings of the National Conference of Charities and Correction*, 345.

Sandel, Michael. 2009. *The Case against Perfection: Ethics in the Age of Genetic Engineering.* Cambridge, MA: Harvard University Press.

Sanders, Frank Knight. 1927. "The Life and Work of Henry Martyn Knight." No page numbers in *Addresses at the Dedication of the Knight Hospital of the Mansfield State Training School and Hospital at Mansfield Depot, Connecticut, October 18, 1926.* New Haven, CT: Yale University Press.

Sarason, Seymour B. 1988. *The Making of an American Psychologist: An Autobiography.* San Francisco: Jossey-Bass.

Sarason, Seymour B., and John Doris. 1969. *Psychological Problems in Mental Deficiency.* 4th ed. New York: Harper and Row.

Sarason, Seymour B., and John Doris. 1979. *Educational Handicap, Public Policy, and Social History: A Broadened Perspective on Mental Retardation.* New York: Free Press.

Schaffer, Kay Bielak. 2014. *"Human Betterment": The Fight for and against 50 Years of Sterilization in North Carolina* [Senior Project]. Annandale-on-Hudson, NY: Bard College. Retrieved September 3, 2015 (http://digitalcommons.bard.edu/cgi/viewcontent.cgi?article=1082&context=senproj_s2014).

Scheerenberger, Richard C. 1983. *A History of Mental Retardation.* Baltimore, MD: Brookes.

Scheerenberger, Richard C. 1987. *A History of Mental Retardation: A Quarter Century of Promise.* Baltimore, MD: Brookes.

Schneider, David M. 1938. *The History of Public Welfare in New York State, 1609–1866.* Chicago: University of Chicago Press.

Schneider, Eric C. 1981. "Mental Retardation, State Policy, and the Ladd School, 1908–1970." *Rhode Island History* 40:133–143.

Schoen, Johanna. 1993. "Interview of Wallace Kuralt." Retrieved July 15, 2015 (https://www.google.com/search?newwindow=1&site=&source=hp&q=wallace+kuralt+sterilization&oq=wallace+kuralt&gs_l=hp.1.1.0j0i22i30l4.1820.7975.0.11661.15.13.0.2.2.0.311.1788.0j12j0j1.13.0....0...1c.1.64.hp..1.14.1683.0.edbcYDEOq8M).

Schoen, Johanna. 2005. *Choice and Coercion: Birth Control, Sterilization, and Abortion in Public Health and Welfare.* Chapel Hill: University of North Carolina Press.

Schrad, Mark Lawrence. 2015. "Does Down Syndrome Justify Abortion?" *New York Times* (4 September). Retrieved July 17, 2015 (http://www.nytimes.com/2015/09/04/opinion/does-down-syndrome-justify-abortion.html?smid=fb-share&_r=1).

Schreiber, Flora Rheta. 1955. "A Retarded Child's Mother." *Cosmopolitan* 138(May):58–61.

Schwartz, Harold. 1956. *Samuel Gridley Howe: Social Reformer, 1801–1876.* Cambridge. MA: Harvard University Press.

Schwartzenberg, Susan. 2005. *Becoming Citizens: Family Life and the Politics of Disability.* Seattle: University of Washington Press.

Schweik, Susan M. 2009. *The Ugly Laws: Disability in Public.* New York: New York University Press.

Scott, Joyce. 2016. *Entwined: Sisters and Secrets in the Silent World of Artist Judith Scott.* Boston: Beacon Press.

Scull, Andrew T. 1977a. *Decarceration: Community Treatment and the Deviant, a Radical View.* Englewood Cliffs, NJ: Prentice-Hall.

Scull, Andrew T. 1977b. "Madness and Segregative Control: The Rise of the Insane Asylum." *Social Problems* 24:335–351.

Scull, Andrew T. 1989. *Social Order/Mental Disorder: Anglo-American Psychiatry in Historical Perspective*. Berkeley and Los Angeles: University of California Press.

Seguin, Edward [Edouard Séguin]. 1839. *Conseils à Monsieur O ... sur l'éducation de son enfant idiot*. Paris: Porthmann.

Seguin, Edward [Edouard Séguin]. 1842. *Théorie et pratique de léducation des enfants arriérés et idiots*. Paris: J. B. Baillière.

Seguin, Edward [Edouard Séguin]. 1843 [1980]. *Hygiène et éducation des idiots*. Reprinted in *Edouard Séguin (1812–1880), "l'instituteur des idiots"* by Yves Pelicier and Guy Thuillier. Paris: Economica. Originally published: Paris: J. B. Baillière.

Seguin, Edward [Edouard Séguin]. 1846a. *Images graduées à l'usage des enfants arriérés et idiots*. Paris: Aubert.

Seguin, Edward [Edouard Séguin]. 1846b. *Traitement moral, hygiène, et éducation des idiots et des autres enfants arriérés ou retardés dans leur développement*. Paris: J. B. Baillière.

Seguin, Edward [Edouard Séguin]. 1847. *Jacob-Rodrigues Pereire, premier instituteur des sourds et muets en France*. Paris: J. B. Baillière.

Seguin, Edward [Edouard Séguin]. 1852a. *Historical Notice of the Origin and Progress of the Treatment of Idiots*. Translated by J. S. Newberry. Cleveland: n.p.

Seguin, Edward [Edouard Séguin]. 1852b. "Letter from E. Seguin to S.G. Howe." Williams College, Chapin Library, Samuel Gridley Howe Papers, Box 6, August 4. Translated by Damon DiMauro and in the author's possession.

Seguin, Edward [Edouard Séguin]. 1856. "Origin of the Treatment and Training of Idiots." *American Journal of Education* 2:145–152.

Seguin, Edward [Edouard Séguin]. 1864. *Idiocy: Its Diagnosis and Treatment by the Physiological Method*. Translated by L. P. Brockett. Albany, NY: VanBenthuysen's Steam Printing House.

Seguin, Edward [Edouard Séguin]. 1866. *Idiocy and Its Treatment by the Physiological Method*. Revised by Edward C. Seguin. New York: W. Wood.

Seguin, Edward [Edouard Séguin]. 1870a. "Idiocy as the Effect of Social Evils and as the Creative Cause of Physiological Education." *Journal of Psychological Medicine* 4:1–27.

Seguin, Edward [Edouard Séguin]. 1870b. "Institutions for Idiots." *Appleton's Journal* 3:182–185.

Seguin, Edward [Edouard Séguin]. 1870c. *New Facts and Remarks Concerning Idiocy, Being a Lecture before the New York Medical Journal Association, October 15, 1869*. New York: William Wood.

Seguin, Edward [Edouard Séguin]. 1873. *Family Thermometry: A Manual of Thermometry for Mothers, Nurses, etc*. New York: Putnam and Sons.

Seguin, Edward [Edouard Séguin]. 1875. *Report on Education. Reports of the Commissioners of the United States to the International Exhibition Held in Vienna, 1873*. Washington, DC: Government Printing Office.

Seguin, Edward [Edouard Séguin]. 1876a. *International Uniformity in the Practice and Records of Physicians*. New York: J. F. Trow.

Seguin, Edward [Edouard Séguin]. 1876b. *Medical Thermometry and Human Temperature*. New York: William Wood.

Seguin, Edward [Edouard Séguin]. 1877. "Monograph of G. C. P." *Proceedings of the Association of Medical Officers of American Institutions for Idiotic and Feeble-Minded Persons*, 11–18.

Seguin, Edward [Edouard Séguin]. 1878a. *Our Parks, To Be or Not To Be*. New York: Brentano's.

Seguin, Edward [Edouard Séguin]. 1878*b*. "Recent Progress in the Training of Idiots." *Proceedings of the Association of Medical Officers of American Institutions for Idiotic and Feeble-Minded Persons*, 60–65.

Seguin, Edward [Edouard Séguin]. 1880*a*. "Psycho-Physiological Training of an Idiotic Eye." *Proceedings of the Association of Medical Officers of American Institutions for Idiotic and Feeble-Minded Persons*, 124–134.

Seguin, Edward [Edouard Séguin]. 1880*b*. "Psycho-Physiological Training of an Idiotic Hand." *Proceedings of the Association of Medical Officers of American Institutions for Idiotic and Feeble-Minded Persons*, 118–123.

Seguin, Edward [Edouard Séguin]. 1880*c*. *Report on Education*. 2d ed. Rev. Milwaukee, WI: Doerflinger Book Pub.

"Séguin, Edouard." 1888. In *Appleton's Cyclopedia of American Biography*, vol. 5, 454. New York: D. Appleton.

"Séguin, Edouard." 1915. In *National Cyclopedia of American Biography*, vol. 15, 151–152. New York: James T. White.

Seguin Physiological School for the Training of Children of Arrested Mental and Physical Development. 1894, 1896, 1905, 1906, 1911. *Catalog*.

Sellen, Betty-Carol. 2008. *Art Centers: American Studios and Gallaries for Artists with Developmental or Mental Disabilities*. Jefferson, NC: McFarland.

Sellers, Charles. 1991. *The Market Revolution: Jacksonian America, 1815–1846*. New York: Oxford University Press.

Semelaigne, René. 1894. *Les grands aliénistes français*. Paris: Steinheil.

Sessions, Mina A. 1918. *The Feeble-Minded in a Rural County of Ohio*. Ohio State Reformatory Printers.

Shaffer, Ellen. 1966. "The Children's Books of the American Sunday-School Union." *American Book Collector* 17:20–28.

Shanks, James. 1970. "The Tragedy of Belchertown." *Springfield Union* (March 17), 1.

Shearer, Ann. 1984. *Everybody's Ethics: What Future for Handicapped Babies?* London: Campaign for Mentally Handicapped People.

Shepard, Edward M. 1884. *The Work of a Social Teacher, Being a Memorial of Richard L. Dugdale*. New York: Society for Political Education.

Shockley, William. 1972. "Dysgenics, Geneticity, Raceology: A Challenge to the Intellectual Responsibility of Educators." *Phi Delta Kappan* 53(January):297–307.

Shorter, Edward. 2000. *The Kennedy Family and the Story of Mental Retardation*. Philadelphia, PA: Temple University Press.

Shriver, Eunice Kennedy. 1962. "Hope for Retarded Children." *Saturday Evening Post* 235:71–75.

Shriver, Timothy P. 2014. *Fully Alive: Discovering What Matters Most*. New York: Sarah Crichton Books.

Sibley, Mulford Q., and Philip E. Jacob. 1952. *Conscription of Conscience: The American State and the Conscientious Objector, 1940–1947*. Ithaca, NY: Cornell University Press.

Sicherman, Barbara. 1967. *The Quest for Mental Health in America*. Ph.D. diss., Columbia University, New York.

Simpson, Murray K. 1999. "The Moral Government of Idiots: Moral Treatment in the Work of Seguin." *History of Psychiatry* 19:227–243.

Simpson, Murray K. 2000. *Idiocy as a Regime of Truth: An Archaeological Study of Intellectual Disability through the Work of Edouard Seguin, William Ireland, and Alfred Binet and Th. Simon*. Dundee, UK: University of Dundee.

Skiba, Russell L., Ada B. Simmons, Shana Ritter, Ashley C. Gibb, M. Karega Rausch, Jason Cuadrado, and Choong-Geun Chung. 2008. "Achieving Equity in Special

Education: History, Status, and Current Challenges." *Exceptional Children* 74(3):264–288.

Sklansky, Jeffrey. 2002. *The Soul's Economy: Market Society and Selfhood in American Thought, 1820–1920.* Chapel Hill: University of North Carolina Press.

Sloan, William, and Harvey A. Stevens. 1976. *A Century of Concern: A History of the American Association on Mental Deficiency, 1876–1976.* Washington, DC: American Association on Mental Deficiency.

Sloss, Robert. 1912. "The State and the Fool." *Harper's Weekly* 56:17.

Smith, J. David. 1985. *Minds Made Feeble: The Myth and Legacy of the Kallikaks.* Rockville, MD: Aspen Press.

Smith, J. David, and K. Ray Nelson. 1989. *The Sterilization of Carrie Buck.* Far Hills, NJ: New Horizon Press.

Smith, J. David, Steven Noll, and Michael L. Wehmeyer. 2013. "Isolation, Enlargement, and Economization: Intellectual Disability in Late Modern Times (1930 CE to 1950 CE)." Pp. 157–185 in *The Story of Intellectual Disability: An Evolution of Meaning, Understanding, and Public Perception,* edited by M. L. Wehmeyer, Baltimore, MD: Brookes.

Smith, J. David, and Michael L. Wehmeyer. 2012. "Who Was Deborah Kallikak?" *Intellectual and Developmental Disabilities* 50(2):169–178.

Society for the Prevention of Pauperism in the City of New York. 1818. *The First Annual Report, to which is added a Report on the Subject of Pauperism.* New York: J. Seymour.

Sokal, Michael M., ed. 1987. *Psychological Testing and American Society, 1890–1930.* New Brunswick, NJ: Rutgers University Press.

Spaulding, Edith, and William Healy. 1913. "Inheritance as a Factor in Criminality: A Study of a Thousand Cases of Young Repeated Offenders." *Bulletin of the American Academy of Medicine* 15:4–27.

Spector, Malcolm. 1985. "Social Problems." Pp. 779–780 in *The Social Science Encyclopedia,* edited by A. Kuper and J. Kuper. London: Routledge and Kegan Paul.

Spector, Malcolm, and John I. Kitsuse. 1987. *Constructing Social Problems.* New York: Aldine de Gruyter.

Spitzer, Stephen. 1975. "Toward a Marxian Theory of Deviance." *Social Problems* 22:638–651.

Spock, Benjamin. 1957. *Baby and Child Care.* New York: Pocket Books.

Spock, Benjamin. 1961. *On Being a Parent of a Handicapped Child* [reprint from parts of several articles in the *Ladies' Home Journal*]. Chicago: National Society for Crippled Children and Adults.

Sprague, E. K. 1913. "Mental Examination of Immigrants." *Survey* 31(17 January):466–468.

Stansell, Christine. 1986. *City of Women: Sex and Class in New York, 1789–1860.* New York: Alfred A. Knopf.

Stein, Michael. 1991. "Sociology and the Prosaic." *Sociological Inquiry* 61:421–433.

Stern, Alexandra Minna. 2005. *Eugenic Nation: Faults and Frontiers of Better Breeding in Modern America.* Berkeley: University of California Press.

Stern, Edith M. 1948. "Take Them off the Human Scrap Heap." *Woman's Home Companion* 75(August):32, 62–64.

Stewart, J. Q. A. 1889. "The Industrial Department of the Kentucky Institution for the Education and Training of Feeble-Minded Children." *Proceedings of the Association of Medical Officers of American Institutions for Idiotic and Feeble-Minded Persons, 1888,* 54–56.

Stewart, William R. 1911. *The Philanthropic Work of Josephine Shaw Lowell.* New York: Macmillan.

Stirling, Nora. 1983. *Pearl Buck: A Woman in Conflict.* Piscataway, NJ: New Century.

Stoddard, Lothrop. 1920. *The Rising Tide of Color against White World Supremacy.* New York: Charles Scribner's Sons.

Stoddard, Lothrop. 1923. *The Revolt against Civilization: The Menace of the Under Man.* New York: Charles Scribner's Sons.

Stoddard, Lothrop. 1924. *Racial Realities in Europe.* New York: Charles Scribner's Sons.

Strait, S. H. 1962. "Bringing Up a Retarded Child." *Parents' Magazine* 37:51–53.

"Struggle to Mend Children's Minds." 1964. *Ebony* 19(September):58–62.

"Summer School for Teachers." 1904. *Journal of Psycho-Asthenics* 8:61.

Sumner, George. 1876. "Letter to S. G. Howe [dated 1 February 1847]." In *Twenty-eighth Annual Report of the Trustees of the Massachusetts School for Idiotic and Feeble-Minded Youth,* 60–72.

Sutton, John R. 1988. *Stubborn Children: Controlling Delinquency in the United States, 1640–1981.* Berkeley and Los Angeles: University of California Press.

Switzsky, Harvey N., and Steven Greenspan. 2006. *What Is Mental Retardation? Ideas for an Evolving Disability in the 21st Century.* Washington, DC: American Association on Mental Retardation.

Szasz, Thomas. 1961. *The Myth of Mental Illness.* New York: Harper and Row.

Talbot, Mabel E. 1964. *Edouard Seguin: A Study of an Educational Approach to the Treatment of Mentally Defective Children.* New York: Columbia University Press.

Talbot, Mabel E. 1967. "Edouard Seguin." *American Journal of Mental Deficiency* 72:184–189.

Tarjan, George, S. W. Wright, H. F. Dingman, and R. K. Eyman. 1961. "The Natural History of Mental Deficiency in a State Hospital, III: Selected Characteristics of First Admissions and Their Environment." *American Journal of Diseases of Children* 65:195–205.

Task Force to Determine the Method of Compensation for Victims of North Carolina's Eugenics Board. 2011. "Preliminary Report to the Governor of North Carolina." Raleigh: North Carolina State Document.

Taylor, Steven J. 2009. *Acts of Conscience: World War II, Mental Institutions, and Religious Objectors.* Syracuse, NY: Syracuse University Press.

"Teachers for the Feebleminded." 1914. *Survey* 32:543.

Thomas, Susan L. 1998. "Race, Gender, and Welfare Reform: The Antinatalist Response," *Journal of Black Studies* 28(March):419–447.

Thomson, Mildred. 1963. *Prologue: A Minnesota Story of Mental Retardation Showing Changing Attitudes and Philosophies prior to September 1, 1959.* Minneapolis, MN: Gilbert.

Thomson, Rosemary Garland. 1996. *Freakery: Cultural Spectacles of the Extraordinary Body.* New York: New York University Press.

Thuillier, Guy. 2011. "Le bicentenaire d'Édouard Séguin (1812–1880): un programme de recherché." *Revue administrative* (septembre n. 383):535–539.

Tomes, Nancy. 1984. *A Generous Confidence: Thomas Story Kirkbride and the Art of Asylum-Keeping.* Cambridge, UK: Cambridge University Press.

"Topics of the Time: The Diseases of Mendicancy." 1877. *Scribner's Monthly* 13:416–417.

Torrey, E. Fuller. 1988. *Nowhere to Go: The Tragic Odyssey of the Homeless Mentally Ill.* New York: Harper and Row.

"Townshend, Norton Strange." 1897. In *National Cyclopedia of American Biography,* vol. 7, 418–419. New York: James T. White.

"The Training School at Vineland, NJ." [ca. 1963]. Supplement to the *Vineland. Times Journal.* Archives of Elwyn Institutes, Elwyn, Pennsylvania.

Trattner, Walter I. 1979. *From Poor Law to Welfare State: A History of Social Welfare in America*. New York: Free Press.

Trattner, Walter I, ed. 1983. *Social Welfare or Social Control? Some Historical Reflections on Regulating the Poor*. Knoxville: University of Tennessee.

Trent, James W., Jr. 1982. *Reasoning about Mental Retardation: A Study of the American Association on Mental Deficiency*. Ph.D. diss., Brandeis University, Waltham, MA.

Trent, James W., Jr. 1986. "Charles Bernstein." Pp. 83–86 in *The Biographical Dictionary of Social Welfare in America*, edited by W. I. Trattner. New York: Greenwood Press.

Trent, James W., Jr. 1987. "A Decade of Declining Involvement: American Sociology in the Field of Child Development, the 1920s." Pp. 11–37 in *Sociological Studies of Child Development*, vol. 2, edited by P. A. Adler and P. Adler. New York: JAI Press.

Trent, James W., Jr. 1998. "Defectives at the World's Fair: Constructing Disability in 1904." *Remedial and Special Education* 19(July/August):200–211.

Trent, James W., Jr. 2001. "'Who Shall Say Who Is a Useful Person?' Abraham Myerson's Opposition to the Eugenics Movement." *History of Psychiatry* 12(1):33–57.

Trent, James W., Jr. 2008. "Essay Book Review of *What Is Mental Retardation? Ideas for an Evolving Disability in the 21st Century*, ed. By H. N. Switzky and S. Greenspan." *Intellectual and Developmental Disabilities* 46:2(April):252–256.

Trent, James W., Jr. 2012. *The Manliest Man: Samuel G. Howe and the Contours of Nineteenth-Century American Reform*. Amherst: University of Massachusetts Press.

Trent, Mary. 2012. '"Many Stirring Scenes': Henry Darger's Reworking of American Visual Culture." *American Art* 26:1(Spring):74–101.

Troyer, Ronald J. 1992. "Some Consequences of Contextual Constructionism." *Social Problems* 39:35–37.

"Tuition of Idiots." 1848. *Living Age* 16:79–82.

Turner, W.W. 1856. "Letter to L.P. Brockett, Esq. [dated 3 March 1856]." *American Annals of the Deaf* 8:250–252.

"Two Immigrants Out of Five Feebleminded." 1917. *Survey* 38(September 15):528–529.

Tyor, Peter L. 1977. "'Denied the Power to Choose the Good': Sexuality and Mental Defect in American Medical Practice, 1850–1920." *Journal of Social History* 10:472–489.

Tyor, Peter L., and Leland V. Bell. 1984. *Caring for the Retarded in America: A History*. Greenwich, CT: Greenwood Press.

Tyor, Peter L., and Jamil S. Zainaldin. 1979. "Asylum and Society: An Approach to Institutional Change." *Journal of Social History* 13(Fall):23–48.

US Department of Commerce. 1919. Bureau of the Census. *Statistical Directory of State Institutions for the Defective, Dependent, and Delinquent Classes*. Washington, DC: Government Printing Office.

US Department of Commerce. 1938. Bureau of the Census. *Mental Defectives and Epileptics in Institutions, 1936*. Washington, DC: Government Printing Office.

United States v. Rhode Island. 2014. US District Court for the District of Rhode Island. Civil Rights Litigation Clearinghouse. Retrieved August 23, 2015 (http://www.clearinghouse.net/detail.php?id=13649).

United States. Supreme Court. 1927. *United States Reports* 27 4(October term, 1924):200–208.

Valenstein, Elliot S. 1986. *Great and Desperate Cures: The Rise and Decline of Psychosurgery and Other Radical Treatments for Mental Illness*. New York: Basic Books.

Vanier, Jean. 1971. *Eruption to Hope*. Toronto: Griffin House.

Vecoli, Rudolph J. 1960. "Sterilization: A Progressive Measure?" *Wisconsin Magazine of History* 43:190–202.

Villager [Amesbury Villager]. 1851. Letters from Jacob Rowell and John Greenleaf Whittier to Samuel G. Howe, March 2, p. 2.

"Visit to the Bicêtre." 1847. *Living Age* 12:606–610.

"Visit to the Bicêtre, etc." 1847. *Chambers Edinburgh Journal* 7(ser. 2):20–22, 71–73, 105–107.

Vogel, Amy. 1995. "Regulating Degeneracy: Eugenic Sterilization in Iowa, 1911–1977," *The Annals of Iowa* 54(Winter):119–143.

Vogt, Sarah. 2012. *Bodies of Surveillance: Disability, Femininity, and the Keepers of the Gene Pool, 1910–1925.* Ph.D. diss., University of Illinois, Chicago.

Wallace, Robert. 1958. "A Lifetime Thrown Away by a Mistake 59 Years Ago: Mental Homes Hold Thousands Like Mayo Buckner." *Life* 44(2 4 March):120–122, 125–26, 129, 133–134, 136.

Wallin, J. E. Wallace. 1914. *The Mental Health of the School.* New Haven, CT: Yale University Press.

Wallin, J. E. Wallace. 1953. "Vagrant Reminiscences of an Oliogophrenist." *American Journal of Mental Deficiency* 58:39–55.

Walsh, Ellen E. 2012. "Conceptions of and Treatments for Cognitive Disability in Antebellum Virginia: John Minson Galt's 'Lecture on Idiocy' (1859)." B.A. Honors Thesis, College of William and Mary, Williamsburg, VA.

Walsh, Kevin K., and Philip McCallion. 1988. *The Training School at Vineland, 1888–1988, Trends of Change: A Collection of Historical Readings from the Archives of the Training School at Vineland.* Vineland, NJ: Training School.

Waterson, Robert C. 1880. "Memoir of George Sumner." *Massachusetts Historical Society Proceedings* 18:189–223.

Watkins, Harvey M. 1930. "Selective Sterilization," *Proceedings and Addresses of the American Association for the Study of the Feeble-Minded,* 51–65.

Watson, Jerome. 1970a. "A Lingering Nightmare: Illinois Care for the Retarded Still Falls Short." *Chicago Sun-Times,* 26 July, sec. 2, pp. 1–3.

Watson, Jerome. 1970b. "Neglect Grips School at Dixon: 'Warehousing' Conditions Held Illinois' Shame." *Chicago Sun-Times,* July 27, pp. 5, 18.

Watson, Jerome. 1970c. "A House of Horror for State's Retarded." *Chicago Sun-Times,* 27 July 27, p. 52.

Watson, Jerome. 1970d. "Bright Side in State's Retardation Jungle." *Chicago Sun-Times,* July 28, p. 59.

Watson, Jerome. 1970e. "Crash Program Urged to Aid Retarded." *Chicago Sun-Times,* July 30, p. 48.

Watson, Luke S., Jr. 1970. "Behavior Modification of Residents and Personnel in Institutions for the Mentally Retarded." Pp. 201–245 in *Residential Facilities for the Mentally Retarded,* edited by A. A. Baumeister and E. Butterfield. Chicago: Aldine.

Waugh, Joan. 1998. *Unsentimental Reformer: The Life of Josephine Shaw Lowell.* Cambridge, MA: Harvard University Press.

"We Committed Our Child." 1945. *Rotarian* 76:1920.

Wehmeyer, Michael, Wil H. E. Buntinx, Yves Lachapelle, Ruth A. Luckasson, Robert L. Schalock, and Miguel A. Verdugo, with Sharon Borthwick-Duffy, Valerie Bradley, Ellis M. Craig, David L. Coulter, Sharon C. Gomez, Alya Reeve, Karrie A. Shogren, Martha E. Snell, Scott Spreat, Marc J. Tassé, James R. Thompson, and Mark H. Yeager. 2008. "The Intellectual Disability Construct and Its Relation to Human Functioning." *Intellectual and Development Disabilities* 46:4(August):311–318.

Wehmeyer, Michael L., and Robert L. Schalock. 2013. "The Parent Movement: Late Modern Times (1950–1980 CE)." Pp. 187–231 in *The Story of Intellectual*

Disability: An Evolution of Meaning, Understanding, and Public Perception, edited by M. L. Wehmeyer. Baltimore, MD: Brookes.

Wembridge, Eleanor Rowland. 1926*a*. "Morals among the Unmoral." *American Mercury* 9:467–471.

Wembridge, Eleanor Rowland. 1926*b*. "The People of Moronia." *American Mercury* 7:1–7.

Wembridge, Eleanor Rowland. 1927. "Dwellers in Neurotica." *American Mercury* 10:460–465.

Wembridge, Eleanor Rowland. 1931. *Life among the Lowbrows*. Boston: Houghton Mifflin.

Wharton, Don. 1939. "Birth Control: The Case for the State." *The Atlantic Monthly* 164:10 (October):463–467.

"Where Toys Are Locked Away." 1965. *Christian Century* 82(September 29):179.

White, William A. 1917. *The Principles of Mental Hygiene*. New York: Macmillan.

Whitney, E. Arthur. 1945. "Our Horizon" [presidential address to the American Association on Mental Deficiency]. *American Journal of Mental Deficiency* 50:218–230.

Whitney, Leon. 1934. *The Case for Sterilization*. New York: Frederick A. Stokes.

"Whitney, Leon Fradley." 1969. P. 1239 in *Contemporary Authors*, vols. 5–8. Detroit, MI: Gale Research.

Whitten, Benjamin Otis. 1967. *A History of Whitten Village*. Clinton, SC: Jacobs Press.

Whittier, John Greenleaf. 1850. "Instruction of Idiots." *National Era* (20 June):1–2.

Whittier, John Greenleaf. 1854. "Peculiar Institutions of Massachusetts." Pp. 20–33 in *Literary Recreations and Miscellanies*. Boston: Ticknor and Fields.

Wickham, Parnel. 2001*a*. "Idiocy and the Law in Colonial New England." *Mental Retardation* 39(2):104–113.

Wickham, Parnel. 2001*b*. "Images of Idiocy in Puritan New England." *Mental Retardation* 39(2):147–151.

Wickham, Parnel. 2002. "Conceptions of Idiocy in Colonial Massachusetts." *Journal of Social History* 35(4:Summer):935–954.

Wickham, Parnel. 2006. "Idiocy in Virginia, 1616–1860." *Bulletin of the History of Medicine* 80(Winter):677–701.

Wickham, Parnel. 2007. "Idiocy and the Construction of Competence in Colonial Massachusetts." Pp. 141–154 in *Children in Colonial America*, edited by J. A. Marten. New York: New York University Press.

Wiggam, Albert E. 1922. *The New Decalogue of Science*. Indianapolis, IN: Bobbs-Merrill.

Wiggam, Albert E. 1925. *The Fruit of the Family Tree*. London: T. Werner Laurie.

Wilbur, Charles T. 1865–80. *Private Letter Book of Dr. C. T. Wilbur*. Vols. 1 and 2. Illinois State Archives, Lincoln Developmental Center Records, record no. 254.2, Springfield.

Wilbur, Charles T. 1870–81. *Scrapbook*. Illinois State Archives, Lincoln Developmental Center Records, record no. 254.40, Springfield.

Wilbur, Charles T. 1877. *An Address on Idiocy and the Treatment of Idiots Delivered to the Legislature of the State of Michigan*. Lansing, MI: W. S. George.

Wilbur, Charles T. 1888. "Institutions for the Feeble-Minded: The Result of Forty Years of Effort in Establishing Them in the United States." *Proceedings of the National Conference of Charities and Correction*, 106–113.

"Wilbur, Charles Toppan." 1900. In *National Cyclopedia of American Biography*, vol. 10, 451. New York: James T. White.

Wilbur, Hervey B. 1865. "Object System of Instruction as Pursued in the Schools of Oswego." *American Journal of Education* 39:189–208.

Wilbur, Hervey B. 1872. "Materialism in Its Relations to the Causes, Conditions, and Treatment of Insanity." *Journal of Psychological Medicine* 6:29–61.

Wilbur, Hervey B. 1876. "Governmental Supervision of the Insane." *Proceedings of the National Conference of Charities and Correction,* 82–90.

Wilbur, Hervey B. 1877. "Buildings for the Management and Treatment of the Insane." *Proceedings of the National Conference of Charities and Correction,* 134–160.

Wilbur, Hervey B. 1881. "Remarks by Dr. H. B. Wilbur of Syracuse, New York." In *In Memory of Edouard Seguin, M.D.,* supplement to the *Proceedings of the Association of Medical Officers of American Institutions for Idiotic and Feeble-Minded Persons,* 25–36.

"Wilbur, Hervey Backus." 1883. *Journal of Nervous and Backward Diseases* 10:658–662.

"Wilbur, Hervey Backus." 1928. Pp. 1302 in *Dictionary of American Medical Biography,* edited by H. A. Kelly and W. L. Burrage. New York: D. Appleton.

Wilbur, Robert C. 1969. *Rome State School, 1894–1969.* Rome, NY: State School.

Wilentz. Sean. 2005. *The Rise of American Democracy: Jefferson to Lincoln.* New York: W.W. Norton.

Wilkinson, Harmon. 1946. "Letter to the Editor." *Christian Century* 63(April 20):466.

Williams, Doone, and Greer Williams. 1978. *Every Child a Wanted Child: Clarence James Gamble, M.D. and His Work in the Birth Control Movement.* Boston: Francis A. Conway Library of Medicine.

Williams, Frankwood E. 1917. "Dr. Samuel G. Howe and the Beginnings of Work with the Feeble-Minded in Massachusetts." *Boston Medical and Surgical Journal* 177:481–484.

Williams, Theodore C. 1887. "James B. Richards." *Proceedings of the Association of Medical Officers of American Institutions for Idiotic and Feeble-Minded Persons, 1886,* 413–417.

Willrich, Michael. 1998. "The Two Percent Solution: Eugenic Jurisprudence and the Socialization of American Law, 1900–1930." *Law and History Review* 16(Spring):63–111.

Wilmarth, A. W. 1892. "The Medical Organization of the General Institution for the Feeble-Minded." *Proceedings of the Association of Medical Officers of American Institutions for Idiotic and Feeble-Minded Persons,* 293–303.

Wilmarth, A. W. 1894. "Causation and Early Treatment of Mental Disease in Children." *Journal of the American Medical Association* 23(7):271–274.

Wilmarth, A. W. 1902. "Report of Committee on Feeble-Minded and Epileptics." *Proceedings of the National Conference of Charities and Correction,* 152–161.

Wilmarth, A. W. 1918. "The Practical Working Out of Sterilization." *Proceedings and Addresses of the American Association for the Study of the Feeble-Minded,* 22–24.

Wilson, Howard E. 1928. *Mary McDowell, Neighbor.* Chicago: University of Chicago Press.

Wilson, W. F. 1892. "Some Notes on the Treatment of Epilepsy." *Proceedings of the Association of Medical Officers of American Institutions for Idiotic and Feeble-Minded Persons,* 304–308.

Wines, Frederick H. 1881. *The Defective, Dependent, and Delinquent Classes of the Population of the United States.* United States Census. Tenth Census, 1880. Washington, DC: Government Printing Office.

Wines, Frederick H. 1888. *American Prisons in the Tenth United States Census.* New York: Putnam.

Winkler, Helen, and Elinor Sachs. 1917. "Testing Immigrants." *Survey* 39(November 10):152–153.

Winship, Albert E. 1900. *Jukes-Edwards: A Study in Education and Heredity.* Harrisburg, PA: R. L. Myers.

Wolf, Theta H. 1973. *Alfred Binet.* Chicago: University of Chicago Press.

Wolfensberger, Wolf. 1972. *The Principle of Normalization in Human Services.* Toronto: National Institute on Mental Retardation.

Wolfensberger, Wolf. 1976. "The Origin and Nature of Our Institutional Models." Pp. 35–92 in *Changing Patterns in Residential Services for the Mentally Retarded*, edited by R. B. Kugel and A. Shearer, Rev. ed. Washington, DC: President's Committee on Mental Retardation.

Wolfensberger, Wolf. 1983. "Social Role Valorization: A Proposed New Term for the Principle of Normalization." *Mental Retardation* 21:234–239.

Wolfensberger, Wolf. 1987. "Values in the Funding of Social Services." *American Journal of Mental Deficiency* 92:141–143.

Wolfensberger, Wolf, and Linda Glenn. 1975. *PASS 3: Program Analysis of Service Systems, a Method for the Quantitative Evaluation of Human Services*, 3d ed. Toronto: National Institute on Mental Retardation.

Woodring, P. 1962. "Slow Learners." *Saturday Review* 45(17 February):53–54.

Wordsworth, William. 1952. "The Idiot Boy." Pp. 67–80 in *The Poetic Works of William Wordsworth*, vol. 2, 2d ed., edited by E. DeSelincourt. Oxford, UK: Oxford University Press.

Wright, David. 2011. *Downs: The History of a Disability*. New York: Oxford University Press.

Wright, Frank L., Jr. 1947. *Out of Sight, Out of Mind*. Philadelphia, PA: National Mental Health Foundation.

Wunderlich, C. A., and Edward Seguin. 1871. *Medical Thermometry and Human Temperature*. New York: William Wood.

Wyatt v. Stickney. 1972. 344 F. Supp 387, 395(Middle District of Alabama 1972), sub no m *Wyatt v. Aderholt*, 503 F. 2d 1305(5th cir 1974).

Wylie, A. R. T. 1900*a*. "Taste and Reaction Time of the Feeble-Minded." *Journal of Psycho-Asthenics* 4:109–112.

Wylie, A. R. T. 1900*b*. "A Study of the Senses of the Feeble-Minded." *Journal of Psycho-Asthenics* 4:137–150.

Wylie, A. R. T. 1902. "On Some Recent Work in Mental Pathology." *Journal of Psycho-Asthenics* 7:1–5.

Wylie, A. R. T. 1903. "Contributions to the Study of the Growth of the Feeble-Minded in Height and Weight." *Journal of Psycho-Asthenics* 8:1–8.

Yates, John V. I. 1824. "Report of the Secretary of State on the Relief and Settlement of the Poor." [New York] *Senate Journal*, 47th sess., 95–108.

Yepsen, Lloyd N. 1934. "Newer Trends in the Rehabilitation of the Mentally Deficient." *Proceedings and Addresses of the American Association on Mental Deficiency*, 101–106.

Zahn, Gordon C. 1946*a*. "State School Unnatural, Maltreats Children." *Catholic Worker* 13(July/August):1, 5–7.

Zahn, Gordon C. 1946*b*. "Slaves or Patients? Rosewood and Enforced Labor." *Catholic Worker* 13(September):1, 6.

Zahn, Gordon C. 1946*c*. "Abandon Hope." *Catholic Worker* 13(October):1, 4, 6.

Zenderland, Leila. 1998. *Measuring Minds: Henry Herbert Goddard and the Origins of American Intelligence Testing*. New York: Cambridge University Press.

Zenderland, Leila. 2004. "The Parable of *The Kallikak Family*: Explaining the Meaning of Heredity in 1912." Pp. 165–185 in *Mental Retardation in America: A Historical Reader*, edited by S. Noll and J. W. Trent Jr. New York: New York University Press.

Zigler, Edward, Robert M. Hodapp, and Mark R. Edison. 1990. "From Theory to Practice in the Care and Education of Mentally Retarded Individuals." *American Journal of Mental Retardation* 96:1–12.

INDEX

Note: Page references followed by *f*, or *t* denote figures, or tables, respectively. Numbers followed by n indicate notes.